Cochlear Implants
Audiological Foundations

Cochlear Implants
Audiological Foundations

Edited by

Richard S. Tyler, Ph.D.
The University of Iowa
Iowa City, Iowa

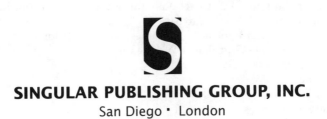

SINGULAR PUBLISHING GROUP, INC.
San Diego · London

Singular Publishing Group, Inc.
401 West "A" Street, Suite 325
San Diego, California 92101-7904

19 Compton Terrace
London, N1 2UN, U.K.

e-mail: singpub@mail.cerfnet.com
Website: http://www.singpub.com

© 1993 by Singular Publishing Group, Inc.
Second Singular Publishing October 1996
Third Singular Publishing April 1998

Typeset in 10/12 Palatino by So Cal Graphics
Printed in the United States of America by McNaughton & Gunn

Library of Congress Cataloging-in-Publication Data

Cochlear implants: audiological foundations / edited by Richard S. Tyler.
   p. c.
  Includes bibliographical references and index.
  ISBN 1-879105-81-0
  1. Cochlear implants.   2. Deaf—Rehabilitation.   3. Hearing impaired—
    Rehabilitation.   I. Tyler, Richard S.
  [DNLM: 1. Cochlear Implant.   2. Deafness—Rehabilitation.
  3. Speech Perception—Physiology. WV 274 C6617]
  RF305.C6292 1992
  617.8'82—dc20
  DNLM/DLC   92–19404
  for Library of Congress   CIP

Contents

Preface   vii
Contributors   xi

Chapter 1   1
Profound Deafness
Arthur Boothroyd

Chapter 2   35
Signal Processing
Blake S. Wilson

Chapter 3   87
Aural Rehabilitation and Patient Management
Nancy Tye-Murray

Chapter 4   145
Speech Perception By Adults
Michael F. Dorman

Chapter 5   191
Speech Perception By Children
Richard S. Tyler

Chapter 6   257
Speech Production
Emily A. Tobey

Chapter 7   317
Electrophysiology
Paul J. Abbas

Chapter 8   357
Psychophysics
Robert V. Shannon

Index   389

To Jack R. Tyler
(1914–1968)

Preface

The utilization of cochlear implants in the rehabilitation of profoundly hearing-impaired patients is now firmly established. The purpose of this book is to provide foundational principles to assist students, audiologists, and speech and language pathologists with their understanding of cochlear implants. A basic comprehension of these principles will allow us to appreciate the entire process involved in cochlear-implant rehabilitation, and therefore help us to provide a better service to our patients. This book can be used as a textbook for classes and seminars on the topic, as a reference book for advanced classes in audiology, and by practitioners as a resource.

In Chapter 1, Arthur Boothroyd describes the deaf population for whom the cochlear implant is intended. Postlingually deafened adults face great communication hardships. Lipreading rapid conversational speech is extremely difficult, and writing notes on paper is cumbersome. Parents of deaf children have critical decisions to make about educational placements that will affect their childrens' future. The Deaf remind us that they have their own culture, including a unique and complete language system—American Sign Language; some don't see the need for cochlear implants. It is important to understand this diverse population so that we can appreciate how cochlear implants fit into the larger picture of the lifestyle of the profoundly hearing impaired.

In Chapter 2, Blake Wilson discusses a variety of signal processing strategies that have been developed for the electrical coding of auditory information. Designing signal processing algorithms that attempt to replace the sophisticated and complex human hearing system is no minor task. However, using what we know about the speech signal and the normal processing of sound, several viable algorithms have been developed. It is important to understand the rationale behind each of the different strategies, and to appreciate the different electrical, biological, and physiological constraints that must be considered. This chapter reviews the important issues about electrical stimulation and how they influence signal processing.

In Chapter 3, Nancy Tye-Murray describes an overall approach to cochlear-implant patient management. Having a well-designed cochlear implant in place is only the first step. It must be adjusted for each patient to optimize the information provided. Furthermore, a complete aural-rehabilitation program is necessary to guide and facilitate the subsequent learning process. With new computer-based technology, efficient individualized training programs are possible.

In Chapter 4, Michael Dorman reviews the speech perception ability of adults using cochlear implants. It is difficult to appreciate what patients perceive with their cochlear implants. Why are some able to have conversations as if they had no hearing loss at all? Others receive limited benefit. We must go beyond quantifying the percent correct word recognition and probe deeper to fully understand what speech features they recognize. This is most easily accomplished by studying the errors that they make. Understanding speech perception in adults is important for fitting the device, planning rehabilitation, and designing better implants in the future.

In Chapter 5, I review the speech perception ability of children with cochlear implants. Speech perception tests represent the foundation for selecting children who are appropriate candidates for a cochlear implant, and are essential to documenting progress. Although a variety of tests are available, an appreciation of their advantages and disadvantages is critical. There are now preliminary results from several groups describing the performance of prelingually and postlingually deafened children. This chapter reviews these findings and discusses their important implications.

In Chapter 6, Emily Tobey describes speech production in adults and children with cochlear implants. One of the most apparent effects of prolonged profound hearing loss can be unclear speech production. Are the perceptual improvements provided by cochlear implants sufficient to make speech intelligible to the laymen? Biomechanical, radiographical, acoustical, and perceptual studies have been utilized to quantify changes in speech production brought about by the cochlear implant.

In Chapter 7, Paul Abbas discusses the electrophysiological responses to electrical auditory stimulation. These studies provide a unique opportunity to objectively explore how the auditory system responds to electrical stimulation. By comparing and contrasting the responses to acoustical and electrical stimulation, we can discover the limitations of electrical stimulation. There is hope that this information will help us adjust the implant for young children and predict preoperatively which patients will benefit from certain cochlear implants.

In Chapter 8, Bob Shannon reviews the psychophysical studies performed on cochlear implant patients. These procedures help us learn more about the particular percepts produced by very specific types of electrical stimulation. They define the capabilities and limitations of performance for adapting speech processors to individuals, and are the key to the design of improved speech-coding algorithms.

We hope that this book will contribute to the broader understanding of cochlear implants, which will, in turn, allow us to serve patients better.

Richard S. Tyler
Iowa City, Iowa

Contributors

Arthur Boothroyd, Ph.D.
Speech and Hearing Science
City University of New York
Graduate Center
New York, New York

Blake S. Wilson, Ph.D.
Head, Neuroscience
Research Triangle Institute
Research Triangle Park, North Carolina

Nancy Tye-Murray, Ph.D.
Department of Otolaryngology—Head & Neck Surgery
University of Iowa
Iowa City, Iowa

Michael F. Dorman, Ph.D.
Speech and Hearing Science
Arizona State University
Tempe, Arizona

Richard S. Tyler, Ph.D.
Department of Otolaryngology—Head & Neck Surgery
University of Iowa
Iowa City, Iowa

Emily A. Tobey, Ph. D.
Louisiana State University
Department Communication Disorders
1900 Gravier Street
New Orleans, Louisiana

Paul J. Abbas, Ph.D.
Department of Speech Pathology
University of Iowa
Iowa City, Iowa

Robert V. Shannon, Ph.D.
House Ear Institute
Los Angeles, California

CHAPTER 1

Profound Deafness

ARTHUR BOOTHROYD

Profound deafness is defined here as **the condition of a person with a sensorineural hearing loss of 90 dB, or more, in both ears.** This loss is based on the average of the pure tone thresholds at 500, 1000, and 2000 Hz, expressed with reference to American National Standards Institute norms (ANSI, 1989).

This is not the only possible way of defining profound deafness (Erber, 1974, 1979; Lloyd & Kaplan, 1978), but it is the one most commonly used. It also has the virtue of being operational. Threshold is relatively easy to measure, the methods are well standardized, the necessary equipment is commercially available, and national and international norms and standards exist (Wilber, 1979).

For many years, profound deafness, as just defined, was beyond the reach of hearing aids and "profound deafness" was synonymous with "total deafness," in terms of the possibilities of prosthetic management. But times have changed. For the past 30 or 40 years we have had the technology needed to provide effective amplification for a large proportion of the profoundly deaf population (Boothroyd, Springer, Smith, & Schulman, 1988; Byrne, Parkinson, & Newall, 1991). The impact, especially on the educational management of profoundly deaf children has been dramatic. Many children who, in earlier years, would have been effectively totally deaf have been enabled to function as if hard-of-hearing by a combination of amplification and appropriately tailored education (Ling & Milne, 1981). The terms "profound deafness" and "total deafness" are no longer synonymous.

1

In the past 10 years, cochlear implants have had a further impact on the prosthetic management of profound deafness. Thousands of profoundly deaf people who were unable to benefit from modern hearing aids have been provided with significant auditory capacity via implants (Watson, 1991). In deafened adults, this capacity has often restored many of the speech perception abilities that were present before the profound deafness was acquired (Owens & Kessler, 1989; Staller, Beiter, & Brimacombe, 1991). In young profoundly deaf children, it has often facilitated the acquisition of spoken language skills and knowledge (Boothroyd, Geers, & Moog, 1991; Dawson et al., 1992; Hasenstab & Tobey, 1991; Tobey & Hasenstab, 1991).

The successes among cochlear implant users have led many professionals to assume that possession of profound deafness is the sole criterion for implant candidacy. But this is not so. The population of profoundly deaf people, as defined here, is far from homogeneous. Its members differ markedly in terms of auditory capacity and many are already able to gain more benefit from hearing aids than can reasonably be expected from a cochlear implant. Its members also differ in terms of several nonauditory variables such as their current developmental status, spoken language abilities, and cultural identity. These variables affect the need for enhanced auditory capacity, the probable outcome of implantation, and the need for specialized educational management in the event an implant is provided.

This chapter reviews the auditory and nonauditory characteristics of the profoundly deaf population and shows how these characteristics relate to issues of implant candidacy and management.

AUDITORY CHARACTERISTICS OF THE PROFOUNDLY DEAF AND THEIR RELEVANCE TO COCHLEAR IMPLANTS

AUDITORY CAPACITIES OF PROFOUNDLY DEAF PERSONS

Profoundly deaf persons differ from each other in terms of **auditory capacity** which is defined here as **the capacity to detect and differentiate sound patterns.** Auditory capacity has three basic components: hearing loss, dynamic range, and resolution (see Figure 1–1).

The **hearing loss** of an individual is usually defined as **the average of the pure tone thresholds at 500, 1000, and 2000 Hz in the better ear, expressed in dB with reference to normal thresholds.** In the profoundly deaf, hearing loss can range from a low of 90 dB (by definition) to a high in the region of 120 dB. People with 120 dB hearing losses are probably totally deaf and respond to sound only through the sense of touch (Boothroyd & Cawkwell, 1970; Nober, 1967). Although we commonly use a three-frequency average to express hearing loss, it is important to remember that hearing loss is usually different at different frequencies and that the function relating hearing loss to frequency also influences auditory capacity.

The importance of hearing loss magnitude is twofold. First, it provides a general index of the extent and integrity of surviving inner-ear structures and is, therefore, predictive of other aspects of auditory capacity. Second, it determines the amount of gain that a hearing aid must provide if the person is to hear (i.e., detect) the quieter sounds of speech. If that gain cannot be provided, then hearing loss magnitude determines how much of the speech signal can be made audible.

Dynamic range is defined here as **the decibel difference between the thresholds of audibility and discomfort.** Normal hearing people have a

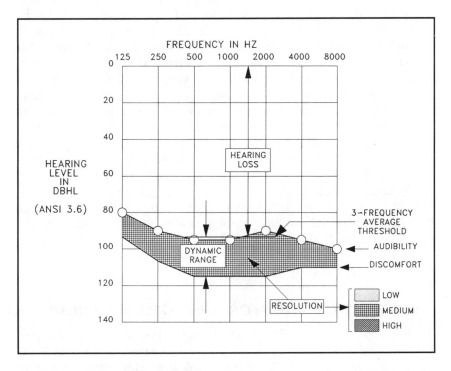

Figure 1–1. The auditory capacity of a profoundly deaf individual is determined by three parameters: (a) hearing loss magnitude, which is an index of the amount of sensorineural damage and also determines hearing aid gain requirements; (b) dynamic range, which is the difference between the thresholds of audibility and discomfort and which provides the target range within which amplified speech must be kept; and (c) auditory resolution, which is a measure of how well patterns of neural stimulation reflect the temporal and spectral detail in the acoustic input and which limits the person's ability to perceive contrasts among amplified speech sounds. Proper amplification and adequate listening experience are required to convert auditory capacity, in the profoundly deaf, into auditory performance.

dynamic range of approximately 90 dB. In the profoundly deaf, this range is seldom more than 30 dB and can be as low as a few dB. Dynamic range tends to fall with increasing hearing loss and, like hearing loss, it can vary with frequency. Unlike hearing loss, however, dynamic range appears to be affected by experience. An ear that has had long-term exposure to amplification tends to have a higher discomfort threshold than one that has not.

The importance of dynamic range in the profoundly deaf lies in the extreme demands it places on the design and fitting of hearing aids. Special steps must be taken to preserve audibility of the quieter sounds of speech while avoiding discomfort from the louder sounds. Moreover, the designer must allow for the 20 or 30 dB range of average intensity accompanying changes of talker, talker effort, and talker distance. Dynamic range may also set an effective limit to the frequency range over which sounds can be made comfortably audible to a profoundly deaf person.

Auditory resolution is defined here as **the ability of the inner ear structures and their associated neural systems to generate patterns of neural activity that reflect spectral and temporal differences among sound patterns.** Profoundly deaf people have poor auditory resolution. Nevertheless, it is often good enough to permit useful speech perception performance. At best, profoundly deaf people have the resolution needed to perceive the rhythm and intonation of speech together with most vowel contrasts and many consonant contrasts. At worst, they can resolve only gross patterns of variation of intensity over time.

The importance of auditory resolution lies in its effect on the perception of speech after the problems of amplification and dynamic range have been addressed. Auditory resolution also has a direct effect on the ability to deal with the interfering effects of noise. The poorer the auditory resolution, the harder it is to maintain speech perception performance in the presence of ambient noise.

AMPLIFICATION ISSUES FOR THE PROFOUNDLY DEAF

As indicated earlier, the design and fitting of hearing aids for the profoundly deaf is not easy. The problems become particularly severe in the case of profoundly deaf children (Ross & Seewald, 1988). Because of acoustic feedback, it is seldom possible to provide more than 60 dB of gain in a personal aid (Boothroyd, 1978; Walden, 1984). The quieter sounds of conversational speech, at a distance of about 4 to 6 feet, are at about 30 dB above the normal threshold of hearing (or 30 dBHL). With 60 dB of amplification, these sounds can be raised to 90 dBHL and, therefore, made audible to a person with a 90 dB hearing loss (Boothroyd, 1992a). Profoundly deaf people with losses in excess of 90 dB, however, cannot hear the quieter sounds of conversational speech via personal hearing aids. They can, nevertheless, hear the louder sounds of conversational speech, which are approximately 60 dB above the normal threshold of hearing and which can be amplified to about 120 dBHL (Boothroyd, 1992a). Most can also hear the quieter sounds of their own speech which, because of proximity, are at about 50 dB above normal threshold and which can be amplified to about 110 dBHL.

There are two basic ways to overcome the 60 dB gain limitation of hearing aids. One is to reduce acoustic feedback with a combination of high frequency attenuation and physical separation of the microphone from the rest of the hearing aid, as in a body aid or a CROS fitting (Skinner, 1988). The other is to use a remote microphone for picking up conversational speech close to the mouth of the talker. The microphone is connected to the rest of the hearing aid by cable or by an FM wireless link. With a remote microphone, full audibility (i.e., including the quieter sounds of speech) can be provided for people with hearing losses as high as 110 dB (Boothroyd, 1992b).

Because of their narrow dynamic range, the profoundly deaf need hearing aids in which the output power is carefully limited so that thresholds of discomfort are not exceeded. Peak clipping accomplishes this with a minimum of circuitry and is appropriate if the clipping level is only infrequently reached. For those people whose narrow dynamic range requires frequent limiting of the louder sounds, fast-acting compression can be used to avoid the nonlinear distortion and reduced signal-to-noise ratio that accompany peak clipping (Boothroyd et al., 1988). Alternatively, the designer can use full-range compression to reduce the dynamic range of the output signal (Preves, 1991).

For all profoundly deaf people, it is difficult to maintain comfortable audibility of speech when there are variations of talker, talker effort, and talker distance. The two solutions to this problem are automatic gain control (which is, essentially, slow-acting compression) and a remote microphone. Note, also, that the remote microphone enhances signal-to-noise ratio for the speech of others by 20 dB or more and can virtually eliminate the interfering effects of ambient noise (Boothroyd, 1992b).

All of the foregoing solutions to the problems of amplification for the profoundly deaf involve acoustic, cosmetic, or logistic compromises. Nevertheless, many profoundly deaf people have enough auditory capacity to justify these compromises.

SPEECHREADING AS AN ADDITIONAL SOURCE OF INFORMATION

In face-to-face communication, profoundly deaf people can supplement auditory input with **speechreading** which is defined here as **the perception**

of spoken language using only the visible movements of speech as a source of sensory data. The problem with speechreading is that most of the essential movements of speech are invisible. Those movements that are visible permit fairly good differentiation of stressed vowels (e.g., "pill" vs. "pull") and of consonants that differ in terms of place of articulation (e.g., "pill" vs. "till"). But intonation patterns are invisible, as are contrasts between consonants that differ in terms of voicing (e.g., "pill" vs. "bill") or manner of articulation (e.g., "bill" vs. "mill") (De Filippo & Sims, 1988; Sanders, 1982). In spite of the sparseness of the visual information in speech, the typical untrained person can usually recognize about 40% of the individual phonemes in lists of single syllable words (Hanin, 1988). Experienced speechreaders perform a little better, recognizing about 50% of the phonemes (Hanin, 1988). Basically, however, the amount of information available in the visual stimulus is the same for everyone, regardless of speechreading experience or competence (Owens & Blazek, 1985).

There are, however, some people who attain excellent speechreading performance when dealing with whole sentences and especially in a conversational context. These excellent speechreaders appear to be particularly adept at taking advantage of the syntactic, semantic, and topical redundancy of speech so as to compensate for the limited sensory data (Boothroyd, 1988a; Hanin, 1988). In formal tests, these excellent speechreaders typically recognize 70% or more of the words in sentences of known topic. For comparison, the typical normally hearing person, with no special experience in speechreading, recognizes only about 30%. Interestingly, one does not have to be deaf to be an excellent speechreader; and, unfortunately, profound deafness does not guarantee excellent speechreading (Hanin, 1988). Moreover, although there is evidence that poor speechreaders improve with training and practice, there is no evidence to show that they become excellent speechreaders (Walden, Erdman, Montgomery, Schwartz, & Prosek, 1981; Walden, Prosek, Montgomery, Scherr, & Jones, 1977). The skills of excellent speechreading appear to be a function of either innate perceptual capacity, established perceptual style, or some combination of the two (Summerfield, 1983). One thing is clear, however. In people whose deafness was acquired early in life, excellent speechreading is only found in those who developed excellent knowledge of spoken language and of the world to which it refers (De Filippo, 1982; Geffner & Levitt, 1987).

AUDITORY CAPACITY VERSUS AUDITORY PERFORMANCE

To return to the issue of auditory capacity in the profoundly deaf, it is important to recognize the distinction between auditory capacity and auditory performance. Profoundly deaf persons need two things if auditory capacity is to be revealed in auditory performance—hearing aids and listening experience. Hearing aids make it possible to detect sound patterns. Listening experience makes it possible to learn the relationships between sound patterns and the objects and events that produce them. In some cases, the listening experience is acquired before the onset of deafness. In others, it must be acquired afterward via hearing aids and limited hearing. Only if one can be sure that a profoundly deaf person has the right hearing aids, and has had adequate experience, can auditory performance be assumed to reflect auditory capacity. Because clinical tests rely on measurement of auditory performance, the clinical assessment of auditory capacity is by no means a simple matter, especially in profoundly deaf children.

CATEGORIES OF PROFOUND DEAFNESS

In terms of auditory capacity, the profoundly deaf can be divided, roughly, into four qualitatively different groups. This grouping is explained below and outlined in Figure 1–2.

1. Profoundly deaf people with considerable auditory capacity usually have hearing losses in the 90 dB region and a dynamic range of around 30 dB. They can be provided with relatively full audibility of speech, both their own and other's, via personal hearing aids. They usually have enough auditory resolution to permit perception of the rhythm and intonation of speech, most vowel contrasts, and many consonant contrasts. Their greatest difficulty is with the place of articulation of consonants (e.g., "pill" vs. "till"). Given proper amplification, adequate listening experience, and good language knowledge, they recognize roughly 40% of the individual phonemes in lists of single syllable words. When the words are in conversational context, these people can recognize, perhaps, 60% of them. For some, this level of performance is high enough to permit open-ended conversations over the telephone, though with difficulty. In face-to-face conversation, those with excellent speechreading skills make few errors. Those with poor speechreading skills can, nevertheless, use vision to enhance hearing in face-to-face conversation, recognizing about 70% of the words.

2. Profoundly deaf people with moderate auditory capacity usually have hearing losses in the 100 dB region and dynamic ranges around 20 dB. With personal hearing aids, they can hear most of their own speech sounds but they need a remote microphone to hear the quieter sounds of the speech of others. Auditory resolution is usually good enough to permit full perception of speech rhythm and partial perception of intonation, vowels, and consonants. In lists of monosyllabic words, they are likely to recognize only about 25% of the phonemes. In conversational context, their auditory recognition of words is not likely to exceed 20%.

Hearing can, however, be a valuable supplement to vision in face-to-face conversation, especially for the excellent speechreader.

3. Profoundly deaf people with minimal auditory capacity typically have hearing losses in the region of 110 dB and a dynamic range of about 10 dB.

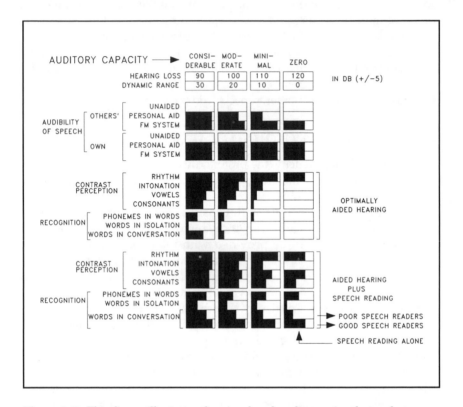

Figure 1–2. This figure illustrates the visual and auditory-visual speech perception performance to be expected from four subgroups of profoundly deaf persons, divided according to auditory capacity. The first two rows show the typical hearing loss and dynamic range for each group. The next six rows indicate, in black, what percentage of the spectrum of speech should be audible with and without amplification. The next four rows show how well the individual should be able to perceive phonologically significant contrasts among speech sounds, and the next three show how well the subjects should be able to recognize phonemes in words, words in isolation, and words in conversational context. The last eight rows show the contrast perception and item recognition data for a combination of hearing and speechreading. Note that the expected recognition of words in conversation is shown for both excellent and poor speechreaders. The numbers are based on the results of several empirical studies but they are approximate and are used for illustration only. Note, also, that the speech perception data assume optimal amplification, adequate listening experience, and normal adult language and world knowledge.

Hearing aids with remote microphones can provide full access to the speech of others. Auditory resolution permits the perception of some of the rhythm and intonation patterns of speech but provides little differentiation among vowels and consonants. Phoneme recognition in single syllable lists is close to chance levels (around 10%). This is not enough to permit recognition of whole words, even in conversational sentence context. If hearing aids are used in face-to-face conversation, however, hearing can enhance speechreading by a small but significant amount—perhaps 10 percentage points.

4. **Profoundly deaf people with no auditory capacity** usually have hearing losses in the region of 120 dB and dynamic ranges close to zero. Even with remote microphones, they can detect only the louder sounds of speech. They are most probably totally deaf and perceive sound via the sense of touch. The tactile sense provides them with access to some of the rhythmic properties of speech but little else. These people must rely entirely on speechreading for the perception of speech.

The foregoing information on auditory speech perception capacity is mostly derived from studies of profoundly deaf teenagers who had been well trained in the use of hearing and spoken language (Boothroyd, 1984, 1985; Erber 1972; Erber & Alencewicz, 1976). The numbers are approximate and are for illustrative purposes only.

LIMITED PREDICTIVE POWER OF PURE TONE THRESHOLD

The classification just given represents an attempt to impose qualitative categories on a population defined by continuously variable quantities. Its purpose is to emphasize the wide range of auditory capacity that can be found in the profoundly deaf population. It should not, however, be taken too literally. Note, in particular, that pure tone threshold, although it is a fairly good index of the extent of sensorineural damage, is not a perfect predictor of either dynamic range or auditory resolution. It is not uncommon to find profoundly deaf people with hearing losses close to 90 dB who have poor auditory resolution, or people with losses in the region of 110 dB who have good resolution. The possible reasons for a lack of perfect correlation between pure tone threshold and other aspects of auditory capacity are several. For example:

- Different underlying pathologies can have differential effects on threshold, loudness perception, and auditory resolution.
- Small conductive hearing losses often go undetected in the presence of a profound deafness, leading to an overestimation of the sensorineural component.
- Young deaf children often give behavioral thresholds that are 5

to 10 dB above their true thresholds until they have had adequate listening experience.

NEED FOR AUDITORY PERFORMANCE MEASURES

Because pure tone threshold is an imperfect predictor of other aspects of auditory capacity, it is important that audiological evaluation of potential implant candidates include empirical measures of auditory resolution and benefit from hearing aids. Unfortunately, such measures are difficult to obtain in a profoundly deaf population for several reasons. For example:

- Psychophysical tests of spectral and temporal resolution are difficult to apply to a clinical population (Davidson & Melnick, 1988; Grant, 1987).

- Even if we could apply them, the relationship of psychophysical parameters to speech-perception capacity is not well understood (Tyler, 1986).

- The results of speech-perception tests depend not only on the subject's auditory resolution but also on his or her auditory and linguistic knowledge (Boothroyd, 1992a). Because this knowledge tends to be very variable in the profoundly deaf population, the validity of speech perception-tests as measures of auditory resolution in these people is limited.

These problems are especially acute in profoundly deaf children because of their auditory, cognitive, and linguistic immaturity. Several research teams, however, have developed clinically useful tests that use speech stimuli, but in a test format that maximizes the role of auditory resolution while minimizing the contribution of linguistic and cognitive factors (Boothroyd, 1991, 1992c; Osberger et al., 1991).

If formal tests of speech perception and hearing aid benefit are not feasible, they may be replaced with the behavioral observations of an experienced teacher or clinician in a diagnostic teaching environment. In fact, such informed observations should be part of the evaluation process for all profoundly deaf children who are being considered for implantation.

COMPARISON OF AIDED AND IMPLANTED PERSONS

We now turn to a key question: "How do cochlear implants compare with hearing aids in terms of their ability to provide profoundly deaf people with sensory data from speech?" The first thing to be noted is that the issue of audibility is more easily addressed in cochlear implants than in currently available hearing aids. Because the cochlear implant does not deliver an acoustic signal, the problem of acoustic feedback is eliminated. It is, therefore, possible to provide audibility of the quieter sounds of conversational speech without worrying about the device becoming unstable. Unfortunately, however, the interfering effects of noise are as serious for implant users as they are for hearing aid users (Hochberg, Boothroyd, Weiss, & Hellman, 1992). Consequently, some of the benefits of improved hearing for remote speech may be lost in a noisy acoustic environment.

A second benefit of cochlear implants is their ability to convey information about the higher frequencies in speech. Hearing aids must generate their acoustic output via electroacoustic transducers. The upper frequency limit of these transducers, when used in hearing aids for the profoundly deaf, is seldom above 3.5 kHz. One reason is the technical difficulty of combining high power and high bandwidth in the same transducer. A second is the acoustic feedback problem, which is particularly acute at high frequencies. Unfortunately, there is useful speech information at frequencies as high as 10 kHz (Boothroyd & Medwetsky, 1992). There are no technical barriers to the coding of these frequencies in cochlear implants (Patrick, 1991).

A third inherent benefit of cochlear implants is that the issue of dynamic range is automatically addressed in their design. The sound input is recoded in the electrical output. During adjustment of the parameters of that code, the fitter "maps" a wide range of input sound levels into the range of electrical currents over which the stimulus is audible and comfortable (Wilson, Lawson, Finley, & Wolford, 1991).

Freedom from gain, bandwidth, and dynamic range limitations are inherent benefits of cochlear implants, regardless of their concept and design. The technology exists, however, to solve these problems within hearing aids (Boothroyd, 1990). The crucial question is how much auditory resolution can be provided by an implant and how this might compare with existing auditory resolution.

To answer this question, my colleagues and I at the City University of New York have been administering a range of speech perception tests to both implant users and hearing aid users. The results of some of this work are illustrated in Figure 1–3. What these and other data show is that the most successful implant users acquire auditory resolution similar to that of the typical hearing aid user with a hearing loss in the 80 to 90 dB range. In other words, they perform as well as, or a little better than, the profoundly deaf person with considerable auditory capacity. This level of implant success often includes the ability to hold unstructured conversations over the telephone. The least successful implant users, however, perform no better than the typical hearing aid user with a hearing loss in the region of 110 to 120 dB. In other words, they have minimal or no auditory capacity. In the data shown in Figure 1–3, the average cochlear implant user performs like the average hearing aid user with a hearing loss in the region of 100 dB. In other words, the average cochlear implant user demonstrates moderate auditory capacity. Note that, although the data shown in Figure 1–3 were obtained with children, we have previously obtained similar results from adult users of hearing aids and cochlear implants (Boothroyd, 1988b).

AUDITORY CRITERIA FOR IMPLANT CANDIDACY

Figure 1–3 includes our attempt to convert the performance data into likelihood ratios. Given no information other than a three-frequency average pure tone hearing loss, we estimate that the relative probabilities of performing better with an implant or performing better with a hearing aid are no better than 1:1 when the hearing loss is around 100 dB. This ratio rises to a more favorable 4:1 when the loss is in the region of 110 dB. On the strength of these data, it would be difficult to advocate the use of a cochlear implant unless the hearing loss were 110 dB or more.

Note, however, the earlier comment about the inadvisability of basing decisions on pure tone threshold data alone. If a person has failed to develop demonstrable auditory capacity in spite of good pure tone thresholds, proper amplification, and adequate listening experience, then the possible benefits of a cochlear implant should be given more weight. One should think very carefully, however, about the interpretation of "proper amplification" and "adequate listening experience." One should also ask whether the failure to develop measurable auditory performance might be attributable to central difficulties of perceptual learning and integration—problems that would still be present after implantation.

SUMMARY

In summary, when examined solely in terms of auditory capacity, profoundly deaf persons differ markedly. Using hearing loss, dynamic range, auditory resolution, and hearing aid benefit as criteria, we can distinguish four subgroups: (a) those with considerable auditory capacity; (b) those with moderate auditory capacity; (c) those with minimal auditory capacity; and (d) those with no auditory capacity. Typical hearing losses for these groups are in the region of 90, 100, 110, and 120 dB, respectively. Compared with hearing aids, cochlear implants offer inherent advantages in terms of freedom from feedback, bandwidth, and dynamic range limitations. There are, however, technical solutions to these problems in hearing aids. In terms of auditory performance, the most successful cochlear

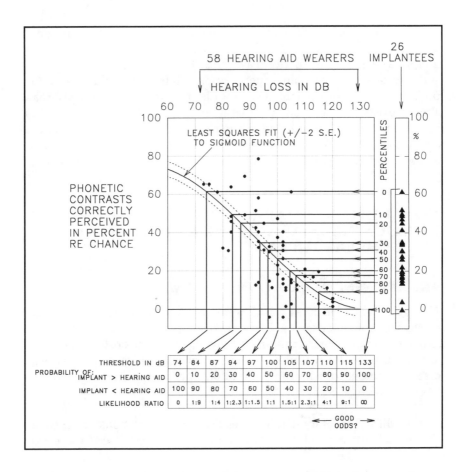

Figure 1–3. These data are from work in progress and show how speech perception performance data can be used to develop an actuarial approach to implant candidacy decisions. In the main graph, speech perception performance is shown as a function of three-frequency average hearing loss for 58 severely and profoundly deaf children who wear hearing aids. The speech perception scores were obtained using a three-interval oddity test of the perception of vowel and consonant contrasts (Boothroyd et al., 1988). The curved line shows the least-squares fit to a sigmoid function. Every tenth percentile of the distribution of corresponding scores for 26 child users of the Nucleus implant, shown on the right, is converted to an equivalent hearing loss using the sigmoid function. The chart at the bottom shows these "equivalent hearing loss" values, together with estimates of the probabilities that a subject with a given loss would be expected to score: (a) better with an implant than with a hearing aid; and (b) better with a hearing aid than with an implant. The ratio of these two probabilities is shown in the bottom row. On the strength of these data, it would be difficult to justify the implantation of an ear with a three-frequency average hearing loss of less than 110 dB, unless candidacy were to be supported by empirical speech perception data, obtained after adequate listening experience with proper amplification.

implant users perform similar to, or somewhat better than, hearing aid users with losses in the region of 90 dB. The average cochlear implant user, however, does not perform as well as this and some demonstrate no auditory capacity. Using an actuarial approach (based on the ratio of the probability that an implant will provide more auditory capacity than already exists, to the probability that it will provide less), it is difficult to justify implantation unless the hearing loss is 110 dB or more. Implant decisions should not, however, be based on hearing loss alone but should involve more extensive assessment of auditory capacity and performance.

NONAUDITORY CHARACTERISTICS OF THE PROFOUNDLY DEAF AND THEIR RELEVANCE TO COCHLEAR IMPLANTS

AGE AT ONSET OF PROFOUND DEAFNESS

The age at which deafness was acquired has a major effect on the consequences of profound deafness. The issue is not so much one of age, however, as of the developmental status of the individual when he or she became profoundly deaf (Boothroyd, 1988c). In the present context, development can be discussed under four headings: audition, speech, spoken language, and world knowledge.

- **Auditory development** involves learning the relationships between sound patterns and the nature and locations of the objects and events that cause them.

- **Speech development** involves learning the relationships between the sound patterns of speech and the movement patterns that cause them. It also involves acquiring control over those movements.

- **Spoken language development** has several components:
  (a) **phonological**, which involves learning the sound system of spoken language and the way sounds are modified and combined to produce words and sentences,
  (b) **lexical**, which involves learning words, their meanings and their associations,
  (c) **syntactic**, which involves learning how words are selected, modified and combined to make meaningful sentences, and
  (d) **pragmatic**, which involves learning how sentences are used to express meaning and to satisfy communicative intent.

- The development of **world knowledge** (or cognition) involves learning about the objects and events of the physical world, their attributes and relationships, the properties of the spatial and temporal dimensions within which they exist, and the physical laws by which these objects, events, attributes, and dimensions are governed. A special component of cognitive development is the development of **social cognition**. This involves learning about people, the events and attributes that are peculiar to people, and the social rules that govern their interactions. General and social cognition are important to our present discussion for three reasons. First, language has no inherent meaning but serves only as a code by which we can refer to the world we know. Second, language has no inherent purpose except as a vehicle for interactions among people. And third, once language is established, it becomes the principal means for furthering world and social knowledge.

We usually subdivide age of onset into prelingual and postlingual, with the dividing age at around 3 to 4 years. Profound deafness that is acquired before basic spoken language skills are established has far more severe and far-reaching consequences than the same profound deafness acquired after those skills are established. We can, however, identify qualitatively different ages-at-onset within these two basic categories.

1. Postlingual

Adult (18+): When profound deafness is acquired in adult life, the psychological and communicative effects are serious and can have devastating social and vocational consequences. But in dealing with the deafness, and adapting to sensory assistance, the deafened adult can take advantage of well established auditory, speech, language, world, and social knowledge. Moreover, the language competence usually includes reading and writing skills.

Late childhood (7 to 18): Postlingually acquired deafness occurring in childhood, however, presents more serious problems, mostly because world knowledge and the corresponding vocabulary are far from complete. In other words, there is more to be learned and less established knowledge to support that learning. In addition, there can be serious psychological consequences when the appearance of a hearing loss collides with the turmoil of adolescence.

Early childhood (3 to 7): When the deafness occurs in the early postlingual years, speech production skills, though apparently complete, are not consolidated. There is, therefore, a serious risk of deterioration that must be addressed through conservation. To make matters worse, the bulk of formal education lies ahead and must now be completed in spite of the limitations of speechreading and limited residual hearing. Nevertheless, there is a considerable auditory, linguistic, and cognitive base from which this education can proceed.

2. Prelingual

Late (1 to 3): Profound deafness acquired between 1 and 3 years of age is certainly prelingual, but the auditory, speech, and pragmatic development that has already taken place can greatly facilitate subsequent learning, including the adaptation to hearing aids or cochlear implants.

Congenital and early (birth to 1): Only when a child is born profoundly deaf, or becomes profoundly deaf during the first year of life, can it be assumed that no prior knowledge is brought to the task of continuing development. This is not to say that no auditory or phonological development occurs during the first year of life. In fact, there is evidence to show that it does. But current practices in identification and intervention do not appear to capitalize on this early knowledge.

The information just presented is summarized in Figure 1–4.

CURRENT AGE

Current age determines the profoundly deaf individual's needs in relation to both sensory assistance and educational or rehabilitative intervention. The adult's needs are mostly social and vocational in nature. The older child's needs are social and educational. In the younger child of school age, the educational needs include the development of reading and writing skills. In the preschool child, the educational needs extend to the development of basic spoken language skills, or to the provision of some alternative to spoken language.

Perhaps the most important issue relating to current age is the relative roles of sensory and educational or rehabilitative management (Alpiner & Garstecki, 1989; Alpiner & McCarthy, 1987; Boothroyd, 1988c; Sanders, 1982; Watkins & Schow, 1989). The profoundly deaf adult who receives sensory assistance in the form of a hearing aid or cochlear implant may need rehabilitative intervention to facilitate adjustment to, and increase the effectiveness of, the device (Rubinstein & Boothroyd, 1987). In contrast, the young profoundly deaf child who is in the process of acquiring spoken language skills needs sensory assistance in order to facilitate learning and to enhance the outcome. In other words, for the adult, the sensory assistance is primary and the rehabilitative training is supportive. In the young child, education is primary and it is the sensory assistance that is supportive. The importance of this distinction is easily overlooked.

DURATION OF PROFOUND DEAFNESS

The third important age-related variable is the duration of the profound deafness, that is, the difference between the current age and the age of onset. In general, a shorter duration of profound deafness means greater potential for successful adaptation to sensory assistance, whether it be by hearing aid, cochlear implant, or some other sensory device. There are two possible problems associated with long durations of deafness. One is the loss of skills and knowledge that were in place at the time deafness was acquired. The other is the development of behaviors that work against the adaptation to sensory assistance.

The problem of duration of deafness is particularly important in the case of individuals with prelingual age-at-onset. If such individuals have been in an educational environment that has promoted the acquisition of

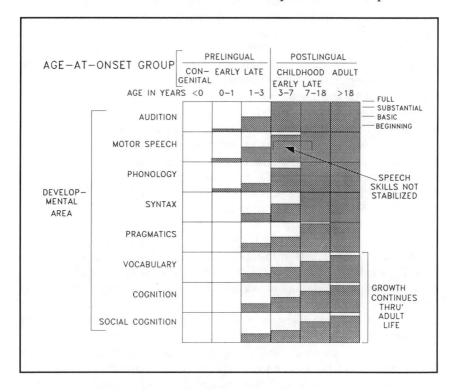

Figure 1–4. This figure illustrates the skills and knowledge that may be assumed to be established, and available to the deaf subject, for six subgroups, based on age-at-onset of deafness. Although the major difference is between subjects with prelingual and postlingual ages-at-onset, qualitative differences also exist within these two groups. These differences affect both what is to be learned and the skills and knowledge that can be called on to support that learning.

spoken language skills and the use of amplified hearing, then the probability of successful adaptation to a cochlear implant is increased, even if several years have elapsed since the profound deafness was acquired. Those individuals who have not developed spoken language or auditory skills, or who have lost whatever they had developed at the time of acquisition, are less likely to benefit from cochlear implants at a later date.

EDUCATIONAL ENVIRONMENT

The impact of profound deafness on the developing child is severe and far-reaching and, if adequate education is not provided, it can be devastating. Professionals disagree, however, about the form that education should take (Bowe, 1988). In particular, they disagree about the feasibility of developing effective spoken language skills or about the advisability of devoting a major portion of the available educational resources and time to the pursuit of that goal. There are several current options (Maestas-Moores & Moores 1989; Moores, 1978; Musselman, Lindsay, & Wilson, 1988; Powell, Finitzo-Hieber, Friel-Patti, & Henderson, 1985; Quigley & Kretschmer, 1982; Schwartz, 1987). They include:

• **The ORAL approach**, in which the primary goal is the development of spoken language skills in spite of the profound deafness. Sensory input involves a mixture of speechreading and aided hearing, with early reliance on written English as an unambiguous code (Gatty, 1987). An important component is the creation of a "spoken language immersion" environment in which speech is used for both instruction and communication throughout the day. Once they have acquired adequate command of spoken language, students from oral programs often transfer to schools with hearing children to finish their education.

• **The AUDITORY-VERBAL approach.** This is an extreme version of the oral approach in which the damaged sense of hearing is expected to play its normal role in the acquisition of spoken language skills. Intense effort is spent on converting auditory capacity into auditory performance. The use of vision and print as supplements to hearing is discouraged. Those children who have the necessary auditory capacity often develop remarkably good speech production and perception skills via an auditory-verbal approach and many transfer at an early age to schools for hearing children. Other intensely auditory approaches go by such names as the VERBO-TONAL method and the ACOUPEDIC approach.

• **The CUED SPEECH approach.** Cued speech is an oral approach in which the segmental ambiguities of speechreading are removed by supplementing them with hand gestures, thus facilitating face-to-face communication.

• **The TOTAL-COMMUNICATION (TC) approach.** In TC programs, a mixture of signed and spoken English is used for instruction and interpersonal communication. Individual instruction in spoken language may also be provided. Partly to avoid conflicts between nonparallel messages and partly to facilitate reading acquisition, the signed language is usually adapted so that its structure and sequence follow that of spoken English. In theory, a TC program should provide the profoundly deaf child with all of the benefits of an oral program, plus a pace of learning that is not slowed by a disparity between cognitive and linguistic development. In practice, it has proved very difficult for profoundly deaf children to develop spoken language skills without the kind of emphasis, and immersion, available in an oral program (Geers, Moog, & Schick, 1984).

• **The AMERICAN SIGN LANGUAGE (ASL) approach.** American Sign Language is the name given to the language most commonly used for face-to-face communication among prelingually deafened adult Americans who do not use spoken language (Fischer, 1982; Mayberry, 1978). It is a signed language that bears no structural relationship to spoken language. Word order usually follows a sequence from high to low in terms of information content, and syntactic relationships are often conveyed spatially rather than in terms of inflection and sequence. Proponents of the ASL approach to education argue that the development of spoken language skills in profoundly deaf children is neither feasible nor desirable. Observing: (a) that most profoundly deaf children grow up to be part of a deaf culture in which American Sign Language is the primary medium of communication; (b) that ASL has a unique structure that does not parallel spoken English; and (c) that the deaf children of deaf ASL users develop both cognitively and linguistically at a rate that equals that of hearing children, it is suggested that ASL should be used as the sole medium of instruction and communication, starting in the home and continuing through school. Although this appears to be a new approach, it is, in fact, a return to one of the methods that was used when the first schools for the deaf were founded in Europe in the 18th century (Lane, 1976).

• **MAINSTREAMING.** Mainstreaming involves placing the deaf child in a school with normally hearing children, with additional support where necessary (Ross, 1990). The concept became popular a few years ago when there was a general shift away from special schools and institutions (Ross, Brackett, & Maxon, 1982). The term "least restrictive environment" was introduced in the laws surrounding special education, and this was often interpreted to mean the child's local school (Tucker, 1984). As indicated earlier, orally trained profoundly deaf children often transfer to public school after they have developed spoken language skills that are good enough to permit them to function in that environment. They will often use FM wireless microphones so that they can hear the teacher's speech and they may also have individual instruction to help them "keep up." Occasionally they will use an "oral interpreter" in class. This is an adult who sits in front of the child and repeats what the teacher or other students are saying, but in a clearly articulated manner that the profoundly deaf child can speechread. There has also been a trend toward mainstreaming deaf children who use sign language. In such cases, a sign language interpreter is mandatory (Witter-Merithew & Dirst, 1982). Use of the term "least restrictive" to describe an environment in which all instruction and interpersonal communication must take place through an interpreter is, obviously, open to question (Ross, 1978).

There is disagreement among proponents of these various approaches. Unfortunately, the debate is seldom driven by objective data. More typically, an advocate will point to the strengths of one approach, using its more successful products for illustration, while emphasizing the weaknesses of another, using its least successful products for illustration. This is an emotionally charged issue driven by a simple fact. Namely that the loss of a major sense creates enormous problems for the developing child. Each of the basic approaches to solving these problems has strengths, weaknesses, benefits, costs, and risks. Each involves compromises. Each is vulnerable to the realities of professional preparation, the variability of professional competence, and the resulting gaps between educational principles and educational practice. Moreover, none represents the optimal compromise for all profoundly deaf children. The problems created by profound deafness are multidimensional. They do not respond to unidimensional solutions.

This is not the place for an in-depth examination of the issues surrounding educational intervention for deaf children. As a starting point for such a review, the interested reader is referred to a recent presidential commission report (Bowe, 1988). Suffice it to say, implant decisions for young children must be made in light of their educational environment. In particular, there is little point in seeking to improve auditory capacity with a cochlear implant unless the child is to be given an opportunity to use that capacity for the development of spoken language skills and competence.

CULTURAL IDENTITY

A common concept of deafness is that it is a loss that needs to be restored, a handicap that needs to be overcome, a condition that needs to be treated, or a barrier that needs to be removed. Most adults who were born deaf, however, do not consider themselves deprived, handicapped, sick, or excluded (Lane, 1992a). In fact, there is a vigorous deaf culture, with its own language, history, social mores, social organizations, even its own humor (Neisser, 1990; Vernon & Andrews, 1990). The deaf children of deaf parents usually enter that culture as infants. Many of the deaf children of hearing parents do so via school or college.

Members of the deaf culture obviously do not perceive a need to enhance their auditory capacity with cochlear implants. More importantly, however, many are also opposed to the implantation of deaf children, whom they see as younger versions of themselves and future members of their culture (Lane, 1992b).

GROUPINGS

In terms of the nonauditory variables just listed, profoundly deaf people can be divided into seven qualitatively different groups.

1. Adults with recently acquired profound deafness are likely to be dealing with the dramatic psychological impact of loss of auditory contact with the environment. Their most important problem, however, is the loss of speech perception ability and the resulting interruption of communication. This loss impacts on social life and on the ability to sustain gainful employment (Knutson & Lansing, 1990; Vernon & Ottinger, 1989). Even when there is considerable auditory capacity, it is so much worse than normal hearing, and the problems of noise and loudness discomfort are so severe, that amplification is unlikely to be successful. Those who have a natural aptitude for speechreading may quickly learn to understand speech with tolerable success. The majority, however, do not, and their problems are compounded by anxiety in situations requiring face-to-face communication. Many choose to solve these problems by avoiding communication or, when forced into it, by asking people to write. Note, however, that the speech of recently deafened people remains virtually intact. The only problems likely to be noticed in their speech are a strained voice quality and difficulty with the control of loudness. Moreover, these individuals retain full auditory, linguistic, and world knowledge. They do not consider themselves to be deaf in a cultural sense. Rather, they are hearing people who have lost their hearing. This group has a great need for the kind of improved sensory capacity that may be available from a cochlear implant. It also has the best chance of successful adaptation to the implant's novel sensory code. An implant will not, however, eliminate the pressing need for counseling and support in relation to the new and unwelcome status (Orlans, 1985).

2. Adults with long-standing, postlingually acquired profound deafness fall into two categories. The members of one continue to perceive themselves as hearing people without hearing. They are generally good speechreaders and they have overcome their initial problems with hearing aids and find them to be somewhat beneficial. If they were deafened in childhood, they have most probably continued their education either in schools with hearing children or in oral schools for deaf children. Issues of social and vocational adaptation have been dealt with.

Many have become active in organizations such as the Alexander Graham Bell Association for the Deaf that promote the development and use of spoken language for communication. These individuals, however, are acutely aware of the limitations imposed by their profound deafness and of the potential benefits that improved sensory input could provide. Moreover, although they may have lost much of the auditory knowledge acquired before deafness was acquired, the chance of successful adaptation to an implant is high, especially if they have continued to use hearing aids.

Members of the second category of adults with long-standing profound deafness perceive themselves as culturally "deaf." If the deafness was acquired during childhood, they most probably continued their education in special programs for the deaf in which sign language was the primary medium for instruction and communication. They will generally have developed friendships with prelingually deafened peers, and acquired a "deaf" identity. Their social circle is likely to consist mostly of deaf persons and they may well work with other deaf people. They may belong to social clubs for the deaf and to organizations that promote the welfare of deaf people. Because of the spoken language skills and knowledge that were acquired via normal hearing, these individuals often become leaders and spokespersons in the deaf community. Some have good speechreading skills but prefer the security and accuracy of a sign language interpreter in face-to-face communication. They usually have retained excellent speech skills, although numerous uncorrected distortions may have crept into their articulation. These individuals are unlikely to feel a need for the kind of increased sensory input that might be provided by a cochlear implant. To the extent that they enquire about the possibilities, it will often be under pressure from others, especially parents who are still seeking to undo what was done by the deafness. These people are unlikely to benefit from cochlear implants.

3. **Adults with prelingually acquired deafness** also fall into two categories. A minority have been successfully educated in oral schools. Most of these have used hearing aids and continue to do so. Speech production may be difficult to follow until the listener is familiar with its characteristics. Speech perception via a combination of speechreading and hearing aids or, in some cases by speechreading alone, may be quite good. Often these individuals have also developed competence in sign language and may count both hearing and deaf people among their friends. They do not, however, perceive themselves as belonging exclusively to a deaf culture. Rather, they perceive themselves either as deaf members of a predominantly hearing culture, inconvenienced but not excluded, or as bicultural. If these individuals have been able to use hearing aids successfully in the past, they may be able to adapt to the

novel sensory input provided by a cochlear implant. The prognosis is not good, however.

The second category of adults with prelingually acquired deafness consists of those whose education was based primarily on the development and use of a sign language for both instruction and communication. Few will have intelligible speech or viable speech perception skills. Face-to-face communication with nonsigning persons will require a sign language interpreter or the use of writing. Even the latter may be difficult because most prelingually deafened people fail to acquire high levels of competence with either reading or writing (Bowe, 1988). These individuals will most likely perceive themselves as culturally deaf. Some members of the deaf culture are very militant in seeking increased rights, considerations, and accessibility. This militancy extends to a negative attitude to cochlear implants, which are seen as a symbol of the "deviancy" model of deafness. To them, deafness is not an illness that needs to be cured, but a characteristic that creates a cultural difference. As indicated earlier, not only would they not seek cochlear implants for themselves, but they object to the implantation of deaf children whom they see as future members of the deaf culture. They would no more approve of surgery to make deaf children into hearing children than a black person would approve of surgery to make black children white. Needless to say, this group of prelingually deafened adults is not rich in implant candidates.

4. Children with recently acquired postlingual profound deafness face all the psychological trauma of the adult and, perhaps, more. Older children may be able to understand what has happened to them. Younger postlingually deafened children, however, may not realize that it is they who have changed but may believe, instead, that the world has turned sound off. Consider, also, that a common cause of postlingually acquired deafness in children is meningitis which can affect the sense of balance. These children may be learning to use vision and proprioception to compensate for the loss of balance at the same time as they are attempting to adjust to the loss of hearing. Beyond these problems, however, are the need to conserve speech and other spoken language skills and the need to continue the acquisition of world knowledge and vocabulary in spite of the deafness. As with adults, the need for increased sensory input, of the type potentially available from a cochlear implant, is high. So, also, is the probability of successful outcome. In fact, the increased adaptability of children may make those with recently acquired postlingual deafness even more suitable candidates than otherwise similar adults.

5. Children with long-standing, postlingually acquired profound deafness may still be able to capitalize on the auditory, speech, and language knowledge that was learned though normal hearing, even if several years have elapsed since they became deaf. Much will depend on the child's educational experience in the intervening years. To the extent that he or she has continued to use spoken language as the primary means of instruction and communication so the probability of successful outcome from a cochlear implant is increased.

6. Children with long-standing, prelingually acquired deafness differ according to their educational experience. To the extent that spoken language has been developed and used for instruction and communication, with as much help from hearing as possible, there may be some virtue in seeking to enhance sensory input with a device such as a cochlear implant. Such a step would need to be followed, however, by a period of training focused on adaptation to sound and hearing. Essentially, the child would need to acquire knowledge of sounds and their causes, and of the relationship between speech sounds and speech movements, at an age when the normal developmental process is much more advanced. Without the means and commitment to ensure this follow-up, there is not much point in trying to enhance sensory input.

7. Children with recently acquired prelingual profound deafness pose a serious question in relation to the commitment that is to be made to the development and use of spoken language as a medium for communication and instruction. If the commitment, and the means to meet it, are present, then enhancement of sensory input becomes a high priority. Moreover, the probability of successful adaptation to enhanced sensory input is high, especially if the profound deafness was acquired after 1 year of age, when basic auditory knowledge and skills are established. Whether a cochlear implant might have more to offer in this regard than a hearing aid, however, is not always easy to determine in children of preschool age. It is hard to derive valid pure tone thresholds from very young children, and even harder to derive valid estimates of auditory resolution. Decisions about the benefits to be obtained from hearing aids require a period of diagnostic teaching and careful observation. If there is no commitment to the development and use of spoken language, or if the means to meet that commitment are lacking, then the possible enhancement of auditory capacity by cochlear implantation is pointless.

As with categorization based on auditory variables, the foregoing analysis is somewhat artificial. Nevertheless, it serves to emphasize the heterogeneous nature of the profoundly deaf population and the many complex issues that impinge on decisions about sensory and educational or rehabilitative management.

SUMMARY

In summary, profoundly deaf persons differ in terms of the age-of-onset of deafness, current age, duration of deafness, educational experience, and cultural identity. These differences exist independently of, but may interact with, the differences of auditory capacity discussed earlier. In terms of the probability of successful implant use (and assuming that the implant provides significant auditory capacity), the most promising candidates are adults or children with postlingually acquired deafness of recent origin. The next most promising are adults and children with postlingually acquired deafness of long standing. Children with prelingually acquired deafness of recent origin may be expected to take advantage of cochlear implants, but only if they are in a program that fosters the development of auditory and spoken language skills. Children and adults with prelingually acquired deafness of long standing might be considered for candidacy if they have been orally educated and have benefited from hearing aids in the past, but the prognosis is not good. Most prelingually deafened adults perceive deafness as a culturally defining condition. Not only would they not seek implants for themselves, but many are strongly opposed to the implantation of deaf children.

OTHER ISSUES

TACTILE AIDS

Before implants were developed, there was a long history of efforts to develop sensory aids for the deaf by converting sound patterns into patterns of tactile stimulation (Levitt, Pickett, & Houde, 1980; Sherrick, 1984) and, in spite of the relatively greater success of cochlear implants, tactile aid researchers are still active (Levitt, 1988). Experimental devices have used both mechanical vibrations and electrical stimulation. Some have used a single stimulator, others have used several. Some have been designed to encode as much of the acoustic signal as possible, others have transmitted selected speech features. Currently, a handful of tactile sensory aids is commercially available (Roeser, 1989).

In controlled studies using closed-set tasks, both deaf and hearing participants have been shown to be capable of perceiving phonologically significant contrasts with these devices (Pickett, & Pickett, 1963; Hnath-Chisolm & Kishon-Rabin, 1988). In one study, participants were even able to identify isolated words from a pool of 200, after many hours of training (Engleman & Rosov, 1975). Moreover, it has been shown repeatedly that speechreading performance improves by a significant amount when tactile information derived from the acoustic speech signal is combined with the visible movements of the face (e.g., Blamey, Cowan, Alcantara, Whitford, & Clark, 1989; Hanin, Boothroyd, & Hnath-Chisolm, 1988; Skinner et al., 1988).

In contrast to the results obtained with cochlear implants, however, no subject has ever been able to hold an unstructured conversation using only a tactile aid for input, and the speechreading enhancement effect, with sentence input, has been consistently small. With novel coding schemes, and/or improved training techniques, we may yet see tactile "stars" who perform as well as the best implantees. To date, however, the performance of tactile aids at the sentence level suggests that even the more complex devices have only provided their users with access to gross temporal patterns.

On the positive side, it should be noted that most studies of tactile aids used for the perception of sentence-length material have found speechreading enhancements of about 10 percentage points (Blamey et al., 1989; Hanin, Boothroyd, & Hnath-Chisolm, 1988; Skinner et al., 1988). This level of performance is better than that of the least successful implant user. Another point in favor of the tactile aid is that it is noninvasive. Its use does not, therefore, involve the risk of destroying usable hearing in the hope of providing something better. Although these devices have not yet had the dramatic impact of cochlear implants, they may yet do so, and even now they can play a significant role in the management of profound deafness.

SEVERELY DEAF PERSONS

Several implant professionals have been so encouraged by the results of the more successful implant users that they have advocated the use of implants with severely deaf persons (that is, those with hearing losses in the 60 to 90 dB range). The argument is that, if implants can give totally deaf people auditory capacity similar to that of severely deaf people, then they should be able to give severely deaf people even more. There is no evidence, however, that postimplant performance is correlated with preimplant hearing loss. In fact, there is evidence to suggest that the two are unrelated (Boothroyd, Geers, & Moog, 1991). If the auditory capacity provided by a cochlear implant is, indeed, independent of preimplant thresholds, then the implantation of severely deaf ears cannot be justified on the basis of results obtained so far. The severely deaf ear already has as much capacity as that provided to the most successful implant users. This argument does not extend, however, to the implantation of a profoundly deaf ear in a person who has a severe hearing loss in the better ear. In this case, there is a possibility of providing roughly equivalent auditory capacity in the two ears without risking the loss of useful auditory capacity in the poorer ear.

COMBINING IMPLANTS AND HEARING AIDS

The last point raises the more general question of the continued use of a hearing aid in the nonimplanted ear of an implant user. Such a step is probably justified if the aided and implanted ears have similar auditory capacities. Moreover, depending on its design, the implant may well provide access to certain phonetic features that are not accessible via the hearing aid. In the studies that my colleagues and I are conducting, for example, we have found that in aided and implanted people with similar overall levels of performance, the hearing aid users tend to have better perception of voicing and intonation cues while users of the Nucleus implant tend to have better perception of vowel and consonant place cues. Such an outcome might have been predicted on the basis of the design features of the Nucleus speech processing system (see Wilson, Chapter 2).

PROGRESSIVE HEARING LOSS

The implication throughout this chapter has been that profound deafness is acquired suddenly. In fact, many individuals suffer a gradual, or stepwise reduction of auditory capacity over a period of years. These people are often in an excellent position to benefit from cochlear implants because they have had the opportunity to adapt to the problems of perceiving speech with a reduced sensory input. As with all the comments about probable success made earlier, however, this one is contingent on the implant's ability to provide the individual with significant auditory capacity.

IMPROVED AIDS AND IMPLANTS

The comments in this chapter about the absolute and relative performance of hearing aids, cochlear implants, and tactile aids are specific to the time of writing. Researchers and engineers are continually striving to improve the design of cochlear implant electrode assemblies, speech processors, and coding systems. We may well, therefore, see significant improvements of performance in the next few years, calling for a revision of criteria for implantation and expectations for outcome. It should be noted, however, that similar improvements may occur in hearing aids. In fact, much of the signal processing technology that was essential to the development of effective implants has yet to be applied to hearing aids for the profoundly deaf (Boothroyd, 1990). When it is, we may well see parallel improvements of hearing aid performance. And, as just mentioned, there remains the possibility that the current barriers to improved performance of tactile sensory aids will be discovered and overcome.

NEED FOR MORE ACTUARIAL DATA

Among the many needs related to profound deafness and cochlear implants, one of the more pressing ones is for better actuarial data. Potential candidates, or the parents of potential candidates, need to be given reliable information about the probabilities of various outcomes. This information must come from careful performance assessment of implant users and hearing aids users, supplemented by exact specifications of their characteristics and learning opportunities.

NEED FOR PREDICTION OF IMPLANT OUTCOME

A second pressing need is for methods of predicting outcome with implant users. Experience has shown that the auditory capacity provided by an implant can range from considerable to zero. The differences are believed to reflect such factors as the number and proximity of stimulable neurons, but the exact causes are not known and we do not, at the present time, have ways of determining, beforehand, how much auditory capacity an individual person will obtain. If reliable predictive measures become available, they will greatly reduce the need for probability-based predictions derived from actuarial data.

CONCLUSION

The cochlear implant has had a dramatic impact on the management of profound deafness. It has expanded the range of available prosthetic options and it has provided considerable auditory capacity to many individuals who were unable to benefit from hearing aids. Not all profoundly deaf persons, however, are candidates for cochlear implants. Many already have as much auditory capacity, accessible via hearing aids, as an implant can reasonably be expected to provide. Even among those profoundly deaf persons who meet auditory criteria for implantation, there are many who are not implant candidates for various nonauditory reasons. Moreover, even among profoundly deaf persons who meet both auditory and nonauditory criteria for implantation, the resulting auditory capacity is likely to vary considerably in ways that cannot yet be predicted from preimplant data. Finally, even among the most successful implant users, the auditory capacity provided by the implant is no better than that of a person with a borderline severe-to-profound hearing loss wearing hearing aids.

The population of profoundly deaf persons is heterogeneous. The consequences of profound deafness are serious and far-reaching. The management of profound deafness is complex and multidimensional. Cochlear implants in no way represent a "cure." They do, however, represent a valuable addition to the available options for the sensory component of management.

ACKNOWLEDGMENTS

Preparation of this chapter was supported, in part, by NIH grant #2PO1DC00178. The assistance of my colleague, Laurie Hanin, is gratefully acknowledged.

REFERENCES

Alpiner, J. G., & Garstecki, D. C. (1989). Aural rehabilitation for adults. In R. L. Schow & M. A. Nerbonne (Eds.), *Introduction to aural rehabilitation.* Austin, TX: Pro-Ed.

Alpiner, J. G., & McCarthy, P. A. (1987). *Rehabilitative audiology: Children and adults.* Baltimore, MD: Williams & Wilkins.

ANSI. (1989). *Specifications for audiometers.* Standard S3.6. New York: American National Standards Institute.

Blamey, P. J., Cowan, R. S. C., Alcantara, J. I., Whitford, L. A., & Clark, G. M. (1989). Speech perception using combinations of auditory, visual, and tactile information. *Journal of Rehabilitation Research and Development, 26,* 15–24.

Boothroyd, A. (1978). Speech perception and sensorineural hearing loss. In M. Ross & T. G. Giolas (Eds.), *Auditory management of the hearing impaired child.* Baltimore, MD: University Park Press.

Boothroyd, A. (1984). Auditory perception of speech contrasts by subjects with sensorineural hearing loss. *Journal of Speech and Hearing Research, 27,* 134–144.

Boothroyd, A. (1985). Auditory capacity and the generalization of speech skills. In J. Lauter (Ed.), *Speech planning and production in normal and hearing-impaired children* (ASHA Reports No. #15, pp. 8–14). Rockville, MD: American Speech Language Hearing Association.

Boothroyd, A. (1988a). Linguistic factors in speechreading. In C. L. De Filippo & D. G. Sims (Eds.), *New reflections on speechreading.* Washington, DC: Alexander Graham Bell Association for the Deaf.

Boothroyd, A. (1988b). *Evaluating the performance of cochlear implantees: Equivalent hearing loss.* Paper presented to the 1988 annual convention of the American Speech Language Hearing Association, Boston, MA.

Boothroyd, A. (1988c). *Hearing impairments in young children.* Washington, DC: Alexander Graham Bell Association for the Deaf.

Boothroyd, A. (1990). Signal processing for the profoundly deaf. *Acta Otolaryngologica, 469,* 166–171.

Boothroyd, A. (1991). Assessment of speech perception capacity in profoundly deaf children. *American Journal of Otology, 12,* 67s–72s.

Boothroyd, A. (1992a). Speech perception, sensorineural hearing loss, and hearing aids. In G. Studebaker & I. Hochberg (Eds.), *Acoustic factors affecting hearing aid performance.* Austin, TX: Pro-Ed.

Boothroyd, A. (1992b). The FM wireless link: An invisible microphone cable. In M. Ross (Ed.), *FM auditory training systems: Characteristics, selection, and use.* Parkton, MD: York Press.

Boothroyd, A. (1992c). Speech perception measures and their role in the evaluation of hearing aid performance. In J. A. Feigin & P. G. Stelmachowicz (Eds.), *Pediatric amplification* (pp. 77–91). Omaha, NB: Boys Town National Research Hospital.

Boothroyd, A., & Cawkwell, S. (1970). Vibrotactile thresholds in pure tone audiometry. *Acta Otolaryngologica, 69,* 381–387. Also in J. B. Chaiklin, I. M. Ventry, & R. F. Dixon (Eds.) (1982), *Hearing measurement: A book of readings* (2nd ed.). Reading, MA: Addison Wesley.

Boothroyd, A., & Medwetsky, L. (1992). Spectral distribution of /s/ and the frequency response of hearing aids. *Ear and Hearing, 13,* 150–157.

Boothroyd, A., Geers, A. E., & Moog, J. S. (1991). Practical implications of cochlear implants in children. *Ear and Hearing, 12,* 81s–89s.

Boothroyd, A., Springer, N., Smith, L., & Schulman, J. (1988). Amplitude compression and profound hearing loss. *Journal of Speech and Hearing Research, 31,* 362–376.

Bowe, F. G. (Chairman). (1988). *Toward equality: Education of the deaf.* Report of the Commission on Education of the Deaf to the President and Congress of the United States. Washington, DC: U. S. Government Printing Office.

Byrne, D., Parkinson, A., & Newall, P. (1991). Modified hearing aid selection procedures for severe/profound hearing losses. In G. A. Studebaker, F. H. Bess, & L. B. Beck (Eds.). *The Vanderbilt hearing-aid report II.* Parkton, MD: York Press.

Davidson, S. A., & Melnick, W. (1988). A clinically feasible method for determining frequency resolution. *Journal of Speech and Hearing Research, 31,* 299–303.

Dawson, P., Blamey, P. J., Rowland, L.C., Dettman, S.J., Clarke, G.M., Busby, P.A., Brown, A.M., Dowell, R.C., & Rickards, F.W. (1992). Cochlear implants in children, adolescents, and prelinguistically deafened adults: Speech perception. *Journal of Speech and Hearing Research, 35,* 401–417.

De Filippo, C. L. (1982). Memory for articulated sequences and lipreading performance of hearing-impaired observers. *Volta Review, 84,* 134–146.

De Filippo, C. L., & Sims, D. G. (Eds.) (1988). *New reflections on speechreading.* Washington, DC: Alexander Graham Bell Association for the Deaf

Engleman, S., & Rosov, R. (1975). Tactual hearing experiment with deaf and hearing subjects. *Exceptional Children, 41,* 143–153.

Erber, N. P. (1972). Auditory, visual, and auditory-visual recognition of consonants by children with normal and impaired hearing. *Journal of Speech and Hearing Research, 15,* 413–422.

Erber, N. P. (1974). Visual perception of speech by deaf children: Recent developments and continuing needs. *Journal of Speech and Hearing Disorders, 39,* 178–185.

Erber, N. P. (1979). Speech perception by profoundly hearing-impaired children. *Journal of Speech and Hearing Disorders, 44,* 255–270.

Erber, N. P., & Alencewicz, C. M. (1976). Audiologic evaluation of deaf children. *Journal of Speech and Hearing Disorders, 41,* 256–267.

Fischer, S. D. (1982). Sign language and manual communication. In D. G. Sims, G. G. Walter, & R. L. Whitehead (Eds.), *Deafness and communication: Assessment and training.* Baltimore, MD: Williams & Wilkins.

Gatty, J. C. (1987). The oral approach: A professional point of view. In S. Schwartz (Ed.), *Choices in deafness: A parent's guide*. Kensington, MD: Woodbine House.

Geers, A., Moog, J., & Schick, B. (1984). Acquisition of spoken and signed English by profoundly deaf children. Journal of Speech and Hearing Research, *49*, 378–388.

Geffner, D., & Levitt, H. (1987). Communication skills of hearing-impaired children. In *Development of language and communication skills in hearing-impaired children* (ASHA Monograph No. 26, pp. 36–26). Rockville, MD: American Speech Language Hearing Association.

Grant, K. W. (1987). Frequency modulation detection by normally hearing and profoundly hearing-impaired listeners. *Journal of Speech and Hearing Research, 30*, 558–563.

Hanin, L. (1988). *The effect of experience and linguistic context on speechreading.* Unpublished doctoral dissertation, City University of New York.

Hanin, L., Boothroyd, A., & Hnath-Chisolm, T. (1988). Tactile presentation of voice fundamental frequency as an aid to the speechreading of sentences. *Ear and Hearing, 9*, 335–341.

Hasenstab, M.S., & Tobey, E.A. (1991). Language development in children receiving Nucleus multichannel cochlear implants. *Ear and Hearing, 12*, 55s–65s.

Hnath-Chisolm, T., & Kishon-Rabin, L. (1988). Tactile presentation of voice fundamental frequency as an aid to the perception of speech pattern contrasts. *Ear and Hearing, 9*, 329–334.

Hochberg, I., Boothroyd, A., Weiss, M., & Hellman, S. (1992). Effects of noise and noise suppression on speech perception by cochlear implantees. *Ear and Hearing, 13*, 263–271.

Knutson, J. F., & Lansing, C.R. (1990). The relationship between communication problems and psychological difficulties in persons with profound acquired deafness. *Journal of Speech and Hearing Disorders, 55*, 356–364.

Lane, H. (1976). *The wild boy of Aveyron.* Cambridge, MA: Harvard University Press.

Lane, H. (1992a). *The mask of benevolence: Disabling the deaf community.* New York: Alfred Knopf.

Lane, H. (1992b). Cochlear implants are wrong for young deaf children. *The National Association of the Deaf Broadcaster, 14*, 1, 5, 9.

Levitt, H. (1988). Recurrent issues underlying the development of tactile sensory aids. *Ear and Hearing, 9*, 310–305.

Levitt, H., Pickett, J. M., & Houde, R. A. (Eds.). (1980). *Sensory aids for the hearing impaired.* New York: IEEE Press.

Ling, D., & Milne, M. (1981). The development of speech in hearing-impaired children. In F. H. Bess, B. A. Freeman, & J. S. Sinclair (Eds.), *Amplification in education.* Washington, DC: Alexander Graham Bell Association for the Deaf.

Lloyd, L. L., & Kaplan, H. (1978). *Audiometric interpretation.* Baltimore, MD: University Park Press.

Maestas-Moores, J., & Moores, D. F. (1989). Educational alternatives for the hearing impaired. In R. L. Schow & M. A. Nerbonne (Eds.), *Introduction to aural rehabilitation.* Austin, TX: Pro-Ed.

Mayberry, R. I. (1978). Manual communication. In H. Davis & R. S. Silverman (Eds.), *Hearing and deafness* (pp. 400–417). New York: Holt, Reinhart, & Winston.

Moores, D. F. (1987). *Educating the deaf: Psychology, principles and practices* (3rd ed.). Boston, MA: Houghton Mifflin.

Musselman, C. R., Lindsay, P.H., & Wilson, A.K. (1988). An evaluation of recent trends in preschool programming for hearing-impaired children. *Journal of Speech and Hearing Disorders, 49*, 58–64.

Neisser, A. (1990). *The other side of silence.* Washington, DC: Gallaudet University Press.

Nober, E. H. (1967). Vibrotactile sensitivity of deaf children to high intensity sound. *Laryngoscope, 77*, 2128–2146.

Orlans, H. (Ed.). (1985). *Adjustment to adult hearing loss.* San Diego, CA: College-Hill Press.

Osberger, M. J., Robbins, A. M., Miyamoto, R. T., Berry, S. W., Myres, W. A., Kessler, K. S., & Pope, M. L. (1991). Speech perception abilities of children with cochlear implants, tactile aids, or hearing aids. *American Journal of Otology, 12*, 105s–115s.

Owens, E., & Blazek, B. (1985). Visemes observed by hearing-impaired and normal hearing adult viewers. *Journal of Speech and Hearing Research, 28*, 281–393.

Owens, E., & Kessler, D. (1989). *Cochlear implants in young deaf children.* Boston, MA: Little, Brown.

Patrick, J. F. (1991). The Nucleus 22-channel cochlear implant. *Ear and Hearing, 12*, 3s–9s.

Pickett, J. M., & Pickett, B. H. (1963). Communication of speech sounds by a tac–tual vocoder. *Journal of Speech and Hearing Research, 6*, 207–222.

Powell, F., Finitzo-Hieber, T., Friel-Patti, S., & Henderson, F. (1985). *Education of the hearing-impaired child.* San Diego, CA: College-Hill Press.

Preves, D. A. (1991). Output limiting and speech enhancement. In G. A. Studebaker, F. H. Bess, & L. B. Beck. (Eds.), *The Vanderbilt hearing-aid report II.* Parkton, MD: York Press.

Quigley, S. P., & Kretschmer, R. E. (1982). *The education of deaf children.* Baltimore, MD: University Park Press.

Roeser, R. J. (1989). Tactile aids: Development issues and current status. In E. Owens & D. Kessler (Eds.), *Cochlear implants in young deaf children.* Boston, MA: Little, Brown.

Ross, M. (1978). Mainstreaming: Some social considerations. *Volta Review, 80*, 21–30.

Ross, M. (Ed.) (1990). *Hearing-impaired children in the mainstream.* Parkton, MD: York Press.

Ross, M., & Seewald, R. C. (1988). Hearing aid selection and evaluation with young children. In F. H. Bess (Ed.), *Hearing impairment in children* (pp. 190–213). Parkton, MD: York Press.

Ross, M., Brackett, D., & Maxon, A. (Eds.). (1982). *Hard of hearing children in regular schools.* Englewood Cliffs, NJ: Prentice Hall.

Rubinstein, A., & Boothroyd, A. (1987). Effect of two approaches to auditory training on speech recognition by hearing-impaired adults. *Journal of Speech and Hearing Research, 30*, 153–160.

Sanders, D. A. (1982). *Aural rehabilitation: A management model.* Englewood Cliffs, NJ: Prentice Hall.

Schwartz, S. (Ed.). (1987). *Choices in deafness: A parent's guide.* Kensington, MD: Woodbine House.

Sherrick, C. E. (1984). Basic and applied research on tactile aids for the deaf: Progress and prospects. *Journal of the Acoustical Society of America, 71*, 1249–1254.

Skinner, M. W. (1988). *Hearing aid evaluation.* Englewood Cliffs, NJ: Prentice Hall.

Skinner, M. W., Binzer, S. M., Fredrickson, J. M., Smith, P. G., Holden, T. A., Holden, L. K., Juelich, M. F., & Turner, B. A. (1988). Comparison of benefit from vibrotactile aid and cochlear implant for postlinguistically deaf adults. *Laryngoscope, 98,* 1092–1099.

Staller, S., Beiter, A., & Brimacombe, J. (1991). Children and multichannel cochlear implants. In H. Cooper (Ed.), *Cochlear implants: A practical guide.* San Diego, CA: Singular Publishing Group.

Summerfield, A. Q. (1983). Audio-visual speech perception. In M. E. Lutman & M. Haggard (Eds.), *Hearing science and hearing disorders.* New York: Academic Press.

Tobey, E. A., & Hasenstab, M. S. (1991). Effects of a Nucleus multichannel cochlear implant upon speech production in children. *Ear and Hearing, 12,* 48s–54s.

Tucker, B. P. (1984). Legal aspects of education in the mainstream: The current picture. *Volta Review, 86,* 53–70.

Tyler, R. S. (1986). Frequency resolution in hearing-impaired listeners. In B. C. J. Moore (Ed.), *Frequency selectivity in hearing.* New York: Academic Press.

Vernon, M., & Andrews, J. F. (1990). *The psychology of deafness: Understanding deaf and hard-of-hearing people.* New York: Longman.

Vernon, M., & Ottinger, P. J. (1989). Psychosocial aspects of hearing impairment. In R. L. Schow & M. A. Nerbonne (Eds.), *Introduction to Aural Rehabilitation.* Austin, TX: Pro-Ed.

Walden, B. E. (1984). Speech perception of the hearing-impaired. In J. Jerger (Ed.), *Hearing disorders in adults.* San Diego, CA: College-Hill Press.

Walden, B. E., Erdman, S. A., Montgomery, A. A., Schwartz, D. M., & Prosek, R. A. (1981). Some effects of training on speech recognition by hearing-impaired adults. *Journal of Speech and Hearing Research, 24,* 207–216.

Walden, B. E., Prosek, R. A., Montgomery, A. A., Scherr, C. K., & Jones, C. J. (1977). Effects of training on the visual recognition of consonants. *Journal of Speech and Hearing Research, 20,* 430–436.

Watkins, S., & Schow, R. L. (1989). Aural rehabilitation for children. In R. L. Schow & M. A. Nerbonne (Eds.), *Introduction to aural rehabilitation.* Austin, TX: Pro-Ed.

Watson, C. S. (1991). Speech-perception aids for hearing-impaired people: Current status and needed research. Report of the CHABA working group on communication aids for the hearing impaired. *Journal of the Acoustical Society of America, 90,* 637–685.

Wilber, L. A. (1979). Threshold measurement methods and special considerations. In W. F. Rintelman (Ed.), *Hearing assessment.* Baltimore, MD: University Park Press.

Wilson, B. S., Lawson, D. T., Finley, C. C., & Wolford, R. D. (1991). Coding strategies for multichannel cochlear implants. *American Journal of Otology, 12,* 56–61.

Witter-Merithew, A., & Dirst, R. (1982). Preparation and use of educational interpreters. In D. G. Sims, G. G. Walter, & R. L. Whitehead (Eds.), *Deafness and communication: Assessment and training.* Baltimore, MD: Williams & Wilkins.

CHAPTER 2

Signal Processing

BLAKE S. WILSON

The most important function of a cochlear prosthesis is to provide some level of speech recognition for implant users. Thus, the task of representing speech signals as electrical stimuli is central to the design and performance of implant systems. Design considerations include (a) the placement, number, and geometric relationships of the implanted electrodes; (b) the likely variation across patients in the location and condition of surviving auditory neurons in the vicinity of the electrodes; (c) the way in which stimulus information is to be conveyed from an external processor to the electrodes; and (d) how electrical stimuli should be derived from speech and other input signals. The purpose of this chapter is to review these considerations, with emphasis on consideration (d).

PROSTHESIS SYSTEMS

Essential elements of prosthesis systems are shown in Figure 2–1. A microphone senses pressure variations in a sound field and converts these into electrical variations. The electrical signal from the microphone is processed to derive stimuli for an implanted electrode or array of electrodes. The stimuli are sent to the electrodes via a transcutaneous link (top panel in Figure 2–1) or through a percutaneous connector (bottom panel). A typical transcutaneous link includes encoding of the stimulus information for radio-frequency transmission from an external transmit-

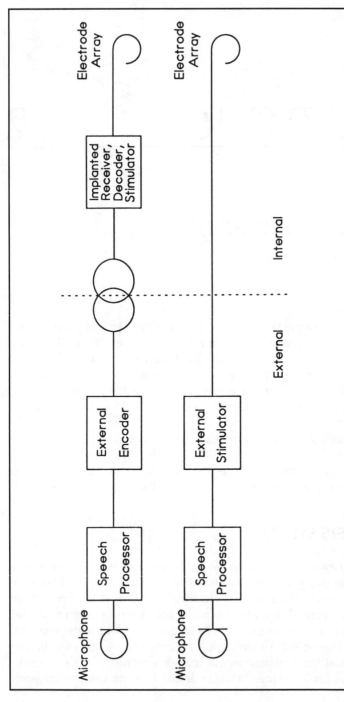

Figure 2–1. Components of prosthesis systems. A microphone senses acoustic pressure variations and converts these to electrical variations. The electrical signal is processed to derive stimuli for an implanted electrode or array of electrodes (bottom panel). A typical transcutaneous link includes encoding of the stimuli for radio-frequency transmission from an external transmitting coil to an internal receiving coil. The signal from the internal coil is decoded to specify stimuli for the electrodes.

ting coil to an implanted receiving coil. The signal from the implanted coil is decoded to specify stimuli for the electrodes.

ELECTRODES

The range of choices in the design of each of these elements, along with potential sources of variation across patients, are indicated in Figure 2–2. Electrodes may be placed on the medial wall or round window of the cochlea ("extracochlear"), in the scala tympani ("intracochlear"), within the modiolus, or on the surface of the cochlear nucleus. Among these, extracochlear placements are the least invasive, and those on the surface of the cochlear nucleus are the most invasive. Cochlear-nucleus implants have been limited to approximately 20 cases of Neurofibromatosis II, where surgical removal of acoustic tumors has severed the auditory nerve (Shannon, Zeng, Wygonski, & Maltan, 1991).

The most common placement by far is within the scala tympani. This placement brings electrodes close to the terminations of auditory neurons, which are spread along the length of the cochlea in an orderly, tonotopic arrangement. For patients with good nerve survival, multiple electrodes can be used to mimic, in a crude way, the "place" representation of frequencies in the normal cochlea. In particular, the presence of high-frequency sounds can be indicated by stimulating electrodes toward the base of the cochlea, whereas lower frequencies can be indicated by stimulating electrodes closer to the apex.

The quality of the place representation presumably depends on the number and spacing of perceptually independent sites of stimulation. Sufficient loss of excitable neurons in particular areas would be expected to degrade or distort the representation. In an extreme case, for example, survival of neurons might be limited to only one tonotopically distinct region of the cochlea. Stimulation with any of the electrodes in an implanted array then would signal to the central nervous system that the same set of peripheral neurons were active, from the same cochlear region. The patient would not be able to discriminate stimuli delivered through different electrodes. For such a patient, one electrode might be as good as a hundred.

At the other extreme, excellent survival of neurons may support an effective representation of frequencies via place of stimulation. Indeed, many implant patients can discriminate electrode positions on the basis of pitch or timbre percepts (see Shannon, Chapter 8). The maximum number of such discriminable positions may depend on how rapidly the electric field drops with increasing distance from each electrode.

Electrodes	Processing Strategy
• extracochlear	• single channel
intracochlear	multichannel
modiolar	• analog
cochlear nucleus	pulsatile
• number and spacing of contacts	• waveform representation
• orientation with respect to excitable tissue	feature extraction

Patient	Transmission Link
• peripheral nerve survival	• percutaneous
surgical placement of electrodes	transcutaneous
function of central auditory pathways	
cognitive and language skills	

Figure 2–2. Principal design options and considerations for cochlear prostheses.

The geometric relationships among electrodes and the target neural tissue can affect the spread of the electric field. Both mathematical modeling (Finley, Wilson, & White, 1990) and electrophysiological measures (Merzenich & White, 1977; van den Honert & Stypulkowski, 1987) have indicated that placements of pairs of bipolar electrodes in close proximity to neural tissue can provide a high degree of spatial specificity. However, more distant placements can substantially degrade such specificity. Monopolar electrodes produce a relatively broad pattern of excitation unless the electrodes are placed within or immediately adjacent to the target tissue.

Present implant devices use both monopolar and bipolar arrangements of electrodes. The Utah/Symbion/Richards device ("Ineraid") uses 6 electrodes spaced 4 mm apart (Eddington, 1980, 1983). In typical clinical applications the 4 most apical of these electrodes are driven in a monopolar configuration, with respect to a remote reference electrode placed in the temporalis muscle. The Melbourne/Nucleus device uses 22 electrodes spaced .75 mm apart (Patrick & Clark, 1991). In typical clinical applications a "bipolar plus 1" configuration is used, in which electrodes 1.5 mm apart are driven as bipolar pairs. Finally, the now-discontinued UCSF/Storz device and the new MiniMed device use bipolar electrodes whose pairs are partially oriented along the radial projections of auditory nerve fibers beyond the spiral ganglion cells and partially oriented along the length of the cochlea (Loeb et al., 1983). These "offset radial" electrodes are spaced at 2 mm intervals, and may provide an especially high degree of spatial specificity for ears in which survival of the peripheral neural processes is good (Merzenich & White, 1977). In typical clinical applications four of the eight pairs are used in the UCSF/Storz device and all eight pairs are used in the MiniMed device. The MiniMed device has the further capability to employ the 16 electrode contacts in a variety of monopolar and longitudinal bipolar configurations (Schindler & Kessler, 1989). All three types of electrode array may be inserted to depths of 20–25 mm within the scala tympani.

While the patterns of electric fields produced by these various arrangements of electrodes are undoubtedly different, the influence of those patterns on perception is largely unknown. For example, it is not known whether the central auditory system requires a sharp, isolated peak in neural responses to infer the position of stimulation in the cochlea. The system might only require relatively shallow skirts on either side of a peak to infer the position. In our experience, a majority of patients using the Ineraid array have little or no difficulty in distinguishing their electrodes on the basis of pitch or sharpness/dullness percepts. Further, there is no obvious difference, with the patients we have studied, of such electrode ranking abilities among patients using the Ineraid, Melbourne/Nucleus, or UCSF/Storz devices. These informal findings suggest the possibility that use of monopolar electrodes may be as effective as use of bipolar electrodes in representing place cues with scala-tympani implants.

TRANSMISSION LINK

Another distinction among implant designs relates to the way in which stimuli are transmitted from an external processor to the implanted electrodes. The Ineraid device uses a percutaneous pedestal, which allows direct transmission through plug connections. The Melbourne/Nucleus, UCSF/Storz, and MiniMed devices use a transcutaneous transmission system, which supports indirect transmission of stimulus information through a radio-frequency link.

A principal advantage of the percutaneous connector is signal transparency; that is, the specification of stimuli is in no way constrained by the unavoidable limitations imposed by any practical design for a transcutaneous transmission system. A further advantage of the percutaneous link is its simplicity. The implanted electronics used in transcutaneous systems are subject to failure, and such failure generally requires surgical removal and replacement of the electronics or of the electronics and electrode array as a unit.

The advantage of the transcutaneous system is that the skin is closed over the implanted components, avoiding a possible pathway for infection. Because the consequences of infection invading the inner ear can be severe, some surgeons prefer devices using a transcutaneous system. However, it is worth noting that experience with the percutaneous pedestal has in general been positive, with a relatively low incidence of infection requiring removal of the device (5 removals in the 153 cases reviewed by Cohen & Hoffman, 1991; 1 removal in the 46 cases reported by Parkin, 1990).

PATIENT

Great variability in outcomes across patients is a common finding in studies of cochlear prosthesis systems. While any of several implant devices can support relatively high levels of speech recognition for some patients, other patients have poor outcomes with each of those same devices. Obviously, characteristics of individual patients can exert a strong influence on performance. Factors contributing to this variability may include differences among patients in the survival of neural elements in the implanted cochlea, surgical placement of the electrodes, integrity of the central auditory pathways, or cognitive and language skills.

Examples of outcomes for two implant devices are presented in Figure 2–3. A histogram of scores for recognition of words in sentences is shown in the top panel for 25 users of the Ineraid device, and a separate histogram of those scores is shown in the bottom panel for 30 users of the Melbourne/Nucleus device (with the "F0/F1/F2" processing strategy). A wide variation in scores is seen across patients for both devices.

Such variability obviously complicates the task of comparing different implant designs. For group comparisons, where a different population of subjects is used to evaluate each design, large variability means that large numbers of subjects will be required to identify differences among designs. Most testing with cochlear implants has involved such group comparisons, and results from those tests do not differentiate effects of patient variables from effects of design variables.

While studies using group comparisons have been of great value in establishing expected levels of performance for contemporary cochlear prosthe-

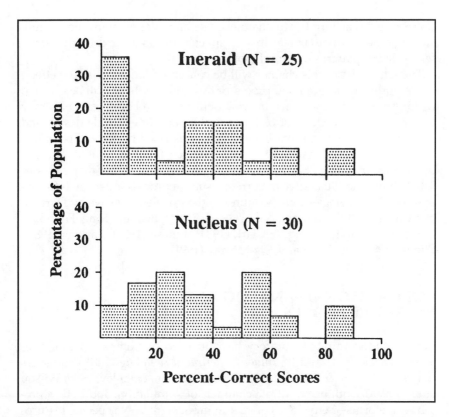

Figure 2–3. Histograms of percent-correct scores for recognition of words in 100 sentences. The top panel shows a histogram for 25 patients using the Ineraid device, and the bottom panel shows a histogram for 30 patients using the Melbourne/Nucleus device (with the "F0/F1/F2" processing strategy). The heights of the bars indicate the percentage of the population with scores in the range of each bin. (Data are from Tyler & Tye-Murray, 1991.)

ses (e.g., Cohen, Waltzman, & Fisher, 1991; Gantz, McCabe, Tyler, & Preece, 1987; Gantz et al., 1988; Tyler, Moore, & Kuk, 1989), within-patients comparisons are most efficient for identifying relative strengths and weaknesses of different prosthesis designs (e.g., Wilson, Lawson, & Finley, 1992).

PROCESSING STRATEGY

A final difference among implant designs is in the strategy used for transforming speech inputs into stimuli for the electrodes. As indicated in Figure 2–2, processing strategies can be broadly distinguished by such characteristics as number of channels, use of analog or pulsatile stimuli, and whether particular features of speech inputs are explicitly represented in the patterns of stimulation.

The remainder of this chapter will be concerned largely with the effects of various differences among processor designs. Emphasis will be given to within-patients comparisons, in which effects of processor variables may be separated from effects of patient variables and of electrode design and placement. While the processing strategies described below will be only a subset of the many that have been developed for implantable auditory prostheses, they have been chosen as representative of the major classes listed above and illustrative of current issues in processor design. Information on other strategies may be found in the excellent reviews by Dorman (see Chapter 4, this volume); Gantz (1987); Millar, Blamey, Tong, Patrick, & Clark (1990); Millar, Tong, & Clark (1984); Moore (1985); Parkins (1986); Pfingst (1986); and Tyler and Tye-Murray (1991).

COMPARISON OF ANALOG AND PULSATILE PROCESSORS

Recent studies in our laboratory have focused on comparisons of *compressed analog* (CA) and *continuous interleaved sampling* (CIS) processors (Lawson, Wilson, & Finley, 1992; Wilson, Lawson, & Finley, 1990; Wilson et al., 1991a). Both use multiple channels of stimulation, and both represent waveforms or envelopes of speech input signals. No specific features of the input, such as the fundamental or formant frequencies, are extracted or explicitly represented. CA processors use continuous analog signals as stimuli, whereas CIS processors use pulses. The CA approach is used in the widely applied Ineraid device (Eddington, 1980, 1983) and in the now-discontinued UCSF/Storz device (with some differences in details of implementation, see Merzenich, Rebscher, Loeb, Byers, & Schindler, 1984; also recall that the electrodes and transmission links are quite different in the two devices). The CIS approach is just becoming available for use in clinical settings.

The designs of CA and CIS processors are illustrated in Figures 2–4 to 2–6. In CA processors microphone signals varying over a wide dynamic range are compressed or restricted to the narrow dynamic range of electrically evoked hearing (Pfingst, 1984; Shannon, 1983) using an automatic gain control. The output of this first stage then is filtered into four contiguous frequency bands for presentation to each of four electrodes. As shown in Figure 2–5, information about speech sounds is contained in the relative stimulus amplitudes among the four electrode channels and in the temporal details of the waveforms for each channel.

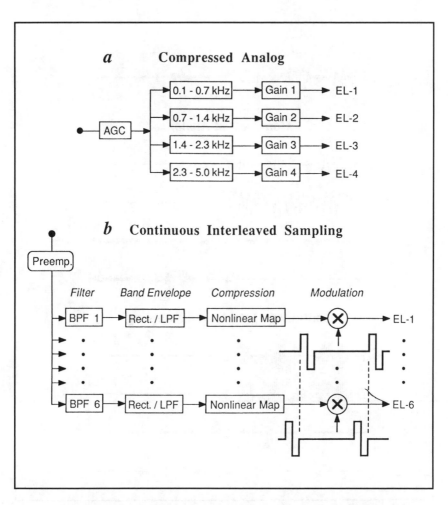

Figure 2–4. Block diagrams of major processing steps in CA and CIS strategies. (a) A CA strategy uses a broadband automatic gain control (AGC), followed by four channels of bandpass filtering (with the indicated frequencies) and adjustable gain controls. The outputs of the gain stages are connected to four intracochlear electrodes (EL-1 through EL-4). (b) A CIS strategy uses a preemphasis filter (Preemp.) to attenuate strong low frequency components in speech that otherwise might mask important high frequency components (high frequency emphasis is accomplished in CA processors by adjustment of the channel gain controls). The preemphasis filter typically is followed by five or six channels of processing. Each channel includes stages of bandpass filtering (BPF), envelope detection, compression, and modulation. The envelope detector consists of a rectifier (Rect.) followed by a lowpass filter (LPF). Carrier waveforms for two of the modulators are shown immediately below the two corresponding multiplier blocks. (Reprinted with permission from *Nature, 352,* 236–238. Copyright 1992 Macmillan Magazines Limited.)

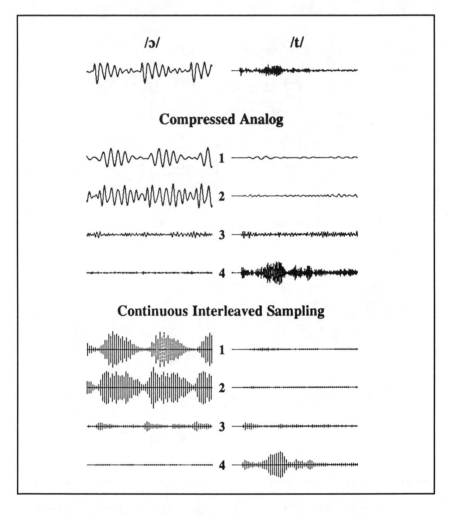

Figure 2–5. Waveforms produced by simplified implementations of CA and CIS strategies. The top panel shows preemphasized (6 dB/octave attenuation below 1.2 kHz) speech inputs. Inputs corresponding to a voiced speech sound ("aw") and an unvoiced speech sound ("t") are shown in the left and right columns, respectively. The duration of each trace is 25.4 ms. The remaining panels show stimulus waveforms for CA and CIS processors. The waveforms are numbered by channel, with channel 1 delivering its output to the apical-most electrode. To facilitate comparisons between strategies, only four channels of CIS stimulation are illustrated here. In general, five or six channels have been used for that strategy. The pulse amplitudes reflect the envelope of the bandpass output for each channel. In actual implementations the range of pulse amplitudes is compressed using a logarithmic or power-law transformation of the envelope signal. (Reprinted with permission from *Nature, 352,* 236–238. Copyright 1991 Macmillan Magazines Limited.)

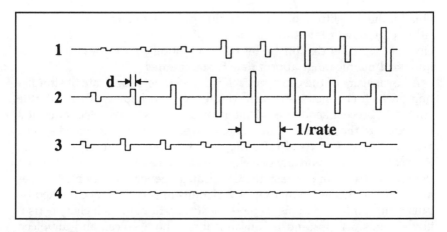

Figure 2–6. Expanded display of CIS waveforms. Pulse duration per phase ("d") and the period between pulses on each channel ("1/rate") are indicated. The sequence of stimulated channels is 4–3–2–1. The total duration of each trace is 3.3 ms. (Reprinted with permission from *Nature, 352,* 236–238. Copyright 1991 Macmillan Magazines Limited.)

A concern associated with this method of presenting information is that substantial parts of it may not be perceived by implant patients (Wilson, Finley, & Lawson, 1990). For example, most patients cannot perceive frequency changes in stimulus waveforms above about 300 Hz (see Shannon, Chapter 8). Thus, many of the temporal details present in CA stimuli probably are not accessible to the typical user.

In addition, the simultaneous presentation of stimuli may produce significant interactions among channels through vector summation of the electric fields from each electrode (e.g., White, Merzenich, & Gardi, 1984). The resulting degradation of channel independence would be expected to reduce the salience of channel-related cues. That is, the neural response to stimuli from one electrode may be significantly distorted, or even counteracted, by coincident stimuli from other electrodes.

The CIS approach addresses the problem of channel interactions through the use of interleaved nonsimultaneous stimuli (Figures 2–4b and 2–6). Trains of balanced biphasic pulses are delivered to each electrode with temporal offsets that eliminate any overlap across channels. The amplitudes of the pulses are derived from the envelopes of bandpass filter outputs. In contrast to the four-channel clinical CA processors, five or six bandpass filters (and channels of stimulation) generally have been used in CIS systems to take advantage of additional implanted electrodes and reduced interactions among channels. The envelopes of the bandpass outputs are formed by rectification and lowpass filtering.

Finally, the amplitude of each stimulus pulse is determined by a logarithmic or power-law transformation of the corresponding channel's envelope signal at that time. This transformation compresses each signal into the dynamic range appropriate for its channel.

A key feature of the CIS approach is its relatively high rate of stimulation on each channel. As described later in this chapter, other pulsatile strategies present sequences of interleaved pulses across electrodes at a rate equal to the estimated fundamental frequency during voiced speech and at a jittered or fixed (often higher) rate during unvoiced speech. Rates of stimulation on any one channel rarely have exceeded 300 pulses per second (pps). In contrast, the CIS strategy generally uses brief pulses and minimal delays, so that rapid variations in speech can be tracked by pulse amplitude variations. The rate of stimulation on each channel usually exceeds 800 pps and is constant during both voiced and unvoiced intervals. A constant, high rate allows relatively high cutoff frequencies for the lowpass filters in the envelope detectors. With a stimulus rate of 800 pps, for instance, lowpass cutoffs can approach (but not exceed) 400 Hz without introducing aliasing errors in the sampling of the envelope signals at the time of each pulse (see Rabiner & Shafer, 1978, for a complete discussion of aliasing and its consequences).

Studies to compare the CA and CIS strategies have been conducted with seven patients selected for their high levels of performance with the CA processor used with the Ineraid device. In addition, studies have been initiated with patients chosen for their relatively poor performances with the clinical processors.

Each patient was studied for a 1-week period in which (a) basic psychophysical measures were obtained on thresholds and dynamic ranges for pulsatile stimuli, (b) a variety of CIS processors (with different choices of processor parameters) were evaluated with preliminary tests of consonant identification, and (c) performance with the best of the CIS processors and the clinical CA processor was documented with a broad spectrum of speech tests. Experience with the clinical processor exceeded 1 year of daily use for all patients. In contrast, experience with the CIS processors was limited to no more than several hours before formal testing.

The comparison tests included open-set recognition of 50 one-syllable words from Northwestern University Auditory Test 6 (NU-6), 25 two-syllable words (spondees), 100 key words in the Central Institute for the Deaf (CID) sentences of everyday speech, and the final word in each of 50 sentences from the Speech Perception in Noise (SPIN) test (here presented without noise). All tests were conducted with hearing alone, using single presentations of recorded material, and without feedback as to correct or incorrect responses.

The results for nine patients are presented in Figure 2–7 (also see Dorman, Chapter 4, for additional results). Scores for the "high performance" patients are indicated by the light lines near the top of each panel, and scores for the two "low performance" patients are indicated by the dark lines closer to the bottom of each panel. (Studies with two additional "low performance" patients have been initiated, but are incomplete as of this writing—see Wilson, Lawson, Finley, & Zerbi, 1992.)

As is evident from the figure, all nine patients scored higher, or repeated a score of 100% correct, on every test, using a CIS processor. The average scores across patients increased from 64 to 86% correct on the spondee test ($p < 0.01$), from 70 to 91% correct on the CID test ($p < 0.02$), from 39 to 76% correct on the SPIN test ($p < 0.001$), and from 34 to 54% correct on the NU-6 test ($p < 0.0002$).

These findings indicate that use of CIS processors can produce large and immediate gains in speech recognition for a wide range of implant patients. Indeed, the sensitivity of some of the administered tests has been limited by ceiling (or saturation) effects: five of the seven "high performance" patients scored 96% or higher for the spondee test using CIS processors; all seven scored 95% or higher for the CID test; and five scored 92% or higher for the SPIN test. Scores for the NU-6 test, while not approaching the ceiling, still were quite high. The 80% score achieved by two of the patients corresponds to the middle of the range of scores obtained by people with mild-to-moderate hearing losses when taking the same test (Bess & Townsend, 1977; Dubno & Dirks, 1982).

Factors contributing to the performance of CIS processors might include (a) reduction in channel interactions through the use of nonsimultaneous stimuli, (b) use of five or six channels instead of four, (c) representation of rapid envelope variations through the use of relatively high pulse rates, (d) preservation of amplitude cues with channel-by-channel compression, and (e) the shape of the compression function. Studies are in progress to evaluate possibilities (a) to (c) and (e). Preliminary results suggest that all of these factors affect performance, and that factors (a) to (c) are especially important. In addition, optimal tradeoffs, among pulse duration, pulse rate, interval between sequential pulses, and cutoff frequency of the lowpass filters in the envelope detectors, appear to vary from patient to patient.

Our comparisons of CA and CIS processors show that use of pulsatile stimuli can be at least as effective as the use of analog stimuli.

EXTRACTION AND REPRESENTATION OF SPEECH FEATURES

Both CA and CIS strategies were designed to convey the *waveforms* of the speech input. CA processors represent the outputs of bandpass fil-

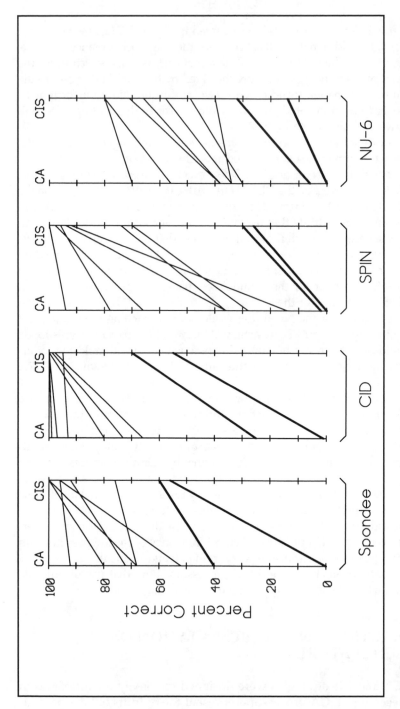

Figure 2–7. Speech recognition scores for CA and CIS processors. A line connects the CA and CIS scores for each patient. Light lines correspond to the seven patients selected for their excellent performance with the clinical CA processor, while the heavier lines correspond to the two patients selected for their relatively poor performance with that processor.

ters, while CIS processors represent envelope signals derived from such bandpass outputs. Variations in the acoustic bands are presented continuously without the extraction of any particular attributes or features of that input.

In contrast, other strategies present different patterns of stimulation based on an explicit analysis of the input signal. For example, the fundamental frequency of voiced speech sounds might be extracted in the analysis and then used to determine stimulus patterns. The aim of this type of processing is to ensure, insofar as possible, the reliable transmission of the selected feature or features. Such reliability may be enhanced by eliminating from the presentation other information that might mask or distort perception of the selected features. Also, restricting the presentation to one or several features may allow an optimal matching of the presented information to the (limited) perceptual abilities of implant patients.

F0/F2 STRATEGY

Examples of the feature-extraction approach may be found in the series of processing strategies developed for use with the Melbourne/Nucleus device (see also, Dorman, Chapter 4; Clark, 1987; Clark, Tong, & Patrick, 1990; Patrick & Clark, 1991). The first strategy, introduced for widespread clinical application in 1982, was designed to represent voicing information and the frequency and amplitude of the second formant (F2). One zero-crossings detector was used to estimate the fundamental frequency (F0) of voiced speech sounds from the output of a 270 Hz lowpass filter. A separate zero-crossings detector was used to estimate the position of the spectral centroid in the output of a bandpass filter spanning the frequency range of F2 (1000–4000 Hz, which also includes substantial portions of the frequency ranges for higher formants). The amplitude of F2 was estimated by detecting the envelope of the second filter's output with a rectifier and lowpass filter. The cutoff frequency for the lowpass filter was set at 35 Hz. This "F0/F2" processor conveyed the estimated frequency of the second formant by selecting the position of excitation in the cochlea (along the length of the implanted electrode array), while it conveyed voicing information by stimulating the selected electrodes at a rate equal to the estimated F0. The amplitudes of stimulus pulses were set to reflect the estimated amplitudes of F2. During unvoiced segments the electrodes were stimulated at quasi-random intervals, with an average rate of around 100 pps.

Performance with this initial processing strategy was encouraging, and its use allowed some patients to understand portions of speech with hearing alone (Clark, 1987; Dowell, Mecklenberg, & Clark, 1986; Patrick & Clark, 1991).

F0/F1/F2 STRATEGY

In late 1985, the F0/F2 strategy was modified to include a representation of the first formant (F1). An additional channel of front-end processing was used to estimate the frequency and amplitude of the spectral centroid in a band encompassing the frequency range of F1 (300–1000 Hz, which also overlaps the low end of the F2 range for male speakers). For each stimulus frame the processor selected two electrode positions for stimulation, one corresponding to the estimated F1 and the other to the estimated F2. As in the F0/F2 processor, the electrodes were stimulated at a rate equal to the estimated F0 during voiced speech, and at random intervals (at relatively low rates) during unvoiced segments. A stimulus frame consisted of stimulation of the selected electrode (pair) for F2 followed by stimulation of the selected electrode for F1. The pulses for each frame were separated by a minimum interval of 800 μs, and again were presented in pairs (for the two electrode positions) at a rate equal to F0 or at quasi-random intervals with an average rate of around 100 pps.

Within-patients comparisons of the F0/F2 and F0/F1/F2 strategies demonstrated improved speech recognition performance with the latter (Dowell et al., 1987a; 1987b; Tye-Murray, Lowder, & Tyler, 1990). All seven patients in the study of Dowell and colleagues, for instance, enjoyed increases in the recognition of key words in the CID sentences (presented with live voice). The average score increased from 30% correct with the F0/F2 processors to 63% correct with the F0/F1/F2 processors ($p < 0.002$). In this study initial experience with the F0/F2 strategy ranged from 3 to 18 months, and subsequent experience with the F0/F1/F2 strategy was fixed at 2 weeks. Some experience with the F0/F1/F2 strategy was deemed necessary inasmuch as many of the patients reported a decrement in intelligibility and naturalness of speech percepts when the strategy was first applied (Dowell et al., 1987a; Dowell, Brown, & Mecklenburg, 1990). Apparently, 2 weeks of experience helped patients to make better use of the new presentation of F1 information.

MIXED FEATURE AND WAVEFORM REPRESENTATIONS

Another major class of processing strategies for multichannel implants combines a feature representation with a waveform representation. In this third class a particular feature (or features) may be emphasized while still providing information on continuous variations in bandpasses of the input signal.

INTERLEAVED PULSES (IP) PROCESSORS

Early and relatively simple examples of the combination of feature and waveform representations were the interleaved pulses (IP) processors (e.g., Wilson et al., 1988a). Two variations have been described. In the first, envelope signals from six bandpass channels were scanned for each frame of stimulation. Pulses then were delivered to electrodes corresponding to the two channels with the highest envelope signals among the six. Electrode channels were assigned to bandpass channels in a tonotopic order, that is, the most apical of the electrodes was assigned to the bandpass channel with the lowest center frequency and the most basal of the electrodes was assigned to the bandpass channel with the highest center frequency. Three hundred μs/phase pulses were used, with 1.0 ms of "dead time" interposed between sequential pulses. The maximum rate on any one electrode channel was 313 pps, which is well below the rates typically used in CIS processors, but comparable to the maximum rates of F0/F2 and F0/F1/F2 processors.

This first type of IP processor was evaluated with one of several studied patients with percutaneous-connector access to an implanted UCSF electrode array (Wilson, Finley, & Lawson, 1985; Wilson et al., 1988a). This patient had extremely narrow dynamic ranges (on the order of 1 dB for pulsatile stimulation at 300 pps) and extremely poor performance with his standard CA processor (using the UCSF design). Indeed, he refused to describe any percepts elicited with the analog strategy as sounding like speech. Application of the pulsatile processor immediately produced speech percepts for this patient, and immediately produced scores significantly above chance on tests of consonant and vowel identification (scores for the CA processor were at chance levels). Unfortunately, medical complications intervened and this patient's implant device had to be removed before he could use the new strategy in his daily life and before we could conduct any more tests.

Note that this first type of IP processor extracts and represents the feature of spectral maxima in the input speech, and also represents envelope signals for the selected bandpass channels. The maximum frequency of envelope variations that can be represented without aliasing, however, is much lower than in CIS processors, the rate of stimulation being much lower in the IP processor.

Waveforms for the second type of IP processor are shown in Figure 2–8. The processing strategy is similar to that described before for the CIS processors, in that the amplitudes of envelope variations are represented on all channels for each cycle of stimulation across electrodes. However, the rates of stimulation vary between voiced and unvoiced segments of the input. During voiced segments cycles are presented at the estimated

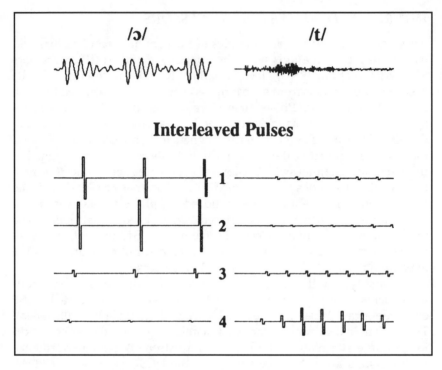

Figure 2–8. Waveforms produced by a simplified implementation of an IP strategy. Inputs, trace duration, and channel numbering are the same as those in Figure 2–5. Note that the prolonged stimulation in the IP processor for the /t/ burst is a consequence of the long time constant of the lowpass filters in the envelope detectors (25 Hz cutoff versus 400 Hz cutoff for the CIS processor implementation shown in Figure 2–5).

F0, while during unvoiced segments they are presented either at a fixed higher rate (e.g., around 300 cycles/s) or at randomly varied intervals (with average rates between 150 and 300 cycles/s). This representation of F0 and voiced/unvoiced segments is similar to the one used in the F0/F2 and F0/F1/F2 strategies, except that rates of stimulation during unvoiced segments generally are higher in the IP processors.

The maximum rate of stimulation in this second type of IP processor approximates 300 pps on any one electrode channel. Thus, to avoid aliasing errors, relatively low cutoff frequencies are used for the lowpass filters in the envelope detectors. A typical choice for the lowpass cutoff has been 25 Hz, which is similar to the 35 Hz cutoff used in the envelope detectors of F0/F2 and F0/F1/F2 processors.

This type of IP processor has been evaluated in tests with one patient using the UCSF percutaneous system (Wilson et al., 1988a), six patients using the UCSF/Storz implant (Wilson et al., 1988b; Wilson, Finley, & Lawson, 1990), and two patients using the Ineraid implant (Wilson et al., 1991b). In all studies, each patient's CA processor was compared with one or more implementations of an IP processor. Implementations for the UCSF/Storz patients were limited by the transcutaneous transmission link used with that device. The principal limitations included (a) inadequate output levels for stimulation with short-duration pulses, (b) a maximum of four electrode channels, and (c) a lack of current control in the stimulus waveforms. All patients except the one using the UCSF percutaneous system had substantial experience (typically a year or more) with their clinical CA processors. The exceptional patient had little experience with CA processors at the time of our tests.

Studies with the first patient, using the UCSF percutaneous system, were limited to tests of vowel and consonant identification. A four-channel CA processor was compared with four- and six-channel IP processors. The lowest scores on both tests were obtained with the CA processor, and the highest with the six-channel IP processor. The four-channel IP processor produced intermediate scores.

Results from the studies with the UCSF/Storz and Ineraid patients are presented in Figures 2–9 and 2–10. Figure 2–9 shows average scores and standard deviations for tests of open-set recognition, and Figure 2–10

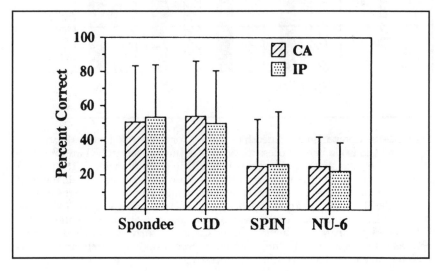

Figure 2–9. Means and standard deviations of scores from tests to compare levels of open-set recognition obtained with CA (striped bars) and IP (stippled bars) processors. Eight patients participated in the comparisons; six patients were implanted with the UCSF/Storz device, and two patients with the Ineraid device. See text for abbreviations.

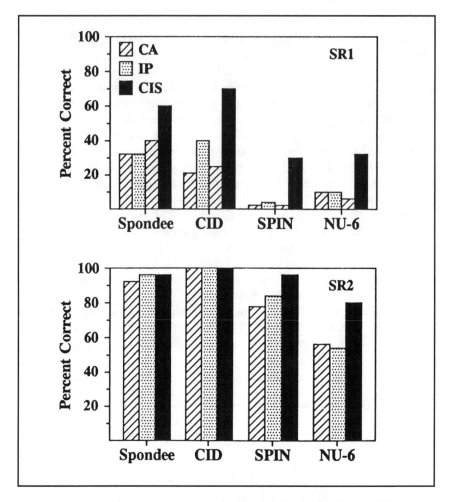

Figure 2–10. Comparisons of speech test scores for CA (striped bars), IP (stippled bars), and CIS (solid bars) processors. Scores for Ineraid patient SR1 are shown in the top panel, and scores for Ineraid patient SR2 in the bottom panel. The two CA scores for each test in the panel for SR1 are those from separate evaluations of that processor. The first evaluation (4/89) was contemporaneous with the evaluation of the IP processor for this patient, and the second evaluation (8/90; see rightmost CA bars for each test) was contemporaneous with the evaluation of the CIS processor. Separate evaluations of the CA processor were not conducted for SR2, as evaluations of both the IP and CIS processors were contemporaneous with the (single) evaluation of the CA processor.

shows individual scores for the two Ineraid patients. Comparison of the average scores demonstrates an equivalence of open-set performances for the CA and IP processors. None of the differences in scores for the two processors is significant. Thus, switching to IP processors did not degrade performance, even though experience with those processors was much less than experience with the clinical CA devices.

While the open-set scores were similar across patients for the CA and IP processors, results among patients appeared to depend, in part, on the quality of fitting for the IP processors. In all cases where at least four channels could be used, along with average pulse durations of 500 μs/phase or less, the scores were equivalent or superior for the IP processors on all four tests (four of the eight patients fulfilled these fitting criteria).

Results for the two Ineraid patients illustrate this point. As indicated in Figure 2–10, IP scores approximate or exceed CA scores for both patients. Each of these patients had percutaneous access to the implanted electrodes, allowing six channels of stimulation with short-duration (100 μs/phase), current-controlled pulses.

Although IP performances might be improved with more favorable fitting conditions and longer durations of use by the patients, these initial results are not as encouraging as the initial results obtained in the comparisons of CA and CIS processors. In the latter comparisons, all patients enjoyed substantial and immediate gains in open-set recognition with use of the CIS processors. In contrast, application of IP processors produced relatively small gains even for the two Ineraid patients, who had the most favorable fittings of IP processors among the eight studied patients. As shown in Figure 2–10, the highest scores on all four tests were obtained with the CIS processors for both patients. The increases in open-set recognition for patient SR1 were especially large, perhaps because his scores did not approach the ceiling on any of the tests.

Comparisons of CA and IP processors again suggest that little, if anything, is lost in substituting pulsatile stimuli for analog stimuli, even with the relatively sparse patterns of pulsatile stimuli used in the IP processors. Further, comparisons of CA and CIS processors suggest that a higher-fidelity representation of envelope signals alone, as supported with higher rates of pulsatile stimulation, may produce significant gains in open-set recognition over CA and IP processors.

MULTIPEAK STRATEGY

In the years 1985 to 1989, Cochlear Pty. Limited (a subsidiary of Nucleus Limited), in collaboration with investigators at the University of Melbourne, redesigned the speech processor for use with the Melbourne/Nucleus device (Patrick & Clark, 1991; Patrick, Seligman, Money, & Kuzma, 1990; Skinner et al., 1991). Digital hardware was substituted for analog hardware, and various aspects of signal processing were refined in the new processor. The refinements included use of a technique originally described by Gruenz and Schott (1949) for a more accurate and robust extraction of F0. In addition, digital processing techniques were applied to improve accuracy and resolution when extracting spectral peaks and amplitudes in the frequency ranges of the first and second formants.

Use of a specially designed integrated circuit for digital signal processing allowed substantial reductions in the size and weight of the new "Mini Speech Processor" (MSP) compared to the previous "Wearable Speech Processor" (WSP III). These reductions helped to make the processor more suitable for pediatric applications.

The MSP can be programmed to implement versions of the F0/F2 and F0/F1/F2 strategies described above. Differences in the implementations include (a) use of refined techniques for feature extraction in the MSP; (b) a change in the "F1 band" from 300 to 1000 Hz in the WSP III to 280 to 1000 Hz in the MSP; (c) a change in the "F2 band" from 1000 to 4000 Hz in the WSP III to 800 to 4000 Hz in the MSP; (d) presentation of pulses in the MSP at rates between 200 and 300 pps during unvoiced segments, as opposed to the average rate of 100 pps used in the WSP III; (e) greatly increased resolution of amplitude coding in the MSP; and (f) use of a more-compressive mapping function to derive pulse amplitudes (or durations, see below) from the bandpass outputs.

In addition to the implementations of the F0/F2 and F0/F1/F2 strategies, the MSP incorporated hardware and processing functions to augment the F0/F1/F2 strategy by a representation of envelope variations in high-frequency bands of the input signal. The bands involved are from 2000 to 2800 Hz (band 3, above the F1 range of band 1 and overlapping the F2 range of band 2), 2800 to 4000 Hz (band 4, also overlapping the F2 range of band 2), and 4000 to 6000 Hz (band 5). In this new "Multipeak" strategy four pulses are delivered in each stimulus frame. During voiced segments these frames (sets of 4 pulses) are presented at a rate equal to the estimated F0, and during unvoiced segments the frames are presented at quasi-random intervals, at an average rate of between 200 and 300 pps. Fixed electrode positions at the basal end of the cochlea are reserved for representation of the amplitudes in the upper three bands, and the remaining (more apical) electrode positions are used for representation of F1 and F2. During voiced segments the electrodes for bands 4 and 3, and for F2 and F1, are stimulated in base-to-apex order. During unvoiced segments the electrodes for bands 5, 4 and 3, and for F2, are stimulated—also in base-to-apex order. Manipulations of both pulse amplitude and pulse duration are used to code loudness (via changes in total charge/phase), primarily to reduce the time required by the transcutaneous transmission system to specify the characteristics for each pulse (it takes much less time to specify and deliver a high-intensity, short-duration pulse than a low-intensity, long-duration pulse of the same charge; e.g., Shannon, Adams, Ferrel, Palumbo, & Grandgenett, 1990). This allows higher rates of stimulation within each frame, and frame rates in excess of 400/s.

Studies have been conducted to compare the F0/F1/F2 strategy, as implemented in the WSP III, the F0/F1/F2 strategy, as implemented in the MSP or a prototype version of the MSP, and the Multipeak strategy, as implemented in the MSP (Dowell et al., 1991; Skinner et al., 1991). In within-patient comparisons with five patients, Dowell and colleagues found significant increases in open-set recognition when the MSP implementation of the F0/F1/F2 strategy was substituted for the WSP III implementation of that strategy, and when the Multipeak strategy was substituted for the MSP implementation of the F0/F1/F2 strategy. In within-patient comparisons with a separate set of five patients, Skinner and colleagues found no significant differences in open-set scores for the two implementations of the F0/F1/F2 strategy but, like Dowell and colleagues, did find significant increases in open-set scores when the Multipeak strategy was used instead of the F0/F1/F2 strategy (here implemented with the WSP III). Average scores for the recognition of NU-6 words, for instance, increased from 13% correct with the F0/F1/F2 strategy to 29% correct with the Multipeak strategy ($p < 0.01$). Thus, the Multipeak strategy was superior to all tested alternatives and, in one of the studies, the MSP implementation of the F0/F1/F2 strategy was superior to the WSP III implementation.

SPECTRAL MAXIMA SOUND PROCESSOR (SMSP) STRATEGY

The most recent in the series of new processing strategies from the University of Melbourne is the "Spectral Maxima Sound Processor" (SMSP) strategy (McDermott, McKay, Vandali, & Blamey, 1991; McKay & McDermott, 1991; McKay, McDermott, Vandali, & Clark, 1991). In this strategy, the amplitudes in each of 16 bands, spanning the range from 200 to 5400 Hz, are estimated using rectifiers and lowpass filters, as above. The cutoff frequency for the lowpass filters is set at 200 Hz. A microprocessor is programmed to scan the outputs of the lowpass filters every 4 ms. At the conclusion of each scan the microprocessor identifies the 6 channels with the highest amplitudes among the 16. It then maps the band amplitude (envelope signal) onto pulse charge (as in the Multipeak strategy) for those six channels. Finally, the pulses are delivered in a nonoverlapping sequence to electrodes whose positions correspond to the identified channels (each of the 16 channels is assigned in tonotopic order to one of 16 electrode positions; in general, the 16 most apical positions are used). The sequence of stimulation follows the ranking of channels in the amplitude scan, that is, the electrode position corresponding to the channel with the highest amplitude is stimulated first, and so on. This processing sequence is repeated every 4.0 ms, and the maximum rate of stimulation on any one electrode cannot exceed 250 pps.

The SMSP strategy is similar in design to the first type of IP processor described above. In that case the greatest 2 of 6 channels are selected for stimulation in each frame, with frames repeated every 3.2 ms.

Initial results obtained in studies with the SMSP strategy have been encouraging (McDermott et al., 1991). For each of three patients, levels of open-set recognition were significantly higher with the SMSP strategy than with the Multipeak strategy. Two of the patients had substantial experience with the Multipeak strategy at the time of the tests, and one of the patients had 12 weeks of initial experience with that processor. Experience with the SMSP processor was 5 weeks or more for all patients.

While additional studies are needed to evaluate the generality of the above results across patients, it appears that performance with the SMSP strategy may be much better than performance with the Multipeak strategy. Also, further improvements in performance might be realized through manipulation of processor parameters, such as the number of channels stimulated in each frame, and through reduction of the cutoff frequency used for the lowpass filters, to reduce or eliminate possible deleterious effects of aliasing errors in the represented envelope signals.

Although the SMSP strategy and the first type of IP strategy have been classified here as having mixed feature and waveform representations, the balance of those representations, compared with the other strategies reviewed in this section, leans heavily toward the waveform representation. That is, representation of only the most intense envelope signals may not be much different from continuous representation of all envelope signals, for a constant total number of stimulus channels and a constant frame rate of channel updates. Inclusion of the least intense signals may not have a large effect on perception (e.g., such signals may be quite small compared to others, or be masked by them). Exclusion of those presumably less-important signals might allow favorable tradeoffs among other processor parameters. For example, a reduction in the number of electrodes selected for stimulation in each cycle allows a corresponding increase in pulse rate on those electrodes. Beneficial effects produced by an increase in pulse rate may outweigh possible deleterious effects produced by a reduction in the number of electrodes stimulated in each cycle. In the context of the SMSP strategy, for instance, rates as high as 300 to 600 pps can be achieved within the constraints of the transcutaneous transmission system used with the Melbourne/Nucleus device if only 6 electrodes are stimulated in each cycle (Dillier, Bögli, & Spillmann, 1992a). Stimulation of all or most electrodes in each cycle would reduce greatly the pulse rate on each channel and (consequently) the highest frequency of envelope variations that could be represented without aliasing.

ADDITIONAL STUDIES INVOLVING CIS PROCESSORS

In current studies, our group has begun systematic investigation of various aspects of CIS performance. These studies include evaluations of CIS performance (a) across numbers of channels, (b) across other manipulations in CIS parameters, and (c) under conditions of noise interference. In addition, Dillier, Bögli, and Spillmann (1992a, 1992b) have begun studies to compare various implementations of CIS processors with each other and with clinical F0/F1/F2 and Multipeak processors used in conjunction with the Melbourne/Nucleus device. Preliminary results from studies (a) and (c) above, and from the studies of Dillier and colleagues, are presented in this section.

MANIPULATIONS IN CHANNEL NUMBER

One of the patients from our "high performance" group (SR2) participated in the studies to evaluate effects of manipulations in channel number and of noise interference. The principal test used in the studies was identification of 24 consonants (/b, d, f, g, dʒ, h, j, k, l, m, n, ɲ, p, r, s, ʃ, t, tʃ, ð, θ, v, w, z, ʒ/) in an /a/-consonant-/a/ context. Multiple exemplars of the /a/-consonant-/a/ tokens were played from laser videodisc recordings of male and female speakers (Tyler, Preece, & Lowder, 1987). A single block of trials consisted of five randomized presentations of each consonant by a single speaker. The tests were conducted with hearing alone and without feedback as to correct or incorrect responses.

Results are presented in Figure 2–11. The top panel shows percent-correct scores for CIS processors with 6, 5, 4, 3, and 2 channels, and for an analogous processor with 1 channel (referred to as a CS processor, since interleaving is not applicable to a single channel). The bottom panels show information transmission scores for various articulatory and acoustic features of consonants (Miller & Nicely, 1955). The features include voicing (Voi), nasality (Nsl), frication (Fric), duration (Dur), place of articulation (Plc), and envelope cues (Env).

Each n-channel processor used the n apical-most electrodes and filtered the same total frequency range into n bands of equal width on a logarithmic scale. For example the three-channel processor used apical electrodes 1, 2, and 3. All processors used 33 μs/phase pulses, presented at the rate of 2525 pps on each channel (delays were interposed between sequential pulses for processors with fewer than six channels to maintain this constant rate). In addition, each processor used 6th order bandpass filters, fullwave rectifiers, and 400 Hz lowpass filters (1st order). For consistency, a fixed base-to-apex update order was used

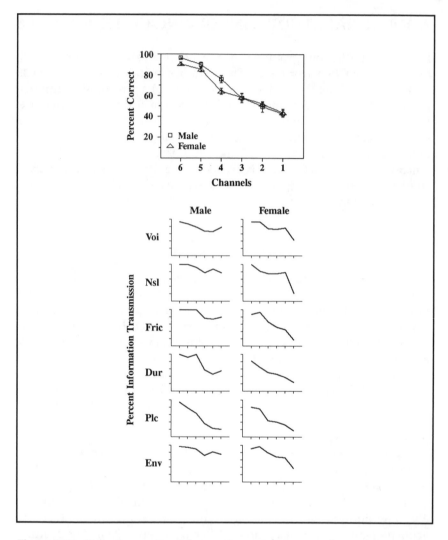

Figure 2–11. Percent correct and feature transmission scores for processors using different numbers of channels. Five presentations of each of 24 consonants by a male speaker, and five presentations of each consonant by a female speaker, were used in the tests with each processor. The presentations were arranged in block randomized order, providing a percent correct score after each set of randomized presentations of all 24 consonants. The square symbols in the top panel show averages of these scores (from five randomized sets) for the male speaker, and the triangles show the averages for the female speaker. Standard errors of the mean are indicated with the vertical bars. The remaining panels show feature transmission scores for the same experimental conditions. The features include voicing (Voi), nasality (Nsl), frication (Fric), duration (Dur), place of articulation (Plc), and envelope cues (Env). Full scale in each panel corresponds to 100% information transfer.

for all processors. For example, the three channel processor stimulated its electrodes in the sequence 3-2-1.

It is worth noting that none of the processors in this series was optimized for the individual patient. The six-channel version, for instance, was inferior to other six-channel processors using a "staggered" order of channel updates (6–3–5–2–4–1; see below and see Lawson, Wilson, & Finley, 1992). Also, processors using fewer than six channels probably would have benefited from use of specific electrodes other than the most apical n (e.g., use of more widely spaced electrodes may have produced a better result). The purpose of this particular study was to evaluate effects of changes in the number of channels, while maintaining a consistency in all other CIS parameters.

The results show a strong effect of channel number on consonant identification. Overall percent-correct scores decline monotonically, for both the male and female speakers, with reductions in the number of channels. Also, transmission of place information declines precipitously for the male speaker as the number of channels is reduced from 6 to 3, and drops precipitously for the female speaker as the number of channels is reduced from 5 to 4. In all cases the transmission of place information declines monotonically as the number of channels is reduced. In contrast, transmission of envelope information is relatively well maintained when the number of channels is reduced, as is the transmission of voicing, frication and nasality information for the male speaker (indeed, the transmission of voicing information remains high even for a single channel). Results for the female speaker are somewhat different in that the transmission of voicing and nasality information drops sharply when the number of channels is reduced from 2 to 1, and the transmission of frication information drops rapidly over the range of channel reductions from 5 to 1.

A consistent finding in the data is the dependence of place transmission on the number of stimulation channels. In addition, results from the female speaker suggest that transmission of frication information may depend on number of channels, at least up to five channels, and at least for certain speakers. Further increases in channel number may improve the transmission of place information and other important cues for the correct identification of consonants. As indicated elsewhere (e.g., Dorman et al., 1990; Tye-Murray & Tyler, 1989; Wilson, Lawson, & Finley, 1990), such identification is highly correlated with open-set recognition of words, sentences and running speech.

EFFECTS OF INTERFERING NOISE

Results from the study to evaluate effects of noise interference are presented in Figure 2–12. Here we show the performances of CIS and CA strategies in noise without any special provisions for noise reduction. A

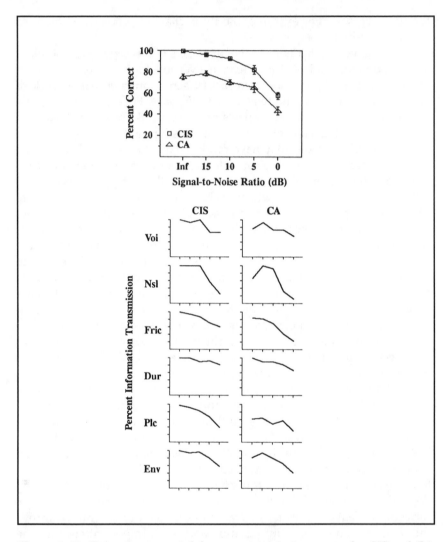

Figure 2–12. Percent correct and feature transmission scores for CIS and CA processors as a function of signal-to-noise ratio (SNR). The SNR of "Inf" refers to presentation of the signal without any accompanying noise. Five presentations of each of 24 consonants by a male speaker were used in the consonant identification tests for each processor at each SNR. The square symbols in the top panel show average percent-correct scores for the CIS processor, and the triangles show the averages for the CA processor. Standard errors of the mean are indicated with the vertical bars. The remaining panels show feature transmission scores for the same experimental conditions. The features include voicing (Voi), nasality (Nsl), frication (Fric), duration (Dur), place of articulation (Plc), and envelope cues (Env). Full scale in each panel corresponds to 100% information transfer.

six-channel CIS implementation was used with the following parameters: 33 μs/phase pulses, 2525 pps rate of stimulation on each channel, staggered update order, 12th-order bandpass filters, fullwave rectifiers, and 400 Hz lowpass filters (1st order).

Consonant identification first was measured under quiet conditions, and then progressively greater amounts of multitalker speech babble were added to the primary speech signal. Signal-to-noise ratios (SNRs) included 15, 10, 5, and 0 dB, with 0 dB corresponding to the babble signal amplitude exceeding the maximum consonant waveform amplitude briefly about once per second on average.

While the presence of noise clearly degrades the performance of both processors, relatively high percent correct scores are maintained down to a SNR of 5 dB. The scores for the CIS processor are higher than those for the CA processor at all SNRs. This is especially encouraging inasmuch as the CA processor in the Ineraid device has been identified as the most resistant to the deleterious effects of noise among several tested implant systems (Gantz et al., 1987; Tyler & Tye-Murray, 1991).

One possible factor underlying the high levels of CIS performance in the presence of interfering speech babble is a good representation of envelope cues. In particular, covariation in envelope information across channels may help maintain high levels of speech recognition in noise (e.g., Hall, Haggard, & Fernandes, 1984; Moore, 1992). Such across-channel information may allow a listener to follow the correlated cues of the primary speech signal, while rejecting the uncorrelated variations produced by the noise.

Another factor that may contribute to the performances found for both the CA and CIS strategies is the fact that neither relies on feature extraction. The accuracy of such extraction can be severely degraded by even modest amounts of noise, as demonstrated in many studies with conventional speech analysis systems (e.g., Rabiner & Shafer, 1978) and in studies with cochlear implant devices (e.g., Gantz et al., 1987).

A key lesson in the present results is that the choice of a basic processing strategy can have large effects on performance in noise.

COMPARISON WITH F0/F1/F2 AND MULTIPEAK PROCESSORS

Dillier, Bögli, and Spillmann (1992a, 1992b) have implemented versions of CIS processors for use with Melbourne/Nucleus device hardware. In general, these versions have much lower pulse rates than CIS processors tested in our laboratory (with Ineraid patients), because the transcutaneous transmission system used in the Melbourne/Nucleus device imposes a minimum time of approximately 300 μs between sequential pulses and a minimum time of approximately 10 μs between the first and second phase of each pulse. This "overhead" limits maximum rates of stimulation to somewhere between 300 and 600 pps (depending on patient thresholds, patient dynamic ranges, choice of electrodes, and choice of pulse parameters) on each channel for a six-channel processor (Dillier, Bögli, & Spillmann, 1992a; Shannon et al., 1990).

Four CIS-like processors were implemented using a specially designed hardware and software system (Dillier, Senn, Schlatter, Stöckli, & Utzinger, 1990). Speech inputs were sampled at 10 kHz (after lowpass filtering to avoid aliasing) and then preemphasized (to accentuate high-frequency components) and windowed into 12.8 ms segments of the sampled data. A Hanning window (see Rabiner & Shafer, 1978) was used to emphasize data in the center of each windowed interval, reducing certain distortions inherent in the use of rectangular windows. Windows were overlapped at the 50% points, for a window rate of 156 Hz (reciprocal of 6.4 ms). Each new window of data was analyzed with a 128-point Fourier transform, which provided power spectra across 64 linearly spaced bands. The band outputs were combined in various ways to estimate energies in logarithmically spaced bands spanning the range from 200 to 5000 Hz. In one combination up to 22 such bands were formed, corresponding to the maximum number of electrodes in the Melbourne/Nucleus array, and in another combination 6 such bands were formed, for use with a subset of the electrodes. The width of bands for the 22–band condition was approximately 1/3 octave, and the width for the 6-band condition was approximately 1 octave.

The four versions of CIS-like processors utilized these combined-band outputs in different ways. The two versions that were most similar to our implementations of CIS processors were named "CIS-NA" and "CIS-WF." In the CIS-NA processor all outputs of the narrow-band filters exceeding a preset "noise threshold" were selected for presentation to a corresponding electrode (between 16 and 22 bands and electrode positions were used, depending on the number of available electrodes for each patient). Thus, a relatively large number of electrodes could be stimulated in each cycle across the electrode array, at a relatively low pulse rate on each channel. In the CIS-WF processor all outputs of the wide-band filters were continuously presented at six widely spaced electrode positions. As in the CIS processors described by our group, band outputs were mapped onto pulse intensities using a nonlinear function, to compress the wide dynamic ranges of processed speech signals into the narrow dynamic ranges of electrically evoked hearing.

Results for the five studied patients are presented in Figures 2–13 and 2–14. Figure 2–13 shows average scores for tests of vowel and consonant identification, and Figure 2–14 shows individual scores for the consonant test. Table 2–1 lists the type of clinical processor used by each patient and his or her experience with it.

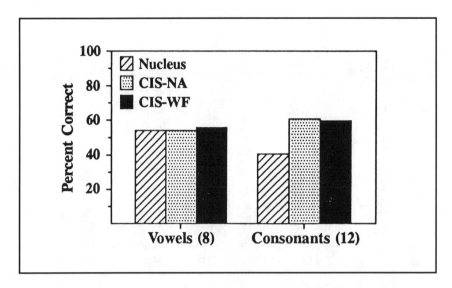

Figure 2–13. Averages of percent-correct scores from tests of vowel and consonant identification used in the studies of Dillier, Bögli, and Spillmann (1992a, 1992b). Average scores for the clinical (Nucleus) processors are shown in the striped bars, those for the CIS-NA processors in the stippled bars, and those for the CIS-WF processors in the solid bars. Chance performance for the vowel test is 12.5% correct, and chance performance for the consonant test is 8.3% correct. Five patients participated in the studies.

The vowel test included 8 vowels and the consonant test 12 consonants (/p, t, k, b, d, g, m, n, l, r, f, s/), presented in an /a/-consonant-/a/ context. Tokens were presented multiple times in random order; each consonant token was presented 12 times (for a total of 144 presentations) for each patient and processor condition. Each of the five patients had substantial experience with his or her clinical processor, ranging from 5 months to 4 years, at the time of testing. In contrast, experience with the alternative CIS-like processors was limited to between 5 and 10 minutes of listening to ongoing speech plus the time taken (presumably another 10 minutes or so) to administer a preliminary 20-item test estimating each patient's ability to identify two-digit numbers.

As indicated in Figure 2–13, use of either CIS-like processor produced a gain in the average percent-correct score for consonant identification. Vowel scores remained unchanged. Individual consonant scores, shown in Figure 2–14, indicated differences in the degree of improvement for the different patients. The CIS-NA processors produced large improvements for patients UT, TH, HS, and SA, and the CIS-WF processors produced large improvements for UT, TH and SA. Performances among

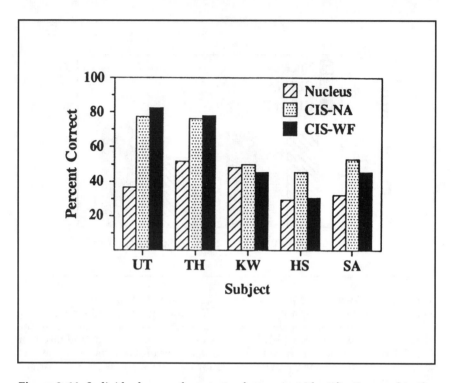

Figure 2–14. Individual scores from tests of consonant identification used in the studies of Dillier, Bögli, and Spillmann (1992a, 1992b). Scores for the clinical (Nucleus) processors are shown in the striped bars, those for the CIS-NA processors in the stippled bars, and those for the CIS-WF processors in the solid bars. Chance performance is 8.3% correct. Table 2–1 lists the type of clinical processor used by each patient and his or her experience with it.

Table 2–1. *Clinical systems used by patients in the studies of Dillier, Bögli, and Spillmann (1992a, 1992b)*

Subject	Processing Strategy*	Hardware*	Experience (Years)
UT	F0/F1/F2	WSP III	4.2
TH	F0/F1/F2	MSP	1.6
KW	Multipeak	MSP	0.4
HS	Multipeak	MSP	2.5
SA	Multipeak	MSP	2.2

*See text for abbreviations.

processors were approximately the same for patient KW. Dillier et al. (1992a) note that this patient also had the least experience among patients with his implant and the longest duration of deafness prior to the implant operation (28 years).

In all, these preliminary results indicate that substitution of a CIS-like processor can produce immediate improvements in consonant identification for at least some users of F0/F1/F2 and Multipeak processors, even with the relatively low rates of stimulation imposed by the transcutaneous link of the Melbourne/Nucleus device. Further studies are needed to (a) evaluate the generality of the preliminary results across a larger number of patients; (b) measure effects of experience on the performance of CIS-like processors; (c) determine, perhaps with Ineraid patients, how much information is lost in reducing rates of stimulation to 300 pps or lower on each channel; and (d) investigate fully the trade-off between number of channels and rate of stimulation.

SINGLE-CHANNEL STRATEGIES

Implant systems using only a single channel of stimulation have the potential advantages of simplicity and lower cost compared with multichannel systems. Therefore, single-channel systems might be preferred if their use could support speech-recognition performances similar to those obtained with multichannel systems.

One indication of possible differences in performance between single-channel and multichannel systems was presented above, in the comparisons of CIS processors with different numbers of channels (see Figure 2–11). In those comparisons reductions in channel number produced a monotonic decline in consonant identification. The lowest scores were obtained with the CS processor, a single-channel variation of CIS processors.

This strong effect of channel number, in the context of CIS processor designs, is generally consistent with the results of other recent studies demonstrating significantly higher average performances with multichannel implant systems compared to performances with single-channel systems (Cohen, Waltzman, & Fisher, 1991; Gantz et al., 1987; Tye-Murray, Gantz, Kuk, & Tyler, 1988; Tye-Murray & Tyler, 1989). However, it is important to note that some patients using single-channel devices have in fact obtained high scores on open-set tests of speech recognition (Banfai, Karczag, Kubik, Lüers, & Sürth, 1986; Hochmair-Desoyer, Hochmair, & Stiglbrunner, 1985; Tyler, 1988a, 1988b; Tyler, Moore, & Kuk, 1989). Such scores have fueled a long-standing (and continuing) debate on the relative merits of single-channel versus multichannel systems.

VIENNA/3M DEVICE

High levels of performance with single-channel systems must result from perception of temporal variations in the stimulus waveform inasmuch as any cues arising from different places of stimulation are discarded. As noted before, variations above 300 Hz (or perhaps somewhat higher for exceptional patients, see Hochmair-Desoyer, Hochmair, Burian, & Stiglbrunner, 1983; Townshend, Cotter, Van Campernolle, & White, 1987) are not generally perceived as changes in pitch or timbre by implant patients. Thus, a single channel of stimulation may be capable of representing F0, voiced/unvoiced distinctions, and temporal variations below 300 Hz or thereabouts in the overall envelope of the speech signal (see, e.g., Dorman, Chapter 4; Rosen, Walliker, Brimacombe, & Edgerton, 1989; Shannon, 1990; Shannon, Zeng, & Wygonski, 1992). In addition, exceptional patients may be able to perceive frequency changes over a portion of the F1 range (see Dorman, Chapter 4).

The Vienna/3M device is designed to make speech sounds over the frequency range of 100 to 6000 Hz audible, using a single channel of analog stimulation (Hochmair & Hochmair-Desoyer, 1983; 1985; Hochmair-Desoyer, Hochmair, & Stiglbrunner, 1985). The speech processor first compresses the input signal into the dynamic range of electrically evoked hearing, as in CA processors. The compressed signal is directed to a frequency-equalization network, and the output of the network to the modulator input of a transcutaneous transmission system. An implanted receiver demodulates the radio-frequency signal of the transmission link, and directs the demodulated stimuli either to a selected pair of electrodes in the scala tympani or to an extracochlear electrode paired with a remote reference electrode.

The equalization network is adjusted for each patient so that input sinusoids with frequencies between 100 and 4000 Hz have equal loudnesses. This helps to ensure that all components of speech with frequencies in this range will be audible. Without equalization, only low-frequency sounds would be heard, inasmuch as low-frequency sinusoids have much lower electrical thresholds than high-frequency sinusoids (see Shannon, Chapter 8).

The combination of appropriate compression and frequency equalization may allow patients to perceive most or all of the information that can be transmitted in a single channel of stimulation. Indeed, some patients using this device have achieved high levels of open-set recognition using hearing alone (Hochmair-Desoyer, Hochmair, & Stiglbrunner, 1985; Tyler, 1988a; Tyler, Moore, & Kuk, 1989). In the study of Tyler, Moore, and Kuk, for instance, nine of the "better" users of this device (as selected by the Vienna implant team) were evaluated with open-set tests of word and sentence recognition. Recognition of monosyllabic words ranged from 0 to 34% correct, with an average score of 15% correct, and recognition of key words in the context of short sentences ranged from 0 to 42% correct, with an average score of 16% correct.

HOUSE/3M DEVICE

One of the earliest and most widely applied of single-channel systems was developed by William House and his associates in the early 1970s (e.g., House & Urban, 1973; House & Berliner, 1982). In the speech processor the input signal is filtered to attenuate frequency components outside of the band between 340 and 2700 Hz (Edgerton & Brimacombe, 1984; Rosen et al., 1989; note that an early version of this device used a filter to attenuate components outside of the band between 200 and 4000 Hz, see Danley & Fretz, 1982). The output of the bandpass filter is used to modulate a 16 kHz carrier signal. Modulation is linear for speech inputs between approximately 55 and 70 dB SPL. For inputs below the lower cutoff the modulation is 100% (producing a small, "residual" carrier output) and for instantaneous inputs above the upper cutoff the modulation is 0% (producing a maximal carrier output). The upper cutoff or "clipping" level can be adjusted over the range of 65 to 75 dB SPL by the user. The modulated carrier signal is applied (after amplification) to an external transmitting coil. Voltages are induced in a separate, implanted coil and the output of the implanted coil is directed (without demodulation or other alterations) to an active electrode in the scala tympani and a reference electrode in the Eustachian tube or temporalis muscle.

As might be expected from the above description, only gross aspects of speech signals are conveyed with the House/3M device. Linear modulation of the carrier over a highly restricted range, as opposed to compressive modulation over a broad range, acts to reduce any opportunity for representing variations in the envelopes of speech waveforms. Also, elimination of sounds with (relatively) low amplitudes, and with frequency components above 2700 Hz, places many consonant sounds outside the perceptual space. Weak fricatives, for instance, are not represented.

An effect of restricting the modulation to a narrow range is to produce an "on/off" pattern of stimulation, with bursts of 16 kHz carrier appearing in synchrony with periods of voiced speech sounds and in synchrony with other relatively-intense segments of the speech input. Thus, information about voicing and other gross temporal details might be contained in the stimuli. Most of the fine detail in temporal variations of speech is, however, discarded or distorted.

Rosen et al. (1989) have conducted tests of consonant identification with four patients using the House/3M device. The average percent-correct score for tests involving 12 consonants was 37% for a "direct input" condition, with feature transmission scores of 53% for voicing, 48% for manner of articulation, and 8% for place of articulation. Rosen and colleagues suggest that these and other results obtained in their study may be explained in large part by perception of periodicity (voicing), randomness (lack of voicing), and silence in the speech inputs. In addition, limited perception of gross envelope cues may have contributed to correct identification of manner distinctions.

Most users of the House/3M device do not enjoy any open-set recognition of speech with hearing alone (e.g., Gantz et al., 1988; Gantz, Tye-Murray, & Tyler, 1989; Tye-Murray et al., 1988; Tye-Murray & Tyler, 1989). Even the exceptional patients have quite modest levels of open-set recognition. In the study of Danhauer, Ghadialy, Eskwitt, and Mendel (1990), for instance, only 5 of 18 patients scored above zero on the NU-6 test. Four of those patients identified 1 of the 50 words (2% correct) and one of the patients identified two of the words (4% correct).

CONTINUOUS SAMPLING (CS) PROCESSORS

A continuous sampling (CS) processor presents a single channel of pulsatile stimulation, with the pulses presented at a constant and relatively high rate (e.g., 2500 pps). The amplitudes of the pulses are determined using a compressive mapping of speech envelope signals, over a wide dynamic range of speech inputs. A typical value for the cutoff frequency of the lowpass filter in the envelope detector is 400 Hz. Thus, envelope variations much above this frequency are not included in the representation.

As indicated in Figure 2–11, relatively high levels of consonant identification and feature transmission can be maintained with a single channel of CS stimulation. For the male speaker transmission scores of 78% or higher were obtained by one "high performance" patient for the features of voicing, nasality, and frication, and a score of 76% was obtained for envelope cues. Overall information transmission, even for this difficult test involving 24 consonants, was 70% for the male speaker and 64% for the female speaker. The percent-correct scores were 43% for both speakers.

In tests with another (highly similar) variation of CS processors this same patient (SR2) demonstrated high levels of open-set recognition with hearing alone, consistent with the consonant results just cited. He scored 68% correct on the spondee test, 36% correct on the CID test, and 20% correct on the NU-6 test (the SPIN test was omitted due to time limitations). These scores are similar to those reported for the better patients using the Vienna/3M device. The NU-6 score of 20% correct, for example, approximates the mean of scores (15% correct) for recognition of monosyllabic words obtained by the nine patients in the study of Tyler, Moore, and Kuk (1989). While the choice of words and language differed in the two studies, the test used in the study of Tyler and colleagues probably was close in difficulty to the NU-6 test.

In a related study, Rabinowitz and Eddington (1990) compared speech reception abilities with one versus four channels of analog stimulation. Tests were conducted with the same patient who participated in our studies with the CS processors (SR2). The standard CA processor of the Ineraid device was used for the four-channel processor, and the four channels were summed into one for the single-channel processor. This summation preserved the loudness balance across frequency ranges achieved in adjustments of channel gains for the four-channel processor, and it preserved the compression characteristics of the automatic gain control.

The comparison demonstrated a large decrement in performance with substitution of the single-channel processor. However, as in our studies of CIS and CS processors, substantial levels of open-set recognition still were obtained with a single channel of stimulation. SR2's score on the NU-6 test, for instance, was 18% correct with the single-channel processor. This score is essentially identical to the score of 20% correct obtained (approximately one year later) by the same patient using a CS processor.

It is worth noting that experience with the alternative CS and single-channel analog processors was limited for SR2. At the time of our studies, for instance, SR2 had more than 5 years of daily experience with his four-channel analog processor, compared with less than two hours of aggregated experience with the CS processor before formal testing.

The apparent similarities in these results, for the Vienna/3M, CS, and combined-channel analog processors, suggest a common substrate for perception of speech sounds. That substrate might include good representations of frequency variations and energies in the range below the "pitch saturation limit" of 300 Hz or so, and of envelope variations for sounds with components at higher frequencies. A restricted or distorted mapping of input levels onto stimulus levels would be expected to limit perception of amplitude variations in speech. Also, deletion of any substantial part of the speech spectrum above 300 Hz would distort the representation of envelope cues. For example, elimination of frequency components above 1000 Hz would eliminate perception of many consonants (e.g., most of the unvoiced consonants) and grossly distort the perceived envelopes of others. This expectation is consistent with the findings of Hochmair and Hochmair-Desoyer (1985), who filtered the output stimulus signal in the Vienna/3M processor to greatly attenuate or eliminate frequency components above 900 Hz for one condition and above 300 Hz for another condition. Elimination of high-frequency components in the stimuli produced marked reductions in speech-reception scores. For one tested patient, for example, elimination of high-frequency components reduced substantially the scores on a test of consonant identification (the test included multiple live-voice presentations of each of 16 consonants, with feedback on the correct response given after each item). The percent-correct score for the normal, wideband condition was 77%, whereas the percent-correct scores for the 900 and 300 Hz conditions were 59 and 33%, respectively.

EMERGING PRINCIPLES OF PROCESSOR DESIGN

The results reviewed in this chapter have illustrated some of the choices listed in Figure 2–2 for the design of processing strategies for cochlear prostheses. In particular, these results provide at least preliminary guidance on the relative merits of single-channel versus multichannel strategies, use of analog versus pulsatile stimuli, and waveform representations versus feature-extraction strategies.

SINGLE CHANNEL VERSUS MULTIPLE CHANNELS

As mentioned above, relatively high levels of open-set recognition have been achieved with the Vienna/3M, CS, and "combined analog" strategies. Each of these strategies provides an appropriate compression of input signals and each of them represents frequency components across the full spectrum and dynamic range of typical speech sounds. The available evidence supports the hypothesis that use of these strategies may allow perception of frequency variations and energies in the range below 300 Hz or so, and of envelope variations for sounds with components at higher frequencies. Indeed, the information presented by the CS processors is restricted to envelope variations below 400 Hz. For frequencies below the 400 Hz cutoff the modulation of stimulus pulses follows individual frequency components, such as F0, and for frequencies above 400 Hz the modulation follows the envelope of all remaining components in the input signal. Performance with CS processors is comparable to the performances of the two analog processors, supporting the above hypothesis.

While high levels of speech recognition can be obtained for some patients using single-channel processing strategies, within-patients comparisons indicate that even higher levels can be achieved with multiple channels of stimulation. Figure 2–11, for instance, shows a large difference in consonant recognition when a six-channel CIS processor is used instead of the single-channel CS processor for patient SR2. For the male speaker, this excellent patient scored 43% correct with the CS processor and 97% correct with the six-channel CIS processor.

Such results indicate that differences in percepts produced by different places of stimulation in the cochlea can be exploited to provide additional information on the spectral content of speech inputs. This additional information should contribute most directly to improved reception of the place-of-articulation feature for consonants. Figure 2–11 indicates a nearly-linear dependence of information-transmission scores for this feature on the number channels used in the tested CS and CIS processors, suggesting that further increases in the number of channels might produce even higher levels of performance.

ANALOG VERSUS PULSATILE

Comparisons of analog and pulsatile processors have not demonstrated any particular advantage of analog stimulation. Among single-channel strategies, results obtained with the Vienna/3M, "combined analog," and CS processors appear to be quite similar. The Vienna/3M and "combined analog" processors (see above and Rabinowitz & Eddington, 1990) use analog stimuli, while the CS processors use pulsatile stimuli. Little, if anything, appears to be lost in discarding the high-frequency details present in analog stimuli.

For multichannel strategies use of pulses has the distinct advantage of allowing nonsimultaneous stimulation across channels. As noted before, such stimulation may help to reduce or eliminate deleterious effects of channel interactions and thereby enhance the salience of channel-related cues.

WAVEFORM REPRESENTATION VERSUS FEATURE EXTRACTION

A major portion of this chapter has been devoted to descriptions and comparisons of different multichannel strategies using waveform representations, extractions and representations of speech features, or mixed feature and waveform representations. A listing of those strategies is presented in Table 2–2. Our studies have involved comparisons of CIS and CA strategies, IP and CA strategies, and CIS and IP strategies. Studies conducted by the Australian team have involved comparisons of F0/F2 and F0/F1/F2 strategies, F0/F1/F2 and Multipeak strategies, and SMSP and Multipeak strategies. In addition, Dillier et al. (1992a) have compared reduced implementations of CIS strategies (as supported with the transcutaneous link of the Melbourne/Nucleus device) with Multipeak and F0/F1/F2 strategies.

In our studies use of CIS processors produced immediate improvements in open-set recognition of words and sentences for every tested patient. As mentioned before, factors underlying these improvements may include (a) reduction in channel interactions through the use of nonsimultaneous stimuli, (b) use of five or six channels instead of four,

Table 2–2. *Strategies used in multichannel cochlear prostheses*

Strategy*	Representation	Device(s)	Citation(s)
CA	Bandpass signals	Ineraid; UCSF/Storz	Eddington, 1980; Merzenich et al., 1984
CIS	Envelope signals	Ineraid	Wilson et al., 1991a
CIS-NA	Envelope signals	Melbourne/Nucleus	Dillier et al., 1992a
CIS-WF	Envelope signals	Melbourne/Nucleus	Dillier et al., 1992a
F0/F2	Spectral peak and voicing features	Melbourne/Nucleus	Tong et al., 1980; Dowell et al., 1986
F0/F1/F2	Spectral peak and voicing features	Melbourne/Nucleus	Dowell et al., 1987a
IP_1	Spectral maxima feature; envelope signals	UCSF, percutaneous	Wilson et al., 1988a
IP_2	Voicing feature; envelope signals	UCSF, percutaneous; UCSF/Storz; Ineraid	Wilson et al., 1988a; Wilson et al., 1991b
Multipeak	Spectral peak and voicing features; envelope signals	Melbourne/Nucleus	Skinner et al., 1991; Dowell et al., 1991
SMSP	Spectral maxima feature; envelope signals	Melbourne/Nucleus	McKay et al., 1991

*See text for abbreviations; note that IP_1 refers to the type 1 IP strategy and IP_2 refers to type 2.

(c) representation of rapid envelope variations through the use of relatively high pulse rates (and corresponding use of relatively high cutoff frequencies for the lowpass filters in the envelope detectors), (d) preservation of amplitude cues with channel-by-channel compression, and (e) the shape of the compression function.

In the studies involving IP processors an immediate equivalence in open-set scores was found for patients using the UCSF/Storz implant system. However, the fitting of IP processors was limited for those patients by characteristics of the transcutaneous link used in their device. Use of IP processors by two patients with percutaneous access to a UCSF electrode array produced large and immediate improvements in consonant and vowel identification. Finally, results from tests with two patients using the Ineraid device indicated similar or somewhat better open-set performance with IP processors. One type of IP strategy was used for the first tested patient using the UCSF percutaneous system, and a second type for all other patients, each using one of three different implant systems. The first type of IP strategy presented sequential pulses to two of six channels in each frame of stimulation, at a constant frame rate, whereas the second presented sequential pulses to all available channels (between 2 and 6, depending on the patient) in each frame, at a frame rate equal to the estimated F0 during voiced segments and at a jittered or fixed higher rate during unvoiced segments.

The relatively large improvements for the two patients with percutaneous access to UCSF electrodes may be attributable in part to their extremely poor performances with standard CA processors. In particular, release from channel interactions, through the use of nonsimultaneous pulses, may have helped these patients. It is worth noting that both of these patients had severe channel interactions with simultaneous stimuli and that one of them had extremely narrow dynamic ranges. Highly variable summations across channels with CA stimuli might be expected to produce substantial distortions in channel-related cues for such patients.

Results from limited comparisons of the CIS and IP strategies, with two Ineraid patients, were consistent with the results of the separate comparisons of both of those strategies with the CA strategy. Open-set scores for the IP processors were generally equivalent to those for the CA processors for the majority of tested patients, while scores for the CIS processors were better than those for the CA processors for all tested patients. In the direct CIS/IP comparisons, higher scores were obtained with the CIS processors. For the same number of channels, and the same type of mapping functions, the CIS processors appear to provide much better speech-recognition performance than the IP processors, for patients who have both high and low levels of performance with clinical CA processors. Factors contributing to the better performances of CIS processors may include (a) use of higher rates of stimulation, which in turn allows representation of higher frequencies in the variations of envelope signals; and (b) no reliance on feature extraction, such as the F0 and voiced/unvoiced features extracted in the IP processors.

It is important to note that accurate extraction of speech features is by no means a trivial task, especially for "real" speech that often is degraded by the presence of noise and reverberation. Accurate extraction of F0 and voiced/unvoiced boundaries in particular is extremely difficult and subject to error even for speech recorded at high signal-to-noise ratios (indeed, an extensive literature exists on approaches to extraction of F0 and voiced/unvoiced boundaries; for examples, see Flanagan, 1972; Hess, 1983; O'Shaughnessy, 1987; Rabiner & Shafer, 1978). Thus, if patients are able to perceive such information from waveform representations, without the help of explicit extraction and representation of selected features, then waveform representations should be preferred inasmuch as they (a) will not contain errors inherent in feature extraction and (b) may contain additional information useful in recognizing speech.

A related danger of a feature-extraction approach is that too few features are included in the representation. That is, information is in general discarded with reductions in the number of selected features. Also, the representation becomes progressively more abstract, and more dependent on models of speech production and perception, as the number of features is reduced.

Such a loss in information was noted in the comparisons of the F0/F2 and F0/F1/F2 strategies, as described by the Australian team (e.g., Dowell, Seligman, Blamey, & Clark, 1987a). In within-patients comparisons, for example, each of seven patients demonstrated better open-set performance with F0/F1/F2 processors. The addition of features related to F1 (spectral centroid and amplitude envelope in the band spanning the range of F1 frequencies) apparently restored some of the information that was discarded in the relatively sparse representation of F0/F2 processors.

The two subsequent strategies in the Australian series, Multipeak and SMSP, provided a mixed feature and waveform representation. The Multipeak strategy retained extraction and presentation of the F0, F1, and F2 features, but also added a waveform representation of amplitude envelopes in three contiguous bands from 2000 to 6000 Hz. The SMSP strategy abandoned the extraction of features related to voicing and formant frequencies and instead selected the six maximum outputs from the amplitude envelopes of 16 bandpasses. The selected maxima then were mapped for presentation to the six corresponding electrodes for each stimulus frame, with frames repeated every 4.0 ms.

As noted before, the balance between feature and waveform representations in the SMSP strategy leans heavily toward the latter. In particular, representation of only the most intense envelope signals may approximate representation of all envelope signals under certain conditions. Also, the "maxima feature" is not derived from a model of speech production or perception; rather, it reflects a relatively simple and modest reduction of information in the short-term spectra of the input waveform.

Within-patients comparisons of F0/F1/F2 and Multipeak strategies demonstrated improved performance with the latter (Dowell et al., 1991; Skinner et al., 1991). Thus, the addition of a waveform representation in the Multipeak strategy appeared to provide greater access to information in the speech input.

Preliminary within-patients comparisons of the Multipeak and SMSP strategies indicate that further gains in open-set recognition might be possible with SMSP processors (see, e.g., McKay et al., 1991). The minimal reliance on feature extraction used in the SMSP strategy, along with higher stimulus rates and higher cutoff frequencies in the lowpass filters for the envelope detectors, may have contributed to the observed improvements. That is, a more direct representation of ongoing envelope variations may allow perception of details in speech that otherwise might be obscured or distorted by a heavy reliance on feature extraction.

An additional trend from the studies comparing the various Australian strategies is that each new strategy produced improvements in speech recognition under conditions of noise interference. Results reported by Dowell, Seligman, Blamey, and Clark (1987b), Franz, Dowell, Clark, Seligman, and Patrick (1987), and Tye-Murray et al. (1990) demonstrate superiority of the F0/F1/F2 strategy compared to the F0/F2 strategy; results reported by Dowell et al. (1991) and Skinner et al. (1991) demonstrate superiority of the Multipeak strategy compared to the F0/F1/F2 strategy; and results reported by McDermott et al. (1991) demonstrate superiority of the SMSP strategy compared to the Multipeak strategy, for the three tested patients. Again, progressively less reliance on feature extraction might be expected to improve the performance of processing strategies in environments with interfering noise. Zero-crossings measures in particular are sensitive to such interference (see, e.g., Rabiner & Shafer, 1978, pp. 129–130), suggesting that performances of the F0/F2 and F0/F1/F2 strategies might be severely degraded by noise.

Taken together, the comparisons presented above suggest a certain convergence of ideas and results. In both the Australian series and ours, improvements in performance were obtained as more information per unit time was added to the representation and as less reliance was placed on feature extraction.

The improvements in performance with increased rates of stimulation are consistent with the findings of two recent studies demonstrating the importance of envelope cues for consonant recognition (Rosen, 1989; Van Tasell, Soli, Kirby, & Widen, 1987). In those studies, noise carriers were modulated by the envelopes of broadband speech signals, and large improvements in the identification of consonants were recorded when the maximum frequency of the envelope variations was raised from 20 Hz to either 200 Hz (Van Tasell et al., 1987) or 2000 Hz (Rosen, 1989; Van Tasell et al., 1987). In the study of Van Tasell and colleagues, for instance, average scores for overall information transmission increased from 22% to 35% when the cutoff frequency of the lowpass filter (in the envelope detector) was increased from 20 Hz to 2000 Hz.

One possible factor underlying the relative increases in performance obtained with the CIS, CIS-NA, CIS-WF, SMSP, and Multipeak strategies is an improved representation of envelope cues. Also, patterns of covariation in envelope modulations across channels may provide additional information on the identity of certain speech sounds and on transitions from one speech sound to another.

In addition, relatively high rates of stimulation can support a representation of high-frequency variations in envelope signals. Envelope variations between 50 and 400 Hz can convey with high fidelity F0; F0 transitions; precise timing of boundaries between voiced, unvoiced, and silent intervals; presence and precise timing of various transient events in speech (such as those associated with plosives); and the presence of speech sounds with mixed voiced and unvoiced components (see Rosen, 1989; Shannon, 1992; Van Tasell et al., 1987).

In broad terms it appears that, for pulsatile processors, the number of channels updated in each frame of stimulation, and the rate at which frames are presented, have strong effects on performance. As indicated in Table 2–3, CIS, CIS-like, and SMSP strategies use the greatest numbers of channels/frame, and the CIS strategy uses the highest rate of frame presentations.

THE FUTURE

This is an exciting time in the development of cochlear prostheses. Much of the excitement stems from the recent progress in signal processing, as

Table 2–3. *Stimulus and channel attributes of strategies used in multichannel cochlear prostheses*

Strategy*	Stimuli	Channels/Frame	Rate on Each Channel
CA	Analog	4	Continuous waveform
CIS	Pulses	6	Fixed at 500 pps or higher
CIS-NA	Pulses	10–20	90–180 pps or higher
CIS-WF	Pulses	6	Fixed at 300 pps or higher
F0/F2	Pulses	1	F0 or random rate around 100 pps
F0/F1/F2	Pulses	2	F0 or random rate around 100 pps
IP_1	Pulses	2	Maximum of 313 pps
IP_2	Pulses	2–6	F0 or fixed or random rate around 250–300 pps
Multipeak	Pulses	4	F0 or random rate around 250 pps
SMSP	Pulses	6	Maximum of 250 pps

*See text for abbreviations; note that IP_1 refers to the type 1 IP strategy and IP_2 refers to type 2.

described in this chapter. Application of new processing strategies has produced unprecedented levels of speech recognition for implant patients. One of the patients participating in our studies (SR2), for instance, now routinely scores at or near 100% correct for the spondee, CID, and SPIN tests using a variety of six-channel CIS processors (with different sets of pulse and other parameters) and also obtains NU-6 percentages in the high 80s or low 90s with those same processors.

While the present results are most encouraging, many important questions remain unanswered, and many possibilities for further improvement remain unexplored. These questions and possibilities are being addressed in ongoing studies in our laboratory and elsewhere. Particularly promising lines of investigation include (a) systematic evaluation of parameter choices for CIS, CIS-like, and SMSP processors; (b) systematic evaluation of how those choices vary across patients; (c) identification of mechanisms underlying patient variability; (d) application of CIS strategies in the MiniMed and other devices, that would allow implementations with more than six channels and with electrode couplings other than the monopolar configuration used in the Ineraid device; (e) evaluation of possible learning effects with extended use of CIS and CIS-like processors; and (f) design and application of new implant devices capable of presenting stimuli at high rates to a large number of electrodes, with a variety of externally controlled coupling configurations.

ACKNOWLEDGMENTS

Many of the results reviewed in this chapter are from studies conducted by the cochlear implant team at Research Triangle Institute and Duke University Medical Center. Team members most involved with the research studies included Charles C. Finley, Dewey T. Lawson, Blake S. Wilson, Robert D. Wolford, and Mariangeli Zerbi. Important scientific contributions also were made by investigators from other institutions. Principal among these investigators were Michael F. Dorman, Donald K. Eddington, F. Terry Hambrecht, Dorcas K. Kessler, Gerald E. Loeb, Michael M. Merzenich, William M. Rabinowitz, Robert V. Shannon, Sigfrid D. Soli, Margaret W. Skinner, and Mark W. White. Finally, it is a pleasure to thank the patients for their enthusiastic participation. Various aspects of this work were supported by NIH projects N01-NS-3-2356, N01-NS-5-2396, and N01-DC-9-2401 through the Neural Prosthesis Program.

REFERENCES

Banfai, P., Karczag, A., Kubik, S., Lüers, P., & Sürth, W. (1986). Extracochlear sixteen-channel electrode system. *Otolaryngologic Clinics Of North America, 19,* 371–408.

Bess, F.H., & Townsend, T.H. (1977). Word discrimination for listeners with flat sensorineural hearing losses. *Journal of Speech and Hearing Disorders, 42,* 232–237.

Clark, G.M. (1987). The University of Melbourne-Nucleus multi-electrode cochlear implant. *Advances in Oto-Rhino-Laryngology, 38,* 1–189.

Clark, G.M., Tong, Y.C., & Patrick, J.F. (1990). *Cochlear prostheses.* Edinburgh: Churchill Livingstone.

Cohen, N.L., & Hoffman, R.A. (1991). Complications of cochlear implant surgery in adults and children. *Annals of Otology, Rhinology and Laryngology, 100,* 708–711.

Cohen, N.L., Waltzman, S.B., & Fisher, S.G. (1991). Prospective randomized clinical trial of advanced cochlear implants: Preliminary results of a Department of Veterans Affairs cooperative study. *Annals of Otology and Laryngology, 100,* 823–829.

Danhauer, J.L., Ghadialy, F.B., Eskwitt, D.L., & Mendel, L.L. (1990). Performance of 3M/House cochlear implant users on tests of speech perception. *Journal of the American Academy of Audiology, 1,* 236–239.

Danley, M.J., & Fretz, R.J. (1982). Design and functioning of the single-electrode cochlear implant. *Annals of Otology, Rhinology and Laryngology,* (Suppl. 91), 21–26.

Dillier, N., Bögli, H., & Spillmann, T. (1992a). Speech encoding strategies for multielectrode cochlear implants: A digital signal processor approach. *Progress in Brain Research,* in press.

Dillier, N., Bögli, H., & Spillmann, T. (1992b). Digital speech processing for cochlear implants. *Oto-Rhino-Laryngology,* in press.

Dillier, N., Senn, C., Schlatter, T., Stöckli, M., & Utzinger, U. (1990). Wearable digital speech processor for cochlear implants using a TMS320C25. *Acta Oto-laryngologica,* (Suppl. 469), 120–127.

Dorman, M.F., Soli, S., Dankowski, K., Smith, L.M., McCandless, G., & Parkin, J. (1990). Acoustic cues for consonant identification by patients who use the Ineraid cochlear implant. *Journal of the Acoustical Society of America, 88,* 2074–2079.

Dowell, R.C., Brown, A.M., & Mecklenburg, D.J. (1990). Clinical assessment of implanted deaf adults. In G.M. Clark, Y.C. Tong, & J.F. Patrick (Eds.), *Cochlear prostheses* (pp. 193–205). Edinburgh: Churchill Livingstone.

Dowell, R.C., Dawson, P.W., Dettman, S.J., Shepherd, R.K., Whitford, L.A., Seligman, P.M., & Clark, G.M. (1991). Multichannel cochlear implantation in children: A summary of current work at the University of Melbourne. *American Journal of Otology, 12* (Suppl. 1), 137–143.

Dowell, R.C., Mecklenberg, D.J., & Clark, G.M. (1986). Speech recognition for 40 patients receiving multichannel cochlear implants. *Archives of Otolaryngology, 112,* 1054–1059.

Dowell, R.C., Seligman, P.M., Blamey, P.J., & Clark, G.M. (1987a). Evaluation of a two-formant speech-processing strategy for a multichannel cochlear prosthesis. *Annals of Otology, Rhinology and Laryngology, 96* (Suppl. 128), 132–134.

Dowell, R.C., Seligman, P.M., Blamey, P.J., & Clark, G.M. (1987b). Speech perception using a two-formant 22–electrode cochlear prosthesis in quiet and in noise. *Acta Otolaryngologica, 104,* 439–446.

Dubno, J.R., & Dirks, D.D. (1982). Evaluation of hearing-impaired listeners using a nonsense syllable test. I. Test reliability. *Journal of Speech and Hearing Research, 25,* 135–141.

Eddington, D.K. (1980). Speech discrimination in deaf subjects with cochlear implants. *Journal of the Acoustical Society of America, 68,* 885–891.

Eddington, D.K. (1983). Speech recognition in deaf subjects with multichannel intracochlear electrodes. *Annals of the New York Academy of Sciences, 405,* 241–258.

Edgerton, B.J., & Brimacombe, J.A. (1984). Effects of signal processing by the House-3M cochlear implant on consonant perception. *Acta Otolaryngologica,* (Suppl. 411), 115–123.

Finley, C.C., Wilson, B.S., & White, M.W. (1990). Models of neural responsiveness to electrical stimulation. In J.M. Miller & F.A. Spelman (Eds.), *Cochlear implants: Models of the electrically stimulated ear* (pp. 55–96). New York: Springer-Verlag.

Flanagan, J.L. (1972). *Speech analysis, synthesis and perception* (2nd ed.). Berlin: Springer-Verlag.

Franz, B.K-H.G., Dowell, R.C., Clark, G.M., Seligman, P.M., & Patrick, J.F. (1987). Recent developments with the Nucleus 22–electrode cochlear implant: A new two formant speech coding strategy and its performance in background noise. *American Journal of Otology, 8,* 516–518.

Gantz, B.J. (1987). Cochlear implants: An overview. *Advances in Otolaryngology, Head and Neck Surgery, 1,* 171–200.

Gantz, B.J., McCabe, B.F., Tyler, R.S., & Preece, J.P. (1987). Evaluation of four cochlear implant designs. *Annals of Otology, Rhinology and Laryngology, 96* (Suppl. 128), 145–147.

Gantz, B.J., Tye-Murray, N., & Tyler, R.S. (1989). Word recognition performance with single-channel and multichannel cochlear implants. *American Journal of Otology, 10,* 91–94.

Gantz, B.J., Tyler, R.S., Knutson, J.F., Woodworth, G., Abbas, P., McCabe, B.F., Hinrichs, J., Tye-Murray, N., Lansing, C., Kuk, F., & Brown, C. (1988). Evaluation of five different cochlear implant designs: Audiologic assessment and predictors of performance. *Laryngoscope, 98,* 1100–1106.

Gruenz, O.O., & Schott, L.O. (1949). Extraction and portrayal of pitch of speech sounds. *Journal of the Acoustical Society of America, 21,* 487–495.

Hall, J.W., Haggard, M.P., & Fernandes, M.A. (1984). Detection in noise by spectro-temporal pattern analysis. *Journal of the Acoustical Society of America, 76,* 50–56.

Hess, W. (1983). *Pitch determination of speech signals: Algorithms and devices.* Berlin: Springer-Verlag.

Hochmair, E.S., & Hochmair-Desoyer, I.J. (1983). Percepts elicited by different speech-coding strategies. *Annals of the New York Academy of Sciences, 405,* 268–279.

Hochmair, E.S., & Hochmair-Desoyer, I.J. (1985). Aspects of sound signal processing using the Vienna intra- and extracochlear implants. In R.A. Schindler & M.M. Merzenich (Eds.), *Cochlear implants* (pp. 101–120). New York: Raven Press.

Hochmair-Desoyer, I.J., Hochmair, E.S., Burian, K., & Stiglbrunner, H.K. (1983). Percepts from the Vienna cochlear prosthesis. *Annals of the New York Academy of Sciences, 405,* 295–306.

Hochmair-Desoyer, I.J., Hochmair, E.S., & Stiglbrunner, H.K. (1985). Psychoacoustic temporal processing and speech understanding in cochlear implant patients. In R.A. Schindler & M.M. Merzenich (Eds.), *Cochlear implants* (pp. 291–304). New York: Raven Press.

House, W.F., & Berliner, K.I. (1982). Cochlear implants: Progress and perspectives. *Annals of Otology, Rhinology and Laryngology,* (Suppl. 91), 1–124.

House, W.F., & Urban, J. (1973). Long-term results of electrode implantation and electronic stimulation of the cochlea in man. *Annals of Otology, Rhinology and Laryngology, 82,* 504–517.

Lawson, D.T., Wilson, B.S., & Finley, C.C. (1992). New processing strategies for multichannel cochlear prostheses. *Progress in Brain Research,* in press.

Loeb, G.E., Byers, C.L., Rebscher, S.J., Casey, D.E., Fong, M.M., Schindler, R.A., Gray, R.F., & Merzenich, M.M. (1983). Design and fabrication of an experimental cochlear prosthesis. *Medical and Biological Engineering and Computing, 21,* 241–254.

McDermott, H., McKay, C., Vandali, A., & Blamey, P. (1991, September). *An improved sound processor for the University of Melbourne/Nucleus multielectrode cochlear implant.* Paper presented at the International Symposium on Natural and Artificial Control of Hearing and Balance, Rheinfelden, Switzerland.

McKay, C.M., & McDermott, H.J. (1991). Speech perception ability of adults with multiple-channel cochlear implants, using the spectral maxima sound processor. *Journal of the Acoustical Society of America, 89* (Suppl. 1), 1959.

McKay, C., McDermott, H., Vandali, A., & Clark, G.M. (1991). Preliminary results with a six spectral maxima sound processor for the University of Melbourne/Nucleus multiple-electrode cochlear implant. *Journal of the Otolaryngology Society of Australia, 6,* 354–359.

Merzenich, M.M., Rebscher, S.J., Loeb, G.E., Byers, C.L., & Schindler, R.A. (1984). The UCSF cochlear implant project. State of development. *Advances in Audiology, 2,* 119–144.

Merzenich, M.M., & White, M.W. (1977). Cochlear implant — The interface problem. In F.T. Hambrecht & J.B. Reswick (Eds.), *Functional electrical stimulation: Applications in neural prostheses* (pp. 321–340). New York: Marcel Dekker.

Millar, J.B., Blamey, P.J., Tong, Y.C., Patrick, J.F., & Clark, G.M. (1990). Speech perception. In G.M. Clark, Y.C. Tong, & J.F. Patrick (Eds.), *Cochlear prostheses* (pp. 41–67). Edinburgh: Churchill Livingstone.

Millar, J.B., Tong, Y.C., & Clark, G.M. (1984). Speech processing for cochlear implant prostheses. *Journal of Speech and Hearing Research, 27,* 280–296.

Miller, G.A., & Nicely, P.E. (1955). An analysis of perceptual confusions among some English consonants. *Journal of the Acoustical Society of America, 27,* 338–352.

Moore, B.C.J. (1985). Speech coding for cochlear implants. In R.F. Gray (Ed.), *Cochlear implants* (pp. 163–179). San Diego, CA: College-Hill Press.

Moore, B.C.J. (1992). Comodulation masking release and across-channel masking. In M.E.H. Schouten (Ed.), *Audition, speech and language.* Berlin: Mouton-de Gruyter, in press.

O'Shaughnessy, D. (1987). *Speech communication: Human and machine.* Reading, MA: Addison-Wesley.

Parkin, J.L. (1990). The percutaneous pedestal in cochlear implantation. *Annals of Otology, Rhinology and Laryngology, 99,* 796–801.

Parkins, C.W. (1986). Cochlear prostheses. In R.A. Altschuler, D.W. Hoffman, & R.P. Bobbin (Eds.), *Neurobiology of hearing: The cochlea* (pp. 455–473). New York: Raven Press.

Patrick, J.F., & Clark, G.M. (1991). The Nucleus 22–channel cochlear implant system. *Ear and Hearing, 12* (Suppl. 1), 3S–9S.

Patrick, J.F., Seligman, P.M., Money, D.K., & Kuzma, J.A. (1990). Engineering. In G.M. Clark, Y.C. Tong, & J.F. Patrick (Eds.), *Cochlear prostheses* (pp. 99–124). Edinburgh: Churchill Livingstone.

Pfingst, B.E. (1984). Operating ranges and intensity psychophysics for cochlear implants. *Archives of Otolaryngology, 110,* 140–144.

Pfingst, B.E. (1986). Stimulation and encoding strategies for cochlear prostheses. *Otolaryngologic Clinics of North America, 19,* 219–235.

Rabiner, L.R., & Shafer, R.W. (1978). *Digital processing of speech signals.* Englewood Cliffs, NJ: Prentice-Hall.

Rabinowitz, W.M., & Eddington, D.K. (1990, June). *Effects of channel-to-electrode mappings with the Symbion cochlear prosthesis.* Paper presented at the Second International Cochlear Implant Symposium 1990, Iowa City, Iowa.

Rosen, S. (1989). Temporal information in speech and its relevance for cochlear implants. In B. Fraysse & N. Cochard (Eds.), *Cochlear implant: Acquisitions and controversies* (pp. 3–26). Toulouse, France: Impasse La Caussade.

Rosen, S., Walliker, J., Brimacombe, J.A., & Edgerton, B.J. (1989). Prosodic and segmental aspects of speech perception with the House/3M single-channel implant. *Journal of Speech and Hearing Research, 32,* 93–111.

Schindler, R.A., & Kessler, D.K. (1989). State of the art of cochlear implants: The UCSF experience. *American Journal of Otology, 10,* 79–83.

Shannon, R.V. (1983). Multichannel electrical stimulation of the auditory nerve in man. I. Basic psychophysics. *Hearing Research, 11,* 157–189.

Shannon, R.V. (1990). A model of temporal integration and forward masking for electrical stimulation of the auditory nerve. In J.M. Miller & F.A. Spelman (Eds.), *Cochlear implants: Models of the electrically stimulated ear* (pp. 187–205). New York: Springer-Verlag.

Shannon, R.V. (1992). Temporal modulation transfer functions in patients with cochlear implants. *Journal of the Acoustical Society of America, 91,* 2156–2164.

Shannon, R.V., Adams, D.D., Ferrel, R.L., Palumbo, R.L., & Grandgenett, M. (1990). A computer interface for psychophysical and speech research with the Nucleus cochlear implant. *Journal of the Acoustical Society of America, 87,* 905–907.

Shannon, R.V., Zeng, F.-G., & Wygonski, J. (1992). Speech recognition using only temporal cues. In M.E.H. Schouten (Ed.), *Audition, speech and language.* Berlin: Mouton-de Gruyter, in press.

Shannon, R.V., Zeng, F.-G., Wygonski, J., & Maltan, A. (1991, September). *Signal processing for electrical stimulation of the human cochlear nucleus.* Paper presented at the International Symposium on Natural and Artificial Control of Hearing and Balance, Rheinfelden, Switzerland.

Skinner, M.W., Holden, L.K., Holden, T.A., Dowell, R.C., Seligman, P.M., Brimacombe, J.A., & Beiter, A.L. (1991). Performance of postlinguistically deaf adults with the Wearable Speech Processor (WSP III) and Mini Speech Processor (MSP) of the Nucleus multi-electrode cochlear implant. *Ear and Hearing, 12,* 3–22.

Tong, Y.C., Clark, G.M., Seligman, P.M., & Patrick, J.F. (1980). Speech processing for a multiple-electrode cochlear implant prosthesis. *Journal of the Acoustical Society of America, 68,* 1897–1899.

Townshend, B., Cotter, N., Van Campernolle, D., & White, R.L. (1987). Pitch perception by cochlear implant patients. *Journal of the Acoustical Society of America, 87,* 106–115.

Tye-Murray, N., Gantz, B.J., Kuk, F., & Tyler, R.S. (1988). Word recognition performance of patients using three different cochlear implant designs. In P. Banfai (Ed.), *Cochlear implant: Current situation* (pp. 605–612). Erkelenz, Germany: Rudolf Bermann.

Tye-Murray, N., Lowder, M., & Tyler, R.S. (1990). Comparison of the F0F2 and F0F1F2 processing strategies for the Cochlear Corporation cochlear implant. *Ear and Hearing, 11,* 195–200.

Tye-Murray, N., & Tyler, R.S. (1989). Auditory consonant and word recognition skills of cochlear implant users. *Ear and Hearing, 10,* 292–298.

Tyler, R.S. (1988a). Open-set word recognition with the 3M/Vienna single-channel cochlear implant. *Archives of Otolaryngology, Head and Neck Surgery, 114,* 1123–1126.

Tyler, R.S. (1988b). Open-set word recognition with the Duren/Cologne extra-cochlear implant. *Laryngoscope, 98,* 999–1002.

Tyler, R.S., Moore, B.C.J., & Kuk, F.K. (1989). Performance of some of the better cochlear-implant patients. *Journal of Speech and Hearing Research, 32,* 887–911.

Tyler, R.S., Preece, J.P., & Lowder, M.W. (1987). *The Iowa audiovisual speech perception laser videodisc.* Laser Videodisc and Laboratory Report, Department of Otolaryngology — Head and Neck Surgery, University of Iowa Hospital and Clinics, Iowa City.

Tyler, R.S., & Tye-Murray, N. (1991). Cochlear implant signal-processing strategies and patient perception of speech and environmental sounds. In H. Cooper (Ed.), *Cochlear implants: A practical guide* (pp. 58–83). San Diego, CA: Singular Publishing Group.

van den Honert C., & Stypulkowski, P.H. (1987). Single fiber mapping of spatial excitation patterns in the electrically stimulated auditory nerve. *Hearing Research, 29,* 195–206.

Van Tasell, D.J., Soli, S.D., Kirby, V.M., & Widen, G.P. (1987). Speech waveform envelope cues for consonant recognition. *Journal of the Acoustical Society of America, 82,* 1152–1161.

White, M.W., Merzenich, M.M., & Gardi, J.N. (1984). Multichannel cochlear implants: Channel interactions and processor design. *Archives of Otolaryngology, 110,* 493–501.

Wilson, B.S., Finley, C.C., Farmer, J.C., Jr., Lawson, D.T., Weber, B.A., Wolford, R.D., Kenan, P.D., White, M.W., Merzenich, M.M., & Schindler, R.A. (1988a). Comparative studies of speech processing strategies for cochlear implants. *Laryngoscope, 98,* 1069–1077.

Wilson, B.S., Finley, C.C., & Lawson, D.T. (1985). *Speech processors for auditory prostheses.* Seventh Quarterly Progress Report, NIH project N01-NS-3-2356.

Wilson, B.S., Finley, C.C., & Lawson, D.T. (1990). Representations of speech features with cochlear implants. In J.M. Miller & F.A. Spelman (Eds.), *Cochlear implants: Models of the electrically stimulated ear* (pp. 339–376). New York: Springer-Verlag.

Wilson, B.S., Finley, C.C., Lawson, D.T., & Wolford, R.D. (1988b). Speech processors for cochlear prostheses. *Proceedings of the IEEE, 76,* 1143–1154.

Wilson, B.S., Finley, C.C., Lawson, D.T., Wolford, R.D., Eddington, D.K., & Rabinowitz, W.M. (1991a). Better speech recognition with cochlear implants. *Nature, 352,* 236–238.

Wilson, B.S., Lawson, D.T., & Finley, C.C. (1990). *Speech processors for auditory prostheses.* Fourth Quarterly Progress Report, NIH project N01-DC-9-2401.

Wilson, B.S., Lawson, D.T., & Finley, C.C. (1992). Importance of patient and processor variables in determining outcomes with cochlear implants. *Journal of*

Speech and Hearing Research, in press.

Wilson, B.S., Lawson, D.T., Finley, C.C., & Wolford, R.D. (1991b). Coding strategies for multichannel cochlear prostheses. *American Journal of Otology, 12* (Suppl. 1), 56–61.

Wilson, B.S., Lawson, D.T., Finley, C.C., & Zerbi, M. (1992). *Speech processors for auditory prostheses.* Eleventh Quarterly Progress Report, NIH project N01-DC-9-2401.

CHAPTER 3

Aural Rehabilitation and Patient Management

NANCY TYE-MURRAY

A cochlear-implant recipient requires support and assistance from a variety of professionals before and after receiving an implant. This chapter considers the patient support and aural rehabilitation that is provided throughout the implantation process. The first half of the chapter describes some of the components of the typical cochlear-implant program and how the key members of the cochlear-implant team contribute to the program. In the second half, considerations for developing a speech perception training program are presented.

PATIENT MANAGEMENT

The seven components of a cochlear-implant program are shown in Figure 3–1. They are: initial contact, a preimplant counseling session, formal evaluation, surgery, fitting, follow-up evaluations, and aural rehabilitation. The key team members who interact with the patient and family are also indicated for each component.

A discussion of the medical evaluation and surgical procedures is beyond the scope of this chapter. The interested reader is referred to Clark, Franz, Pyman, and Webb (1991), Graham (1991), and Webb, Pyman, Franz, and Clark (1990). The formal evaluation of speech perception and speech production will be considered only briefly here, as it is considered by authors Dorman, Tyler, and Tobey (see Chapters 4, 5, and 6, respectively).

INITIAL CONTACT

The first step toward obtaining a cochlear implant is taken by the hearing-impaired adult or a family member. The individual may have read

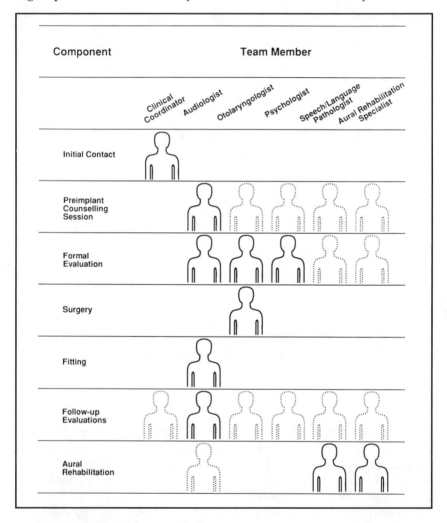

Figure 3–1. The seven components of a cochlear implant program and the professionals involved with each. Solid lines indicate team members who are primarily involved. Dashed lines indicate other team members who may or may not participate, or who may play secondary roles.

a newspaper article or talked to an audiologist and desires more information about cochlear implants and candidacy. The individual contacts the clinical coordinator at the cochlear-implant center, and commonly asks questions like those listed in Table 3–1.

The clinical coordinator attempts to screen out obviously inappropriate candidates by asking questions in return. For instance, the coordinator may ask whether the potential cochlear-implant candidate speaks on the telephone and whether hearing loss was incurred before speech and language were acquired. Persons who successfully use the telephone or adults who have a prelingual, profound hearing loss and rely on sign language (see Boothroyd, Chapter 1) are discouraged from pursuing a formal evaluation, as they either have too much residual hearing or they would be unlikely to benefit from receiving a cochlear implant.

The clinical coordinator sends printed materials and schedules an appointment for a preliminary counseling session or formal evaluation. The printed materials may cover the following topics in a cursory fashion: the functions of a cochlear implant, how the cochlear implant differs from a hearing aid, who is a cochlear-implant candidate, the rea-

Table 3–1. *Questions commonly asked by patients or family members during the initial contact*

a. Will the cochlear implant help me/my relative to hear speech?

b. What will speech sound like?

c. How does a cochlear implant work?

d. Will the cochlear implant be reliable?

e. How does it look when it is on the body?

f. Can people with cochlear implants understand talkers on the television or the telephone?

g. Are cochlear implants waterproof? Can users swim and take a shower?

h. Can a cochlear implant electrocute the user?

i. Will an implant affect tinnitus?

j. What is the difference between a single-channel cochlear implant and a multichannel implant?

k. What happens if someone with a cochlear implant gets hit in the head?

l. How much does an implant cost?

m. What will music sound like?

n. How does somebody get one?

o. (If candidate is a child) Will we have to change our communication mode? Will this help my child to talk better?

sons why some patients may receive more benefit than others, the kinds of benefits that can be expected, and the limitations of the implant.

PRELIMINARY COUNSELING

Counseling for both the patient and family is very important. Counseling provides information about obtaining, maintaining, and using a cochlear implant, and for maximizing its benefits. Counseling is ongoing and occurs throughout the cochlear-implant process. At one time or another, every member of the cochlear-implant team provides counseling. Whether patients and family members are at the stage of determining candidacy or of planning aural rehabilitation (Figure 3–1), they must be aware of what is happening and what will happen, they must be prepared for a variety of outcomes, and they must feel as if they are contributing to the decisions that concern them.

Although counseling is ongoing, a block of time is usually set aside for preliminary counseling, either before or after the formal evaluation. This counseling session is most often conducted by the audiologist. The topics that are included in the preliminary counseling session are summarized in Table 3–2. In the following discussion, we will consider what the audiologist might tell the candidate and family about each of these topics.

Audiological and Medical Candidacy Qualifications

The audiologist reviews audiological and medical candidacy criteria. Some criteria apply to both child and adult candidates, while some apply to one group or the other.

All candidates must have a profound bilateral sensorineural hearing loss. The candidate should receive minimal benefit from amplification;

Table 3–2. *Topics reviewed during the preliminary counseling session*

- a. Audiological and medical candidacy criteria
- b. Cochlear-implant hardware
- c. Costs and insurance reimbursement
- d. Realistic expectations
- e. Commitments
- f. Social considerations
- g. Communication mode and educational placement

for instance, the candidate should not recognize words auditorily. With the exception of 250 Hz, pure-tone thresholds typically should be no better than 95 dB (Mecklenburg et al., 1990).

Good general health, no chronic ear disease, and an unobstructed cochlea are prerequisites for most cochlear implants. The presence of other handicapping conditions, such as blindness or mental retardation, may require special consideration but does not necessarily preclude implantation. For instance, Fryauf-Bertschy (1990) described a congenitally blind boy who suffered a complete hearing loss at age 3, following meningitis. The cochlear-implant team was concerned about whether he would benefit from implantation because he had no means of communicating with the audiologist during the device fitting, and the child had no vision to enhance the use of the electrical speech signal. The child was implanted about a year following deafness. After 12 months of experience, he scored well above chance on an open set word test and was able to understand conversation that was constrained by context. His speech production improved remarkably. Fryauf-Bertschy concluded that children with minimal communication abilities can be fitted with a cochlear implant, and that cochlear implants may serve as a "primary sensory substitute" for some blind postlingually deaf children (also for adults, Ramsden, 1990; Shallop, Dooley, Heller, Arndt, & Blamey, 1991).

The adult candidate should have a postlingual rather than a prelingual hearing loss. In most cases, it is desirable that hearing was present until at least age 6. Results from adults who incurred hearing loss before this age have been disappointing (Clark et al., 1987; Cooper, 1991a).

Typically, the child candidate must be 2 years or older (Graham, 1990). Although there are exceptions, younger children are usually not implanted because hearing status is difficult to determine; ability to benefit from amplification cannot be ruled out. Loeb (1989) presents three other reasons why caution is exercised in implanting very young children: (a) rapid head growth may still be occurring, which may cause an implanted electrode to dislodge or tissue to erode; (b) young children are more prone to middle ear infection than are older children, and infection may lead to explantation and possibly infection of the inner ear or central nervous system; and (c) the child may be unable to participate in the fitting procedure, thereby making electrical thresholds and comfort levels of stimulation difficult to determine. Recent data show a correlation between duration of deafness and benefit, with children who receive cochlear implants after a short period of deafness performing better on measures of speech perception than those who receive one after a longer period (see Tyler, Chapter 5; Staller, Beiter, Brimacombe,

Mecklenburg, & Arndt, 1991). Such findings may lead to more children
below the age of 2 years receiving cochlear implants.

The Cochlear-Implant Hardware

A brief overview of the cochlear-implant hardware is important so that
the candidate will appreciate what the device will look like, how it will
be worn, and what will be involved in maintaining it in good working
order. The external components that are worn outside of the body (for
many implants, the speech processor, the microphone, and the transmitter) are distinguished from the internal components that are implanted
in the mastoid bone (the electrode array and for some cochlear implants,
the internal receiver) using a photograph like that shown in Figure 3–2,
or a model.

The candidate learns how the device will appear, and considers how
he or she might wear it, perhaps with the aid of photographs like those
shown in either Figure 3–3 or Figure 3–4. Figure 3–3 shows an individual wearing the Nucleus cochlear implant and Figure 3–4 shows another
individual wearing the Ineraid device. These two cochlear implants

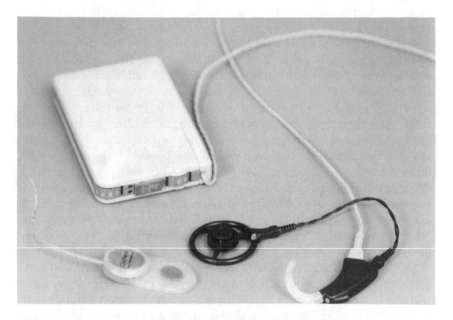

Figure 3–2. A picture of the Nucleus cochlear implant. From top clockwise, the
components are the speech processor, the long cord, the microphone, the short
cord, the transmitter, and the internal receiver.

represent two different means of transmitting the signal from the speech processor to the electrode array. The Nucleus is a transcutaneous system, and the Ineraid is a percutaneous system. The Nucleus transmitter, which is about the size of a quarter, is aligned with the internal receiver by magnetic induction. The Ineraid does not require a transmitter, but has a plug that inserts into the skull.

Costs and Insurance Reimbursement

The cochlear implant and surgery are very expensive. Costs for the formal evaluation, hospitalization, surgery, the device, and fitting may total $35,000. Follow-up visits and aural rehabilitation present additional costs.

The cochlear-implant user should expect some expenses related to cochlear implant maintenance annually since problems with the device hardware are not uncommon (Tyler & Kelsay, 1990). For instance, cords may need to be replaced several times per year, especially with young users. Most cochlear implants have a warranty on the external parts, which may extend from 1 to 3 years. Service contracts need to be pur-

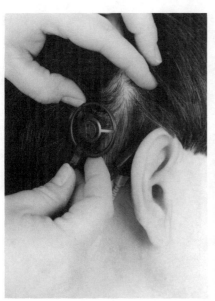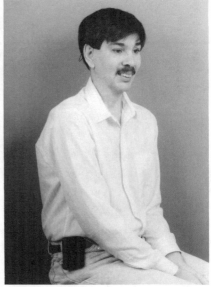

Figure 3–3. The left half of the figure shows a head view of a patient wearing a Nucleus cochlear implant. The Nucleus is an example of a transcutaneous system. In the right half, the patient is shown wearing the speech processor.

chased thereafter. Service contracts may cost from $300–600 annually. These contracts typically cover parts and labor.

In some instances, the candidate's medical insurance policy will pay for some of the costs related to obtaining a cochlear implant (Moora & Wallace, 1991). Since many policies are negotiated individually, and benefits change periodically, it is difficult to generalize with accuracy how much of the total costs might be covered by any particular policy. Preauthorization of insurance benefits should be obtained from the provider before significant costs are incurred. The clinical coordinator and the candidate usually share responsibility in obtaining preauthorization.

Insurance policies can be classified as private, state, and/or federal plans. Private insurance companies (with the exception of many Health Maintenance Organizations [HMOs]) have been the most cooperative in approving coverage of cochlear implants, although there is considerable variability in the extent of authorized benefits. Many state plans such as Blue Cross and Blue Shield provide coverage. Medicaid, which is jointly funded by the state and federal governments, provides some coverage (for those who cannot afford health insurance) in roughly 20 states. Finally, federal programs such as Medicare (which is designed to pro-

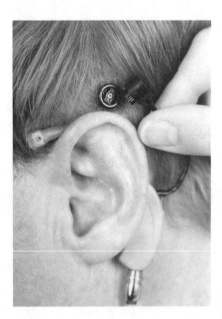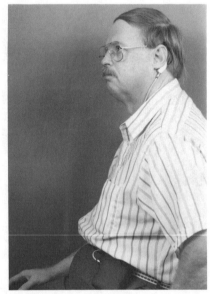

Figure 3–4. In the left half of the figure is shown a head view of a patient wearing an Ineraid cochlear implant. This is how a percutaneous system appears. In the right half, the patient is shown wearing the speech processor.

vide medical coverage for elderly citizens) and Champus (designed for retired and disabled military personnel and their dependents) usually pay for some fraction of the costs incurred for cochlear implantation, often less than half.

Realistic Expectations

The candidate and family members must develop realistic expectations about what the cochlear implant will provide. Otherwise, they may suffer disappointment and frustration and even a sense of betrayal after the patient receives the device. Unmet expectations will dampen enthusiasm to participate in follow-up visits and aural rehabilitation, and may even lead to nonuse of the cochlear implant.

All members of the team help the candidate and family members to develop realistic expectations, beginning with the clinical coordinator during the initial contact. The audiologist's role during the preliminary counseling session is to probe the candidate's and family's expectations, and correct them when necessary. The audiologist makes clear that the candidate will always have a hearing deficit. The cochlear implant is a communication aid and not a bionic ear that will provide normal hearing. The audiologist also explains in laymen's terms how other users perform.

Expectations are probed with such questions as, *Do you think you will be able to talk on the telephone as you did before losing your hearing?* or *Do you think your child will start speaking normally once she receives an implant?*, and corrected when inappropriate. Information about the performance of other cochlear-implant users is often presented in graphic form, as in Figure 3–5. By looking at this figure, the candidate or family members can learn about the average performance of users and their range of performance.

The primary benefit of receiving a cochlear implant is an enhanced ability to speechread (that is, to recognize speech using both the auditory and visual signals; see Dorman, Chapter 4; Tyler, Chapter 5). Almost all multichannel users receive speechreading enhancement, although they vary widely in the amount. Some recipients also recognize speech in an audition-only condition. Almost everyone detects environmental sounds, and many can identify many of them. Some adults use the telephone on a limited basis (Dorman, Dove, Parkin, Zacharchuk, & Dankowski, 1991), and a minority enjoy listening to music (Brown, Dowell, Martin, & Mecklenburg, 1990; Gfeller & Lansing, 1991). Speech through a cochlear implant may sound mechanical, and experience is usually necessary before it sounds natural. Some adults have described speech as sounding like "Donald Duck" or "squawking parrots."

How well a user will perform with a cochlear implant is difficult to predict, and the audiologist must explain that the outcome for the particular patient cannot be surmised. There is some evidence that a combination of factors may influence success. Gantz, Woodworth, Knutson, Abbas, and Tyler (in press) related a number of historical, preimplant audiological, electrophysiological, and psychological measures to the audition-only word recognition scores achieved by 48 experienced multichannel cochlear-implant users. Their analyses suggest that patients with a shorter duration of deafness will achieve better audition-only

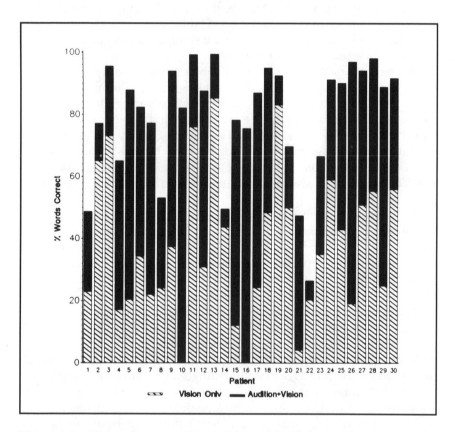

Figure 3–5. The performance of 30 multichannel cochlear implant users on the Iowa Sentence Test Without Context (Tyler, Preece, & Tye-Murray, 1986). Patients completed the test in a vision-only and audition-plus-vision condition after 18 months of experience. The auditory signal was presented at 73dB SPL, a moderately loud conversational level. The test contains 100 sentences, with five sentences each spoken by 20 different talkers. A graph such as this can be used to show the cochlear-implant candidate how users vary in their performance and the average level of lipreading enhancement.

word recognition than patients who have been deafened for more than 6 years. A combined index of the following variables correlated highly with scores on a sentence recognition test and word recognition test: duration of deafness, residual hearing prior to implantation, vision-only speech recognition ability, the ability to process rapidly presented sequences of visual stimuli, the motivation and willingness of the patient to comply with the aural rehabilitation process, and the use of communication strategies. Etiology, measured intelligence (as indicated by Wechsler Adult Intelligence Scale-Revised [WAIS-R] scores), and pre-operative electrophysiological measures were not good predictors of audiological success.

A number of factors may influence a child's performance with a cochlear implant, and the parents will be asked to consider these factors in relation to their child. A child with a postlingual hearing loss will exhibit better listening abilities than one with a prelingual hearing loss, at least for several years following implantation (Staller, Dowell, Beiter, & Brimacombe, 1991). A child who has a hearing loss of short duration will likely show greater benefit than one who has a loss of long duration (Staller et al., 1991). The support system provided by the family, the status of the auditory nerve and cochlea, the child's personality and interest in communicating with speech, and the quality and quantity of aural rehabilitation are other factors that determine benefit (Tyler & Fryauf-Bertschy, 1992).

One potential pitfall in establishing realistic expectations is that parents may come to expect too little and never challenge their child to listen. We have known parents who are delighted that, on receiving a cochlear implant, their child begins to respond to environmental sounds and to recognize his or her own name. They do not expect the child to utilize the electrical signal as a means of enhancing speechreading performance, nor for speech listening, even when audiological testing indicates good benefit from the device. To some extent, parents—and teachers—can limit the child's performance by their own limited expectations.

Commitments

Receiving a cochlear implant requires tremendous commitment from the patient and family in terms of time, effort, and money. The audiologist must take great care that the magnitude of these commitments is fully comprehended.

The patient (and parents) must return to the cochlear-implant center periodically for device adjustments and audiological evaluation. During the first year of implant use, return trips may number three or more for the adult patient and six or more for the child. They usually occur at least annually thereafter. A visit to the cochlear-implant center may require that the patient or parent take leave from work and that the family allocate funds for travel and perhaps lodging, if the cochlear-implant center is far from the home.

Patients or parents must maintain the device. They must learn how to determine when the device is malfunctioning and how to perform minor repairs (such as replacing a cord). They must have the financial wherewithal to replace nonfunctioning hardware. The patient or parents are responsible for handling the device (e.g., placing it on the body, turning it on, and adjusting the level) and storing the device when it is not in use. Unless the child is older, the parents must assume responsibility for ensuring that the child wears the device during all waking hours at the appropriate settings. They may have to instruct the child's teacher about how to handle the device (Fryauf-Bertschy, 1992).

Receipt of a cochlear implant marks the beginning of an aural rehabilitation process that may last for some years. The adult patient must practice listening and speechreading by engaging in conversational interactions and/or formal speech perception training. Parents must ensure that the child has a stimulating auditory environment in both the home and school. Ideally, family members should be willing to direct the child's attention toward sounds in the home environment and label them and consistently integrate speech into their communication mode.

Social Considerations

Parents of cochlear-implant candidates need be aware of the controversy surrounding implantation in children. Many members of the Deaf community and its advocates discourage cochlear implants for young prelingually deaf children. Lane (1990) suggests that a cochlear implant may prevent or delay a hearing-impaired child from becoming acculturated as a member of the Deaf community. After receiving a cochlear implant, the child may not learn American Sign Language or socialize with members of the Deaf community because of the necessity of intense auditory stimulation and an emphasis on aural/oral communication skills during childhood. On the other hand, the child may not develop the aural/oral skills that would allow him or her to integrate easily into the hearing world. Implanted children may someday be "culturally homeless, belonging to neither the Deaf nor the hearing communities" (Evans, 1989, p. 312). A cochlear implant may also delay the parents' acceptance of the child's hearing loss (see Boothroyd, Chapter 1).

Although these are serious concerns, the audiologist might point out that the child who receives a cochlear implant has a peer group in the making: Profoundly deaf children in numerous places around the world are receiving cochlear implants. By the time these children reach adulthood, cochlear implants will be commonplace. Moreover, severely hearing-impaired children who use hearing aids will be members of their peer group since they have similar hearing abilities. Finally, most prelingually deaf children with hearing parents (about 90% of all deaf children) use total communication. Signing does not suddenly disappear after the child receives a cochlear implant; rather, increased emphasis is placed on integrating auditory information into the child's communication mode.

Communication Mode and Educational Placement

As just noted, a cochlear implant need not affect communication mode, especially during the first year. For instance, if parents and child communicate using total communication prior to the child's receiving a cochlear implant, they will continue using total communication afterward. Firszt, Reeder, Zimmerman-Phillips, Tonokawa, and Proctor, (1991) studied 32 children who had an average of 18 months of experience with a multichannel cochlear implant. The children's age at implantation ranged between 2 1/2 years to 18 years, and their duration of deafness prior to implantation ranged between 4 months to 17 years. Thirteen children used oral communication before and after implantation and 17 used total communication. Only two children changed their communication modes: One child changed from an oral educational program to a total communication program after receiving a cochlear implant; another changed from a total communication program to an oral program.

Although communication mode will likely not change, a new emphasis must be placed on aural/oral interactions. The child requires a rich auditory environment and should use aural/oral communication for some part of every day, however brief (Tye-Murray, 1992a). Hearing must become a part of the child's personality and influence his or her self-perception.

The amount of mainstreaming also will not likely change following implantation. Here, the term "mainstreaming" refers to placement in a classroom with normal-hearing children for academic subjects other than art or physical education (Firszt et al., 1991). Firszt and colleagues reported that 17 of their children were mainstreamed for similar amounts of time before and after implantation. Eleven children increased and one child decreased the amount of mainstreaming. The investigators noted that children who increased mainstreaming often used sign language interpreters (thus still relying on total communication), and they suggested that this increase would have occurred without the introduction of cochlear implants, as a result of the subjects' maturation.

Although the educational placement need not change, the child's school should be supportive of sensory aids and provide opportunities for speech-perception training and speech therapy. Tye-Murray (1992b) suggests that implanted children might benefit more from speech perception training in the school than hearing-aid users, since they can learn to use the information provided by the electrical signal, whereas hearing-impaired children typically have adapted to having residual hearing.

Interactions with Other Cochlear-Implant Users and Deaf Adults

The audiologist ensures that the hearing-impaired individual and family have an opportunity to meet with other individuals or parents of children who have received cochlear implants. These meetings allow the candidates to obtain information about implantation from those who have experienced it firsthand. Questions can be asked about the user's satisfactions, disappointments, recommendations, and problems. If possible, the young candidate should have an opportunity to meet with a child of the same age and sex. This will allow the candidate to see how the cochlear implant appears on a contemporary and will lead to an awareness that other children are wearing these devices, and it is quite normal to do so.

Parents may be provided with an opportunity to meet deaf adults who use American Sign Language. This will help them appreciate the rich culture afforded by the Deaf community (Kessler & Owens, 1989), and may lead them to reconsider their decision for cochlear implantation. If their child proves not to benefit very much after receiving a cochlear implant, their awareness of the Deaf community may mollify unrealized hopes.

THE FORMAL EVALUATION

The formal evaluation includes extensive audiological testing and medical examination. It often includes psychological testing and, for children, evaluation of speech and language proficiency. It may last from 1 to 5 days.

The audiological testing usually occurs first. Tests of speech perception must indicate that the individual receives no benefit, or limited benefit, from a conventional hearing aid (see Dorman, Chapter 4 and Tyler, Chapter 5). If the candidate is found to recognize words auditorily while wearing a hearing aid, the formal evaluation is usually terminated at this point and the individual is no longer considered as a candidate.

The medical examination includes a medical history and physical examination to assess general health and to determine whether the individual can undergo general anesthesia. Computerized axial tomography (a CAT scan) determines the status of the cochlea. Ideally, the cochlea should be structurally normal, although there have been reports where children with cochlear deformities have been implanted successfully (Firszt, Novak, Reeder, & Proctor, 1991). It is desirable that the cochlea be free of bone growth. However, there have been instances where existing bone growth has been removed during the surgery and the patient subsequently received benefit from the cochlear implant (Balkany, Gantz, & Nadol, 1988). If the otologist determines that medical reasons exist that preclude implantation of an electrode (such as a cochlea structural anomaly), the remainder of the formal evaluation is canceled.

A psychologist may evaluate cognitive and behavioral status. Some suggest that the results of this assessment help to predict whether the individual will be a successful user and might help in the planning of a rehabilitation program (Downs, 1986; Knutson et al., 1991; McKenna, 1991).

One of the primary purposes of the psychological evaluation is to determine whether the candidate and family have developed realistic expectations about the benefits of implantation. In assessing realistic expectations, the psychologist might separately interview both the candidate and family members and ask them to complete questionnaires. Questions that might be asked of the adult candidate, child candidate, and parents are presented in Table 3–3. If the candidate and family have unrealistic expectations, or if the child or teenage candidate expresses reluctance about receiving a cochlear implant, further counseling may be recommended before the candidate proceeds to surgery.

A speech-language pathologist evaluates the child's language and speech skills. Typically, these measures are not used for determining candidacy, although the language measures may indicate whether the child can participate in the fitting process. Grossly delayed language is cause for concern. This may indicate that the child is not receiving sufficient language stimulation in the home or school environment, which does not bode well for successful cochlear-implant use. The language measures may help the audiologist to select language-appropriate tests for measuring the child's hearing abilities. Both the language and speech measures can be used to design an aural-rehabilitation program following surgery and may indicate secondary benefits of implantation.

Once the candidate has passed through each stage of the formal evaluation, the members of the cochlear-implant team meet and discuss their test results. The patient or parents may be invited to this meeting. In most cases, a decision regarding candidacy is fairly straightforward. If the individual meets the audiological and medical criteria, and realistic expectations are present, implantation is usually recommended. A number of factors can cloud a decision, including the presence of the following: emotional disturbance in the candidate or family members, severe behavioral problems, an unwillingness to commit time and effort

Table 3–3. *Questions asked of candidates and their family members to probe realistic expectations*

Candidates

  a. Do you think you will be able to talk on the telephone?
  b. Do you think the cochlear implant will help you to speechread more easily?
  c. (If the hearing loss is postlingual) Do you think that speech will sound like it did when you had normal hearing?
  d. Do you think that a cochlear implant will help you to speak more clearly, with more appropriate pitch and loudness?
  e. (If the candidate is a child) Do you want this? How do you think this will affect your school activities? What do you think your friends will think about the cochlear implant?

Parents

  a. Will a cochlear implant eventually help your child to develop normal-sounding speech?
  b. Will you stop using sign language after your child receives a cochlear implant?
  c. How will use of a cochlear implant affect your child's educational achievement?
  d. Will your child improve his or her speechreading skills during the first couple months following implantation?
  e. Will the child's use of a cochlear implant relieve family tensions regarding your child's hearing loss or your child's communication problems?

toward making the cochlear implant a successful communication aid, unrealistic expectations, an inability to participate in the fitting procedure (say because of limited language or reduced cognitive functioning), financial difficulties, and/or an unstable home environment (such as the presence of alcoholism or drug abuse). There are no cookbook procedures to follow when these factors are present. Usually a decision is reached after much discussion among the team members, the patient, and the family. Sometimes other professionals are consulted, such as an educator or social worker.

SURGERY

Once an individual's candidacy is established, surgery is scheduled. Cochlear-implant surgery requires general anesthesia and lasts about 2 hours. Afterward, the patient spends one to three nights in the hospital.

Regardless of the counseling that has occurred beforehand, patients and family members often feel anxious before the surgery. Some worry about the anesthesia, potential surgical complications, the aftermath of surgery, and whether they or their child will receive benefit from the device. Some parents may experience guilt for inflicting a surgical procedure on their child. These feelings should be recognized and acknowledged by members of the implant team, and additional counseling provided when necessary.

The patient may feel uncomfortable the day following surgery. Some experience tinnitus or soreness around the ear. On rare occasions, a patient will experience nausea and slight vertigo. Most of these aftereffects disappear quickly.

THE COCHLEAR-IMPLANT FITTING

The patient returns to the cochlear-implant center about 4 to 6 weeks following surgery for the device fitting. Before beginning, the audiologist reviews what will happen and what to expect, and reminds the patient what auditory stimuli might sound like. Since parents usually are permitted to sit in the room and observe, the audiologist may brief them about how to behave. For instance, the audiologist might ask parents not to distract the child while thresholds are being determined, nor signal when electrodes are stimulated.

During the fitting, the external components are placed on the patient and adjusted so that the patient can wear them comfortably. The audiologist then adjusts the stimulus parameters of the speech processor, which determine the signals delivered to the electrodes in the electrode array. Many cochlear implants interface with a personal computer for this process.

Cochlear implants vary in the number of parameters that can be adjusted. The descriptions below apply to most multichannel devices, and concern dynamic range, loudness balancing, pitch ranking, and eliminating electrodes for stimulation.

Dynamic Range

In adjusting the speech processor, each electrode is programmed according to the threshold of stimulation and maximum acceptable loudness level using an ascending approach (to avoid overstimulation). The difference between these two current levels defines a dynamic range. An electrical threshold is the amount of current that must be passed through an electrode so that the individual is just aware of a sound sensation. Maximum loudness level is the maximum current level that can be introduced before the individual experiences discomfort. Threshold and maximum loudness level are determined by the amplitude of the current and current duration (see Shannon, Chapter 8).

The thresholds and maximum loudness levels will vary among electrodes and between patients, as a function of neural survival and current spread. Greater dynamic ranges permit finer amplitude resolution (Brown et al., 1990).

Loudness Balancing

Through loudness balancing, the speech processor is programmed so that stimulation across electrodes preserves the loudness contour of the speech signal. Patients are asked to judge the relative loudness of signals presented to different electrodes in the electrode array. If the electrodes are not balanced, the patient might experience occasional popping sounds and may not hear some speech information.

Pitch and Pitch Ranking

Electrodes situated near the basal end of the cochlea are programmed to represent the high-frequency range and those near the apical end represent the low-frequency range. This representation matches the tonotopic organization of the cochlea.

Pitch ranking determines the ability to discriminate pitch from the basal to the apical electrodes. During pitch ranking, two electrodes are stimulated, one right after the other. The patient's task is to indicate which stimulus pulse has a higher or lower pitch. The pulses are adjusted to sound equally loud since pitch judgments are influenced by the loudness of the stimuli. Sometimes by changing the stimulus parameters of an electrode, the ability to pitch rank can be improved. During pitch ranking, the audiologist sequentially stimulates electrodes across the electrode array from apical to basal end and vice versa (a "sweep"). The patient should hear a signal that rises or falls steadily in pitch.

Exclusion of Stimulating Electrodes

One or more electrodes may not be programmed to provide stimulation to the auditory nerve. The number of electrodes available for stimulation depends in part on how many electrodes were successfully inserted into the scala tympani. Due to unforeseen problems, such as missing or aberrant neurons or ossification or damage to the electrode array, stimulation of an electrode may not result in auditory sensation or may create an unpleasant sound, such as a squeak. It may produce pain, tinnitus, or facial twitching. Although intuitively one might think that an individual who has a relatively large number of active electrodes receives greater benefit from the cochlear implant than one who has a relatively small number, this is not necessarily true (Roberts, 1991). For instance, Roberts (1991) mentions a Nucleus user with only seven channels who achieved open-set word recognition in an audition-only condition.

Time Course of the Fitting.

Fitting may take a few hours for an adult, although some refinement of the device settings may occur during the first few weeks. A young child must learn to detect when sound is present and to indicate when it is soft and comfortably loud. Initial thresholds may be high and maximum current levels low; these may change as the child becomes accustomed to hearing. In addition, due to a limited attention span, only a few electrodes may be programmed during the initial fitting session. Although most children can use their cochlear implant after one or two fittings, an optimum fitting may require several months.

Device Activation

The audiologist activates the device after programming the speech processor and introduces a simple listening task. The patient should have a successful listening experience as soon as possible. With an adult, the audiologist might count and ask the individual to identify how many numbers were spoken. The audiologist may then read a passage from a book as the patient follows along with a copy of the text. The patient will also read aloud and listen to his or her own voice. After this introduction, the new user walks about the center and listens to environmental sounds.

The prelingually deaf child may show no response to sound. Other responses include fright, surprise, rejection, distress, or wonderment. Some children report a sensation in the neck or head. After activating the device, the audiologist might ask the child to detect sound by standing behind the child and speaking his or her name. The child's task is to turn around when the audiologist speaks. The audiologist might have to turn the child physically the first few times.

Patient or Parent Instruction

Before leaving the cochlear-implant center, the patient or parents receive instruction about how to handle the device. Mecklenburg et al. (1990) present a list of topics that the audiologist may review. The authors present the topics in question form, and they are quoted verbatim here.

    a. How is the speech processor turned on and off?
    b. How are batteries changed?

   c. How long should the batteries last?
   d. Can rechargeable batteries be used?
   e. How is the speech processor tested to see if it's working properly?
   f. What does the sensitivity control do?
   g. Can the speech processor be repaired?
   h. How can the speech processor be connected to a radio-frequency or infrared transmission system?
   i. How can the telephone signal be fed into the speech processor?
   j. How can the television sound be fed into the speech processor? (p. 214)

Additional topics of instruction include the warranty, how to put the device on and take it off, how to troubleshoot the device, and how to perform minor repairs.

A schedule for when the patient will wear the cochlear implant is established. The patient begins by wearing the device in a quiet environment. After a period from 1 week to 2 months, the cochlear implant is usually worn during all waking hours. Parents of young users are responsible for enforcing the schedule.

FOLLOW-UP VISITS

After the first year of cochlear-implant use, the patient returns to the cochlear-implant center annually (or more often). Audiological evaluation indicates whether the cochlear implant is functioning properly and whether performance has changed. Decreased performance is cause for concern since it may signal problems with the device or physiological changes in the auditory system. The audiologist may adjust the speech processor to enhance performance. During the annual visit, the patient or parents are advised whether the manufacturer has made new software or other options available for the cochlear implant and may be provided with an opportunity to try them.

Patients should return to the cochlear-implant center whenever problems arise that cannot be fixed by a minor repair. These problems include an intermittent signal, facial stimulation, a change in sound quality, and an abnormal sound sensation, such as popping or squeaking.

AURAL REHABILITATION

After the device fitting, the aural rehabilitation process begins. The involvement of the cochlear-implant aural-rehabilitation specialist varies, depending on the proximity of the patient to the cochlear implant center, the patient's or family's desire for services, and in the case of the child, the amount of support provided by the school system. Specific speech-perception training procedures are considered in the second half of this chapter. Here, we will consider possible contributions of the rehabilitation specialist, who in some cases, may also be the cochlear-implant audiologist or speech/language pathologist.

Adults

An aural rehabilitation program for adults might include speech-perception training, instruction about assistive devices, communication therapy wherein the patient learns to structure the listening environment and use repair strategies, and involvement of family members in the aural rehabilitation process.

The adult patient may return to the cochlear-implant center for formal auditory and speechreading training. The patient may attend 1-hour speech-perception training sessions once or twice a week, for several weeks or months.

In addition or alternatively, the patient might be provided with speech-perception practice materials to use at home. Home materials for auditory training might include audiotaped speech samples and a tape recorder or language master. For speechreading training, the patient might take home audiovisual speech materials that can be played on the home VHS machine (e.g., Greenwald, 1984; Russell, 1987). Sometimes a computerized laser videodisc teaching station is loaned to the patient (Tye-Murray & Kelsay, in press), to be used for providing interactive training with one of the currently available laser videodisc programs (Sims, 1988).

The patient's spouse or other family members may be asked to perform speech-perception training exercises with the patient at home. For instance, the family member might read aloud from the newspaper each morning, while the patient listens and watches. A record-keeping system is usually provided to the patient and family to track their progress. The record-keeping system may consist of a daily log, a checklist, or a weekly questionnaire. An example of a daily log for a family member is presented in Appendix 1. This daily log assesses whether the family member attempted to provide auditory practice to the patient and whether the person used verbal repair strategies (described below).

Information about assistive devices is often provided to the patient, and the patient may have opportunity to use them under the aural-rehabilitation specialist's supervision. Instruction may be provided about using telephone strategies (e.g., Erber, 1985) and if available, telephone adapters for the particular cochlear-implant model. Some cochlear implants can be interfaced with the television with an adapter, and patients may receive instruction about their use (Brown et al., 1990). Another assistive device includes a clip-on lapel microphone to be used when the patient is attempting to converse in the presence of background noise. Apart from assistive devices pertaining specifically to their cochlear implant, patients may also learn about other assistive devices, such as alerting and captioning systems.

The patient may receive instruction about how to structure the listening environment to maximize communication effectiveness (for instance, turning off the radio or ensuring that the talker is well lit) and how to repair communication breakdowns when they occur. For example, Tye-Murray (1991) describes a computerized laser videodisc program that teaches hearing-impaired adults to use repair strategies when they do not recognize a spoken message. In this program, talkers appear on a computer monitor and speak sentences. The patients watch and listen to each sentence. When they do not understand one, patients have the opportunity to ask the talker to repeat the message, rephrase it, simplify it, elaborate it, or speak a keyword. Whatever their request, the talker reappears on the screen and fulfills it right away. This allows patients to experience firsthand the value of repair strategies, and in some cases, allows them to decide which are the most effective repair strategies for them. This program has been shown to alter the way hearing-impaired individuals implement repair strategies and is currently in use with cochlear-implant adults.

Instruction about structuring the environment and using repair strategies may not directly impact the cochlear-implant user's speech perception skills. However, the individual may become more willing to engage in conversational interactions because they become more rewarding as a result of therapy. The individual may thus practice speechreading more talkers and more speech materials. This in turn may develop speech perception skills.

The last responsibility of the aural rehabilitation specialist that will be considered here, and certainly one of the most important, is that of providing instruction and counseling to family members (Tye-Murray & Schum, in press). Family members can learn how to facilitate the patient's efforts to recognize speech. They can learn to use the verbal repair strategies described in Table 3–4 when breakdowns in communication occur. For instance, they might learn to indicate the topic of conversation by speaking (or writing) a key word when their relative misunderstands their message. Family members can learn how to optimize the speechreading environment, for example, by ensuring good lighting. They can learn to speak appropriately using the speaking behaviors listed in Table 3–5. For example, speaking with a moderately slow speaking rate and clear articulation is much better than mumbling and speaking quickly (Picheny, Durlach, & Braida, 1986).

Table 3–4. *Verbal repair strategies that can be taught to parents and spouses by the aural rehabilitation specialist*

Verbal Repair Strategies and Examples of Each

---

a. Repeat: Say the message again.
    Original sentence: My mother called today.
    Repair strategy: My mother called today.
b. Simplify: Use fewer words and/or more commonplace words.
    Original sentence: The black and yellow cardigan is hanging in the closet.
    Repair strategy: The sweater is in the closet.
c. Rephrase: Use different words.
    Original sentence: The television is broken.
    Repair strategy: The T.V. is not working.
d. Keyword: Speak one important word.
    Original sentence: The boys are playing baseball.
    Repair strategy: Baseball.
e. Elaborate: Repeat keywords and/or provide a little more information.
    Original sentence: I made some chicken.
    Repair strategy: I made some chicken. We'll take the chicken to the picnic.
f. Delimit: Limit the responses when asking a question.
    Original question: Where did you go?
    Repair strategy: Did you go home or to the party?
g. Build from the known: Start by presenting information that can be recognized.
    Original sentence: Please put the tray on the table on the porch.
    Repair strategy: Here is the tray (talker hands tray to cochlear-implant user). The table is on the porch (talker gestures toward solarium). Please take the tray to the table.
h. Ask for feedback: Ask the listener to repeat or rephrase what was understood.
    Original sentence: We'll pick Jim up after school.
    Repair strategy: Tell me what you heard (talker then repeats the information that the listener missed).

Adapted from Tye-Murray, 1992a.

Training procedures with relatives might include role-playing with the aural-rehabilitation specialist, watching instructional films[1] (for example, vision-only examples of talkers mumbling and then speaking clearly—a procedure that we have found to be effective in establishing clear articulation), completing interactive laser videodisc instructional programs (Tye-Murray, 1992e), and completing workbook activities. An example of a workbook activity is one that promotes the use of verbal repair strategies. The family member is presented with a list of sentences.

Table 3–5. *Appropriate speaking behaviors for talking to a cochlear-implant user*

a. Ensure that your face is clearly visible. Do not speak with your hand covering your mouth, or while chewing on an object such as a pencil.

b. Use "clear speech." Speak slightly slower than usual and articulate each word carefully. However, do not exaggerate your mouth movements. As Dr. Carol De Filippo (1991) at the National Technical Institute for the Deaf suggests, speak like an elementary school teacher.

c. Use your voice; do not mouth words or sign without speaking. The loudness of your voice should be at a normal conversational level or slightly louder. Shouting will make your speech more difficult to understand.

d. Allow the patient to view your face from a frontal position. If you speak from behind the patient or in profile, your facial movements will not be visible. Try to keep your head fairly still as you speak.

e. Use facial expressions, interesting intonation, and hand gestures.

f. Indicate changes in the topic of conversation. You might pause slightly or use an agreed-on hand gesture, or say, "I'm going to talk about something different now." Some talkers speak a key word when changing the topic. For instance, the talker might say "car," pause, and then say, "Who will pick up the car after work?"

The individual's task is to circle a key word in each sentence that he or she could repeat following a communication breakdown to indicate the topic of conversation.

Children

Much of the above discussion pertaining to adults also applies to children. Children may return to the cochlear-implant center for formal speech-perception training. They and their parents may receive instruction about using assistive devices and structuring the listening environment. Both children (Tye-Murray, 1992c) and parents (Tye-Murray & Kelsay, in preparation) may learn how to repair breakdowns in communication by using verbal repair strategies. In addition to this, parents may be counseled about how to provide informal speech-perception training and occasional aural/oral conversation.

The aural-rehabilitation specialist usually describes informal speech-perception training activities for the parents and child to perform at home. For example, a game of musical chairs can encourage the development of sound detection skills in the young child. Sometimes caution must be exercised in recommending home activities, as some parents become overzealous in providing training (Lisa Tonokowa, personal communication, October, 1991), especially if their child's progress is extremely slow or rapid. Some may view every waking moment as an opportunity for auditory learning. For these parents, it may be necessary to underscore the importance of relaxation and "fun time," and the need to let the child be a child.

The family and child will continue to rely on sign for communication if they did so before implantation. However, the parents may be encouraged to use aural/oral communication occasionally, if only for a brief period a few times a day. Informal conversational interactions are the most effective means for developing a child's ability to use the auditory signal and for increasing his or her reliance on the auditory signal for communication.

Tables 3–6 and 3–7 present handouts that might be reviewed with parents during instruction about aural/oral communication. Table 3–6 lists routine activities that might provide the child with a successful aural/oral communication experience. Parents may be asked to review their typical day, and identify other routine activities where aural/oral communication can be attempted. Table 3–7 lists general guidelines to follow when attempting a brief aural/oral interaction. For instance, the parent is encouraged to talk about the here and now rather than events in the past or future or people and objects not present in the room.

The aural rehabilitation program often extends beyond the boundaries of the family. If the child is of school age, the rehabilitation specialist will interact with the school personnel to varying degrees. The level of interaction may range from simply sharing copies of patient reports to the specialist becoming significantly involved with developing the child's Individualized Educational Plan (IEP).

In many cochlear-implant programs, the aural-rehabilitation specialist provides a 1- or 2-day inservice to the child's school personnel. Information may be provided about the following topics: how the cochlear implant works, how it compares to a hearing aid, how to introduce the cochlear implant to the child's classmates, how to handle and care for the device and troubleshoot it, and how to couple the cochlear implant to a frequency modulated (FM) training unit (see Fryauf-Bertschy & Kirk, 1992).

Often, the specialist will spend time observing the child in the classroom environment. She or he then may make specific recommendations about how the teacher can incorporate informal listening practice into the academic curriculum. For example, Reeder and Firszt (1990) have developed the *Guide for Optimizing Auditory Learning Skills* (GOALS) for elementary school children. GOALS provides suggestions for incorporating auditory-training objectives into lessons of science, social studies,

Table 3–6. *Routine or familiar activities that may provide the child with successful experiences in using aural/oral communication*

The aural-rehabilitation specialist might provide parents with this list of routine activities, and ask the parents to identify other activities wherein they might occasionally attempt aural/oral communication.

- Getting ready for bed
- Getting dressed in the morning
- Taking off the cochlear implant
- Making the bed
- Brushing teeth
- Putting toys away
- Folding the laundry
- Feeding a pet
- Setting the table
- Cleaning the kitchen
- Making cookies
- Shopping for groceries
- Playing familiar games
- Reading favorite books
- Playing with familiar toys
- Coloring
- Mailing a letter
- Wrapping a present

Adapted from Tye-Murray, 1992b.

reading, language, math, and health. Robbins (1990, p. 367) describes a language lesson wherein the teacher attempts to develop the child's comprehension of noun modifiers such as "a," "a few," and "all of the." After reviewing the concepts of "a peanut," "a few peanuts," and "all of the peanuts," the child is asked to respond to the sentence, "You can have _____ peanut(s)," using only audition. The child can learn to identify these sentences, even if the child utilizes only time-intensity cues. During a history lesson, an older child might be asked to identify a word by listening, from a closed-list of content words, such as "taxation, colonists, mountains, and King George" (Nevins, Kretschmer, Chute, Hellman, & Parisier, 1991, p. 203).

Finally, the aural-rehabilitation specialist may demonstrate to the classroom teacher and the speech-language pathologist what kinds of listening skills the child now has and share audiological test results. The

Table 3–7. *Guidelines for occasionally using aural/oral communication*

In describing how to increase the child's reliance on the auditory signal for communication, the aural rehabilitation specialist may provide guidelines for attempting aural/oral communication occasionally. Below is a list she or he might review with the parents, one by one.

- Talk about the here and now. Talk about what you are doing or about objects in the room.
- Attempt aural/oral communication during routine activities, such as getting ready for bed or cleaning the kitchen.
- Use simple, short sentences. This is not a time to introduce new vocabulary.
- Expect your child to respond at a level that he or she is capable of responding.
- Try establishing a context using total communication before speaking without sign. For instance, you might say and sign, "John went to the swimming pool about an hour ago," then say without sign, "Would you like to go swimming too?"
- Before speaking without sign, encourage your child to watch your face.
- Watch for signs of frustration in your child. Aural/oral communication may only be appropriate for a 5 to 10 minute period.
- Be sensitive to the child's focus of attention.Talk about what he or she is interested in at the moment. This will increase the likelihood of your child attending to what you have to say.
- Do not talk too much; encourage turn-taking wherein you talk, then the child talks, you talk, and then the child talks. Let the child share responsibility in shaping and directing the conversation.

Adapted from Tye-Murray, 1992b.

specialist may suggest ways that the teacher and speech-language pathologist can capitalize on these specific skills for teaching academic material and conducting speech therapy.

SPEECH-PERCEPTION TRAINING

Adults and children present somewhat different challenges for aural rehabilitation. Both groups must learn to associate the electrical signal with speech and to interpret it. However, adults and children will have a different baseline level of performance at the beginning of the rehabilitation process.

For adults, memories of how speech used to sound may need to be awakened, depending on the duration of hearing loss. Most have extensive knowledge of the grammar and vocabulary of spoken language.

They can use this knowledge to recognize speech (which likely sounds distorted) through a cochlear implant. For example, an individual probably could deduce the word table if he or she recognized the words, *The _____ and chairs are in the kitchen*. During aural rehabilitation, adults may learn to use the electrical signal to enhance speechreading and to recognize speech in an audition-only condition.

The prelingually deaf child has no memory of spoken language and may have only a rudimentary understanding of grammar. The child likely has limited vocabulary and relies primarily on sign language for communication. Thus, the child cannot draw on memories of how speech should sound or on linguistic knowledge for interpreting the electrical signal. Since the child has limited world knowledge, he or she cannot make deductions as well as adults about words or phrases that were missed. Children must learn how to attend to auditory stimuli before learning to abstract meaning from them. During aural rehabilitation, they learn to relate auditory stimuli to their sign vocabulary and their articulatory behavior and relate the auditory signal to visible facial movements.

The situation of the postlingually deaf child may resemble that of the adult or prelingually deaf child, depending on when the hearing loss occurred and how much speech and language were present at the time.

In the following discussion, we will first consider auditory training and then speechreading training. The following topics will be considered for both: designing training objectives and tasks, materials and procedures for training, and assessment procedures.

AUDITORY TRAINING

The primary goal of auditory training is to develop the patient's ability to recognize speech using the electrical signal. During training, the clinician obscures his or her mouth, either by covering it or by sitting out of view.

Designing Training Objectives and Tasks

In providing auditory training, the aural-rehabilitation specialist first develops a program with specific training objectives and tasks. Although this program should be flexible and revised according to patient performance over time, it provides a systematic, well thought out course of action.

Four sources of information are available that can help with the design of an auditory-training program. They are: the cochlear-implant design, how the patient's speech processor is programmed, developmental models of listening, and how patients with the particular cochlear implant generally perform.

Auditory-training activities should encourage the patient to use the particular kinds of information transmitted by the cochlear implant (Stark, 1986; Tyler, Tye-Murray, & Lansing, 1988). For example, the University of London device codes principally fundamental frequency (Fourcin et al., 1979). An exercise wherein the user must discriminate between syllables varying in initial consonant place of production (such as *pat* vs. *cat*) may have little relevance since signal parameters distinguishing the two syllables are not coded by this cochlear implant. On the other hand, activities centering on voicing contrasts (such as *pat* vs. *bat*) are appropriate.

Consideration of the Nucleus cochlear implant can illuminate how this information might guide the development of the auditory-training program. The Nucleus cochlear implant attempts to code the first five formants (see Wilson, Chapter 2). The amplitude of stimulation is used to code the loudness of speech whereas pulse rate is used to code fundamental frequency. It is, therefore, quite reasonable for training activities to direct a patient's attention toward discriminating sibilants such as [s] and [sh] (Moog & Geers, 1991) and vowels that have similar first formant and different second formant values, such as [i] and [u] (Mecklenburg et al., 1990). These activities would be inappropriate for many profoundly hearing-impaired hearing-aid users, who often do not utilize mid- and high-frequency information well. Since amplitude is coded, a patient's attention may also be directed toward amplitude contrasts in distinguishing different consonants (Mecklenburg et al., 1990).

There is a danger in basing training solely on the design characteristics of the cochlear implant because the patient's potential may be underestimated. Some patients perform remarkably well given the presumably limited information provided by their device. For instance, Tyler (1988) found very good word recognition in a patient wearing the Vienna cochlear implant, a single-channel device. The auditory-training objectives that are appropriate for this patient likely surpass what one might have selected on the basis of the cochlear-implant design. Mecklenburg et al. (1990) offer sage advice on this issue: knowing what speech information the cochlear implant codes should not eliminate speech cues from training, but should help the aural rehabilitation specialist to organize training activities so that easier materials precede more difficult materials.

The second source of information that can be reviewed in establishing auditory-training objectives is that about how the patient's speech processor is programmed (Margaret Skinner, personal communication, September,

1991). This information includes the patient's thresholds and maximum comfort levels of stimulation (i.e., the dynamic range), and the ability of the patient to pitch rank. For example, in the case where a patient has very narrow dynamic ranges, attending to intensity differences of consonants may be an auditory training objective that should be included fairly late (if ever) in the aural-rehabilitation program rather than early on.

A third source of information that can influence the auditory-training program concerns the hierarchical sequence hypothesized to underlie the development of listening skills. The patient's level of functioning is identified through testing, and the objectives and training tasks are designed to advance the patient from one level to the next. The four levels—awareness, discrimination, identification, and comprehension—and training tasks are described below. A number of popular auditory-training programs are based on this sequence, including those described by Erber (1982) and Stout and Windle (1986).

The first level of tasks, awareness training, encourages the patient to distinguish between when sound is present and when it is absent. For example, a child might draw a line across a paper whenever the clinician vocalizes.

Postlingually deafened adults need perform few if any awareness tasks, since most recognize the presence of sound immediately after receiving a cochlear implant. This is not the case for the prelingually deaf child, who may not spontaneously react to sound until 6 or 8 months after the device fitting. The prelingually deaf child must realize that sounds convey information and must learn how to attend to them actively. Only then will the child begin to associate specific sounds with their meaning.

Once sound awareness has been established, auditory training can include discrimination tasks. For example, the individual might initially discriminate monosyllables from multiword utterances, such as *cat* from *a big brown cat*. As skills develop, finer discriminations can be attempted. The patient might discriminate between two monosyllabic words that differ only in initial consonant place of production.

Identification tasks require labeling of words, phrases, and sentences. For example, the patient might recognize the phrase, *That's a bat*, from a closed set of four choices. Fairly soon after receiving a cochlear implant, most adults can identify some words auditorily when limited to a set of four or six choices. After 9 months, most can recognize some words presented in an open-set format, particularly when the words are presented in sentence context. Prelingually deaf children require more experience before they can participate in even elementary identification training, often 18 months or more.

During comprehension training, the patient must understand speech stimuli. The patient demonstrates comprehension by correctly answering a question or following a direction, or by responding appropriately after listening to the clinician.

The final source of information that can influence the development of auditory-training objectives and tasks is information about average patient performance. During the past decade, a plethora of data have become available about how patients perform with various cochlear implants. We now have a fairly clear picture of how well words are recognized in isolation and in sentence contexts, and which speech features are utilized in recognizing consonant and vowel stimuli (see Dorman, Chapter 4 and Tyler, Chapter 5). The auditory-training program described by Tye-Murray and Fryauf-Bertschy (1992) illustrates how this information can be used in ordering auditory-training objectives. For example, most adults with multichannel cochlear implants perceive consonantal voicing distinctions relatively well, they experience more difficulty in distinguishing fricative and nonfricative consonants, and have great difficulty in utilizing information pertaining to place of production. Thus, training tasks centering on voicing contrasts are placed relatively early in the program whereas those that require place discriminations are placed relatively late.

Auditory-Training Materials and Procedures

The training materials and procedures are influenced by a number of factors, including the specific training objectives, the age of the patient, and the setting wherein training occurs. Training materials and procedures are greatly influenced by whether training is formal or informal. Formal training occurs at a designated period of the day and usually includes drill activities. Informal training can occur throughout the day and is incorporated into other activities, such as conversation or academic instruction. Except when the patient is a young child, the optimum program allows for both types of training. Children under the age of 5 years should receive primarily informal training.

General guidelines for formal speech-perception training appear in Table 3–8. During formal instruction, auditory-training objectives may dictate one of two levels of speech stimuli, phonetic level and phrase/sentence level, or preferably both (Stout & Windle, 1986). Phonetic-level stimuli vary in their phonetic composition (e.g., *pop, top, cop*). Stimuli become increasingly difficult to discriminate as training progresses. For example, an early exercise may emphasize the consonants [s], [n], and [b], because they differ in manner of production, voicing, and/or place of articulation. In later training, [p], [t], and [k] might be contrasted, since these sounds are acoustically similar. Phrase/sen-

Table 3–8. *General guidelines for formal speech perception training*

a. *Training stimuli should become more challenging to discriminate over time.* Multichannel cochlear implant users often can determine whether a sound is nasalized or voiced, and less often, whether the sound has frication. They have difficulty in distinguishing place of production. In initial training, patients may be asked to discriminate between sounds that differ in manner or voice. In late training, they can discriminate between sounds that differ only in place.

b. *A variety of talkers should speak training stimuli.* Patients learn that the same sounds or words can be acoustically or visually different when repeated or when spoken by different talkers. This realization allows them to generalize what they learn in therapy to a variety of talkers. Tape recorders, audio tape-card machines, VHS tapes, and laser videodiscs can be used to present stimuli.

c. *Many, many training items should be presented during a relatively short period of time.* Concentrated training focuses patients' attention on listening and maintains their interest, leading to fast learning. Adherence to this guideline means that training reinforcements are provided sparingly, since they may be time consuming and distracting.

d. *Nonspeech training stimuli should be used only with young patients who are prelingually deaf, and only for a short period.* Nonspeech stimuli develop two important concepts: "First, sound conveys meaning and second, action often produces sound" (Tye-Murray & Fryauf-Bertschy, 1992, p. 93). The child might turn on and off a water faucet or clap hands. The exception to this guideline is the patient who is interested in developing his or her ability to appreciate music.

e. *A speech perception exercise can include both phonetic-level and phrase/sentence-level stimuli.* Occasionally the patient's attention is focused on recognizing speech sounds and single words or phrases, and occasionally on recognizing words in a meaningful context.

f. *Training progresses from closed-set to open-set response modes.* A new young user might be asked to color a shape red and have to choose between a red or blue crayon (closed-set). An experienced user might be asked to select the red crayon, when crayons from an entire box are available as options (open-set).

g. *Ten to 15 minutes a day should be devoted to formal speech perception training, preferably at the same time everyday.* Training thus becomes a part of the daily routine.

h. *Formal training objectives should be pursued informally throughout the day.* When opportunity arises during conversation or academic instruction, the patient can be presented with speech recognition tasks that reinforce the formal training objectives.

i. *Training activities must be engaging and interesting.* Otherwise, the adult may simply pass through the motions of training without receiving benefit; the child may not cooperate.

tence-level stimuli might include carrier phrase materials initially such as, "That's a _____." Related and unrelated sentences may be practiced in advanced exercises.

Closely associated with the division of formal training stimuli into phonetic-level and sentence-level categories is the classification of training activities as either analytic or synthetic. Analytic training focuses the patient's attention on recognizing every sound or word in a message. Synthetic instruction focuses attention on recognizing the general idea of a message, but not necessarily every word.

Cooper (1991b) describes training tasks that provide analytic and synthetic training. The analytic tasks include recognizing the number of syllables in a nonsense utterance or word, recognizing the stress pattern of a sentence, and discriminating and then identifying consonant and vowel stimuli. Training for these activities usually progresses from a closed-set response mode to an open-set response mode. For example, for consonant analytic work, the patient might be asked to discriminate between /ama/ and /ana/. Once the patient can reliably make such discriminations, the set of response options increases, to four then six or more. Eventually, sound contrasts are incorporated into sentence recognition. Cooper presents the examples of "I want a new FAN" versus "I want a new VAN," where [f] and [v] are the contrasting sounds (p. 229).

Synthetic training activities include connected discourse tracking (De Filippo & Scott, 1978) and recognizing topic-related sentences, and everyday sentences. Initially, patients may be asked to identify a sentence from a list of five sentences, all relating to a common topic. Later in training, they may only be advised of the topic of the training sentences, but will not be provided with a list of choices.

During informal auditory training, the patient is asked to attend to the speech signal in the context of natural conversation. For instance, a classroom teacher may encourage the child to identify words beginning with [p] and [b] during an art activity such as making a puppet. Before beginning, the teacher may identify several words she or he will speak, such as *puppet, paste, bell,* and *pail.* As they construct the puppet, the teacher will occasionally require the child to identify these words auditorily, in the context of conversation.

Formal training objectives should be pursued informally throughout the day, and formal and informal auditory training should be complementary. For example, a child might be asked to discriminate words from a closed set of three choices during formal auditory training. During the school day the classroom teacher might occasionally speak from behind the child and ask the child to pick up one of three objects on a desk or to circle one of three numbers on the chalkboard.

ASSESSMENT AND AUDITORY TRAINING

The three goals of assessment for auditory training are: (a) to obtain information for developing new auditory training objectives, (b) to determine whether present auditory-training objectives have been achieved, and (c) to evaluate whether overall speech recognition has improved as a result of aural rehabilitation. Although the patient's performance during training will provide useful information toward the first two goals, formal assessment serves to document achievements objectively and ensures that a variety of skills are tapped.

Three measures often used with children to assess training and determine placement in an auditory-training program are the Developmental Approach to Successful Listening Placement test (DASL) (Stout & Windle, 1986), the Glendonald Auditory Screening Procedure (GASP) (Erber, 1982), and the Discrimination After Training (DAT) (Thielemeir, Tonokawa, Petersen, & Eisenberg, 1985) (but see Tyler, Chapter 5). The DASL and GASP indicate which level of the four developmental skills described above have been achieved. The DAT also assesses a hierarchy of skills, from detection of voice, to distinguishing words that differ in number of syllables, to distinguishing words with the same number of syllables.

Traditional audiological tests, such as word and sentence recognition tests, can be used to assess therapy efficacy with adults. One useful measure is a consonant nonsense syllable confusion test, where syllables such as /ata/ and /ada/ are presented auditorily for identification. Information transmission analysis (Miller & Nicely, 1955) can be performed on the confusion matrices that are generated with the test results. This analysis indicates which speech features are well utilized and which are poorly utilized and how the use of speech features changes with training. The results can indicate which features should be targeted for remediation and might indicate which features should be capitalized on for increasing word recognition in sentence contexts.

SPEECHREADING TRAINING

Even though many adults recognize some speech auditorily, the cochlear implant's most important role remains that of speechreading enhancement. Most cochlear-implant users recognize significantly more speech in a vision-plus-audition condition than an audition-only condition. Speechreading training helps the patient relate the electrical signal to the corresponding visible articulatory behaviors.

DESIGNING TRAINING OBJECTIVES AND TASKS

Speechreading training objectives should be ordered such that the patient becomes increasingly reliant on the auditory signal for recognizing speech. For example, in the early stages, the patient might discriminate consonant pairs that differ in place of production, such as *cat* and pat. The [k] and [p] belong to two different viseme groups, and are easily distinguished visually. An advanced exercise might require discrimination of consonant pairs that share voice and place of production, such as *tack* and *sack*. The patient must rely primarily on auditory information to discriminate the initial consonantal contrast. An early exercise may also present the talker full-faced. An advanced exercise may present talkers speaking in profile, thereby obscuring some of the visible facial movements.

Training Materials and Procedures

Training should always present both the auditory and visual signals, regardless of whether the patient has good or poor vision-only speech recognition skills. A number of investigations indicate that it is difficult to improve vision-only speech recognition performance (Binnie, 1977; Heider & Heider, 1940; Lesner, Sandridge, & Kricos, 1987) although there are some exceptions to these findings (Dodd, Plant, & Gregory, 1989; Walden, Erdman, Montgomery, Schwartz, & Prosek, 1981; Walden, Prosek, Montgomery, Scherr, & Jones, 1977). Presenting both the auditory and visual signals teaches the patient to associate and assimilate the electrical signal with visual speech information. If the patient performs extremely well in an audiovisual condition, then background noise can be introduced with the training stimuli to make training more challenging. Alternatively, aural rehabilitation might only provide auditory training.

As with auditory training, speechreading training may be formal or informal. Informal speechreading training is much like informal auditory training, except that the patient is allowed to view the clinician's face while listening. The tasks for formal speechreading training may be somewhat more demanding, as most cochlear-implant users can recognize more speech when speechreading than when only listening.

In the following discussion, five training activities that are included in our speechreading-training program are described (Tye-Murray, 1992d and Tye-Murray, in press, present materials for these activities). The descriptions are condensations from Tye-Murray (in press; Tye-Murray, 1992d). All five can be included in a formal speechreading-training exercise, although the patient's skills will determine whether more emphasis is placed on the simpler activities such as babbling and sound awareness or the more challenging activities, such as related sentence recognition. The five types of training activities are: babbling and sound awareness, same/different discriminations, phrase identification, key word training, and related sentence recognition. The first three activities can be considered more analytic whereas the latter two can be considered more synthetic. The activities have been used with hearing-impaired children as young as 5 years and adults as old as 89 years.

A *babbling and sound awareness activity* can be used to introduce target sounds that will be trained during an exercise and is especially appropriate for children. Patients' awareness of sound is closely linked with their ability to produce it. This activity encourages them to associate the speech sounds that they speechread with their own articulatory behavior. Prelingually deaf children and some children who lost their hearing at a young age may not have established these associations.

With the patient watching, the clinician repeats a series of nonsense syllables with the target sounds, such as "pa ba pa ba." The patient then repeats the string. The next string is presented similarly. Syllables are presented in both homogeneous syllable strings (all syllables are the same) and alternating strings (syllables alternate between two). Syllable strings that might be practiced when the target sounds are [p] and [b] are presented in Table 3–9. The strings are practiced in rapid succession.

The *same/different activity* can be presented following the babbling and sound awareness activity. This speechreading activity allows a small set of sounds to be contrasted and focuses the patient's attention on the differences that exist between sounds that may be acoustically and/or visually similar.

The clinician speaks two words or phrases, using similar loudness and intonation for each. The patient's task is to indicate whether the training items are the *same* or *different*. Examples of word pairs that might be practiced when the target sounds are [p] and [b] are presented in Table 3–10.

The *phrase identification activity* requires patients to recognize phrases from a closed set of options. Recognizing words in a closed set prepares the patient for recognizing them in an open set. The set may include anywhere from two to six or more options, depending on the patient's maturity and speechreading skills.

In a typical phrase identification activity, six pictures are placed before the patient. Before starting, the clinician points to each picture and names it, ensuring that the patient knows the names. The clinician says an item with his or her face visible. The patient's task is to point to the picture that illustrates the item and speak the key word. For

Table 3–9. *Syllable string stimuli for the babbling and sound awareness activity when the target sounds are [p] and [b]*

The clinician speaks a string, then the patient. The strings are presented in rapid succession.

a. pah pah pah pah
b. bah bah bah bah
c. pee pee pee pee
d. bee bee bee bee
e. poo poo poo poo
f. boo boo boo boo
g. pah bah pah bah
h. pee bee pee bee
i. poo boo poo boo
j. bah pah bah pah
k. bee pee bee pee
l. boo poo boo poo

Adapted from Tye-Murray, in press.

Table 3–10. *Word pair stimuli for the same/different activity when the target sounds are [p] and [b]*

The clinician speaks each member of the pair with similar loudness and intonation.

a. pet/pet
b. bell/pail
c. pull/bull
d. push/bush
e. punch/bunch
f. buy/buy
g. beg/peg
h. pet/bet
i. pull/pull
j. bee/bee
k. pie/buy
l. pole/bowl
m. peg/peg

Adapted from Tye-Murray, in press.

instance, the clinician says, "That's a pan," and the patient points to the pan illustration and says, "pan." Table 3–11 presents phrases that might be practiced when the target sounds are [p] and [b]. Figure 3–6 presents the six illustrations that might be available as response options. Orthographically presented words can be used in lieu of pictures when the patient is an adult, and more than six words can be included in the response set.

The *key word request activity* requires the patient to recognize sentences from a closed set of options. Patients speechread a sentence and then touch one of 4 or 6 pictures that illustrate the sentence. If they respond correctly, the next sentence is presented. If they respond incorrectly, the clinician speaks a key word from the sentence and then repeats the sentence. Sentence illustrations can either be photographs or artistic drawings.

This activity is excellent for a number of reasons. First, it allows many training items to be presented during a short period of time. Concentrated training prevents boredom and leads to faster learning. Second, the activity requires patients to speechread for the general idea of a sentence and not necessarily for every word, which is how hearing-impaired listeners generally attend to speech (Tye-Murray, Purdy, & Woodworth, 1992). Third, this task allows even the poorest speechreader to experience successful speechreading occasionally since they are limited to a closed set of responses. Fourth, the activity is easily comprehended by children as young as 5 years old. Finally, patients may learn to use the key word repair strategy (see Table 3–4) when they do not understand a spoken utterance. This is a means of incorporating communication therapy into speechreading training.

Figure 3–7 presents four pictures that might be included in a key word request activity, when the target sounds are [p] and [b]. The figure is placed before the patient and the clinician speaks one of the sentences listed in Table 3–12. The patient touches the one picture that illustrates the sentence. The four pictures have some items in common so more than one or two words must be recognized to identify a sentence illustration correctly. (The patient has a 25% chance of responding correctly by guessing. Occasional success helps to prevent frustration.)

The clinician encourages the patient to provide instructions when the patient cannot recognize a sentence. The clinician suggests that the patient say, "Say an important word" or "Tell me what you are talking about." Following the patient's directive, the clinician then says an important content word and repeats the sentence.

The final training activity that can be included in a speechreading exercise is *related sentences*. This activity encourages the patient to attend to context cues when speechreading and also encourages the patient to provide information to the talker when a communication breakdown occurs

Table 3-11. *Phrase stimuli for the phrase identification activity when the target sounds are [p] and [b]*

Each phrase is presented five or more times during an exercise. When the patient has sufficient speech recognition and reading skills, the target words can rhyme and they need not be words that can be illustrated since response choices can be presented orthographically.

a. That's the pole.

b. That's the boat.

c. That's the *P*.

d. That's the bee.

e. That's the bat.

f. That's the bowl.

Adapted from Tye-Murray, in press.

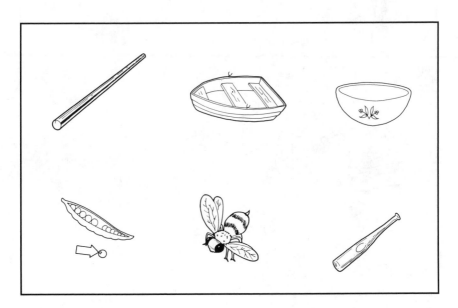

Figure 3–6. Illustrations for the phase-identification activity using a closed-set of six responses. (Reprinted from Tye-Murray, N., in press, *Communication training for hearing-impaired children and teenagers: Speechreading, listening and using repair strategies*, Austin, TX: Pro-Ed, with permission.)

(thereby providing communication therapy in addition to speechreading training).

The patient views a drawing or photograph during a related sentence activity. The picture provides contextual cues for recognizing the training sentences. For instance, Figure 3–8 shows a boy holding a baseball glove and bat. Corresponding sentences appear in Table 3–13. One of the training stimuli is: "Bill has a new baseball glove." The patient's task is to repeat or paraphrase each sentence after speechreading the clinician.

The training sentences are topically related and are appropriate for a commonplace conversational setting; for instance, sentences within an

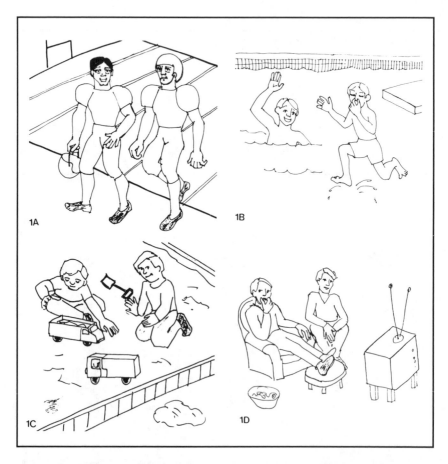

Figure 3–7. Sentence illustrations for the key word request activity using a close-set of four responses. (Reprinted from Tye-Murray, N., in press, *Communication training for hearing-impaired children and teenagers: Speechreading, listening and using repair strategies*, Austin, TX: Pro-Ed, with permission.)

Table 3–12. *Sentence stimuli for the key word request activity when the target sounds are [p] and [b] (sentences correspond to Figure 3–7)*

These sentences were designed for children who have limited language. More sophisticated sentences can be constructed for adult patients. The clinician presents the sentences in random order during training.

Picture 1A
    a. The two boys play with the shovel and *pail*.
    b. The *pick-up-truck* is in the sandbox.
    c. Bob holds a plastic *shovel*.

Picture 1B
    d. One boy *jumps*.
    e. The big boy waves *goodbye*.
    f. The two boys play in the *pool*.

Picture 1C
    g. The big men played *football*.
    h. Peter and Bill are *walking* and talking.
    i. Peter and Bill are on the football *field*.

Picture 1D
    j. Paul and Brian watch *television*.
    k. The big men sit on the *chairs*.
    l. Paul puts his feet on a *footstool*.

Adapted from Tye-Murray, in press.

exercise might relate to a fast-food restaurant, math class, or the school cafeteria for children. For adults, the topics may include a bank setting, a restaurant, or a shoe store. Patients thus practice recognizing sentence materials that are meaningful to their everyday communication demands. The target consonants of the exercise (in this example, [p] and [b]) are well represented in the sentences.

In providing instructions for the related sentence activity, the clinician explains that the patient must "tell me what you think you heard" by repeating or paraphrasing each sentence item. The clinician discusses how knowing what information the patient missed helps the clinician to formulate what to say next. Before beginning an exercise, the clinician and patient discuss the corresponding picture and identify visual context cues that might help the patient recognize the sentence items.

Evaluating the Effects of Speechreading Training

A few tests are available for assessing speechreading skills before and after training. Jorgensen (1991) suggests the following measures for children: the Pediatric Speech Intelligibility (PSI) test, Word Intelligibility by Picture Identification (WIPI) (Ross & Lerman, 1971), the Central Insti-

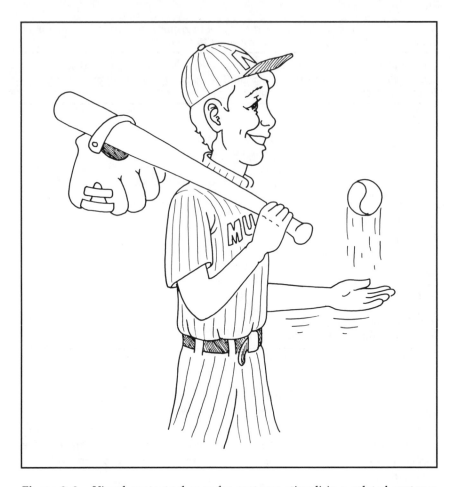

Figure 3–8. Visual contextual cues for sentence stimuli in a related sentence activity. (Reprinted from Tye-Murray, N., in press, *Communication training for hearing-impaired children and teenagers: Speechreading, listening, and using repair strategies*, Austin, TX: Pro-Ed, with permission.)

tute for the Deaf (CID) Everyday Sentences (Davis & Silverman, 1970), and the Connected Discourse Tracking Procedure (De Filippo & Scott, 1978; but see Tye-Murray and Tyler, 1988, and Matthies & Carney, 1988, for a discussion of problems related to using connected discourse tracking). The latter two tests are not appropriate for young children. The Craig Words and the Craig Sentences (Craig, 1975) are also appropriate speechreading measures for children (see Tyler, Chapter 5).

For adults, consonant nonsense syllable tests presented in an audition-only, vision-only, and audiovisual condition can provide valuable infor-

Table 3–13. *Sentence stimuli for the related sentences activity when the target sounds are [p] and [b] (sentences correspond to Figure 3–8*

These sentences were designed for children who have limited language. More sophisticated sentences can be designed for adults.

Bill is going to the playground.
Bill wants to play baseball.
He has a ball and bat.
Bill also has a new baseball glove.
Bill will meet some other boys.

From Tye-Murray, N., in press, *Communication training for hearing-impaired children and teenagers: Speechreading, listening, and using repair strategies.* Austin: Pro-Ed, by permission.

mation. By comparing the difference scores between the audiovisual and audition-only conditions that were obtained prior to and then after training, the clinician can determine whether speechreading enhancement has increased. The vision-only scores and the audiovisual scores will indicate absolute changes in vision-only and audiovisual speech recognition. A feature analysis (Miller & Nicely, 1955) can indicate whether the transmission of feature information has improved in any of the three conditions.

For both adults and children, sentence tests are often used to index training effectiveness. Typically, the clinician presents a list of audiovideotaped sentences before and after training and computes a difference score between the two measures.

Montgomery and Demorest (1988) discuss some of the problems inherent in this methodology. Patients tend to learn the test items on a list with repeated testing, so performance may improve for reasons other than training. Equivalent lists, which bypass the problem of learning, are nearly impossible to construct, especially when three different conditions are evaluated (i.e., vision-only, audition-only, audiovisual). Finally, patients show day-to-day variability in their performance: On some days, they may score higher than on others. This is especially problematic with children who may vary dramatically from day to day in their willingness and motivation to participate in testing.

We evaluate the efficacy of our speechreading training intervention program with four sentence lists, which comprise The Repeated Sentence Frame Test (Appendix 2).[2] Lists A and B are presented in an audition-plus-vision condition, and lists C and D are presented in a vision-only condition. Lists A and C are completed on one day and lists B and D on the next day. Speechreading training begins thereafter. On completion of the training program, the tests are administered again during a 2-day period. The tests are scored by the number of keywords repeated verbatim.

By testing on two separate days, some information about performance variability is obtained. Also, two scores within a test condition are available. Before audiovisual speech recognition performance is considered improved, scores on both lists A and B must improve following training; likewise for visual speech recognition and lists C and D.

The lists in The Repeated Sentence Frame Test each contain 24 sentences, with six sets of four. Each set of four sentences share syntactic structure and differ only in two or three keywords. The keywords within a set are interchangeable and are approximately equally probable in the sentence context. They also have the same number of syllables. The use of sentence sets is meant to minimize the learning effects associated with repeated testing. For instance, if the patient recognizes the words *in the sky* in list A, the keywords will not be known due to prior exposure to the list. *Three stars, ten birds, six clouds,* and *eight kites* are all possible elements of the test sentence. The sentences within a list are randomly presented.

Posttherapy performance on a test list is compared to pretherapy performance using a within-subject statistical procedure (Tye-Murray, Tyler, Woodworth, & Gantz, 1992; Woodworth, submitted). The number of words correct in each sentence is tabulated and then a paired t statistic is computed, with the sentences paired to compare performance pre- and posttherapy. A paired t test is appropriate because the same sentences are presented before and after aural rehabilitation therapy. Since a list contains 24 sentences, each t-test statistic has 23 degrees of freedom.

THE BENEFITS OF SPEECH-PERCEPTION TRAINING

Many adults improve their speech-recognition abilities with experience (Clark et al., 1984; Dorman, Dankowski, McCandless, Parkin, & Smith, 1990; Spivak & Waltzman, 1990; Tye-Murray, Tyler, Woodworth, & Gantz, 1992), particularly during the first year of cochlear-implant use. This suggests that they learn to use the electrical signal. Anectodal reports attest to the importance of speech-perception training. For example, Shirley Ackehurst in her book, *Broken Silence* (1989), describes how she diligently pursued listening experiences after receiving a Nucleus cochlear implant. During formal practice sessions, her husband would speak from behind her or read simple stories while Mrs. Ackehurst listened with her eyes closed. She listened to books on tape while following the printed text. She purposefully alerted to new sounds and asked family and friends to identify them. During her first 9 months, her auditory skills developed rapidly. She noted that she felt more self-confident and assertive and no longer had to strain to speechread.

Although many speech and hearing professionals suggest that speech-perception training accelerates and enhances the learning process (Abberton et al., 1985; Bergeron, Ferron, Gobeil, & Desgague, 1990; Cooper, 1991b; Eisenberg & Berliner, 1983; Lansing & Davis, 1988; Owens & Raggio, 1987), few investigators have evaluated intervention effects with adults, and in particular, children. Those who have present different pictures about the effectiveness of training.

The work of Lansing and her colleagues (Lansing, 1990; Lansing & Davis, 1988) and Cook (1991) address the value of speech-perception training for adult cochlear implant users. Lansing provided a 10-day intensive aural rehabilitation program to a large group of adults wearing the Nucleus cochlear implant and the Ineraid cochlear implant. The program included training in discriminating phonemes, recognizing sentences, and speech tracking (De Filippo & Scott, 1978). Some patients received training 1 month following cochlear-implant fitting, and others received training after 9 months. The results suggest that aural rehabilitation improved consonant recognition, especially when it was provided early on. The training effects were still evident after 18 months of cochlear implant use. Lansing (1990) noted that patients differed in their ability to benefit.

Cook (1991) describes the aural-rehabilitation program developed by members of the Department of Audiology at Sodersjukhuset, Stockholm. The program includes training at the cochlear-implant center and home-based training. Patients receive audiovisual speech training with a computer-controlled audiovisual tape player. Patients also engage extensively in continuous discourse tracking (De Filippo & Scott, 1978), and receive telephone training. Sixteen adult patients, 10 who use a single-channel cochlear implant (the Vienna device) and 6 who use a multichannel device (the Nucleus device), have enrolled in the program. Cook (1991) summarizes the results of those who have completed the program as follows: "Improvement in perception and understanding of spoken language using the auditory signal alone or the auditory/visual signals, is present to a greater or lesser degree as a result of the rehabilitation program" (p. 247). Audiological data from two patients are presented to support this conclusion.

At least two studies have not shown speech-perception training to effect dramatically speech-recognition skills. Boothroyd, Hanin, and Waltzman (1987) found that sentence training was beneficial for a small group of adult Nucleus cochlear-implant patients, but that the benefits were very small in comparison to those provided by receipt of the device. The authors also noted large intersubject differences in training benefits.

Gagné, Parnes, La Rocque, Hassan, and Vidas (1992) provided 36 hours of aural rehabilitation to four adult Nucleus patients, using a single-subject experimental protocol. Training activities were presented during a 12-week interval, and included phoneme recognition, sentence recognition, and continuous discourse tracking (De Filippo & Scott, 1978). Patients also received telephone practice and communication strategy training. Speech-perception skills did not change as a result of aural rehabilitation. The authors speculated that the length of training may have been too brief to effect an improvement. They also noted that their test battery did not assess whether telephone skills or communication behaviors improved.

These different findings, indicating speech perception to be more or less valuable, might relate to differences in training procedures, differences in patient population (especially since almost all investigations conclude that patients differ in their ability to benefit), and differences between the time at which aural rehabilitation was provided. Certainly, an avenue for future research is systemic evaluation of aural rehabilitation addressing the following issues: the most effective training stimuli and procedures, the value of aural rehabilitation for children and adults, the characteristics of patients who are most likely to benefit, and the optimum time course for intervention.

SUMMARY

The decision to receive a cochlear implant requires a tremendous commitment from the hearing-impaired individual and his or her support system (cochlear-implant center, family, friends, school, and workplace). This chapter reviewed the components of a cochlear-implant center program, which include initial contact, preimplant counseling, candidate selection, surgery, fitting, follow-up, and aural rehabilitation. The two components of speech-perception training were considered: auditory and speechreading training. Means for developing training objectives, training activities, and assessment procedures were presented for both.

ACKNOWLEDGMENTS

This work was supported in part by a National Institute of Health grant DC00242; grant RR59 from the General Clinical Research Center Program, Division of Research Resources, NIH; and a grant from the Lions Club of Iowa. I thank Mary Lowder, Holly Fryauf-Bertschy, Ruth Severson, Jill Firszt, Margaret Skinner, and Lisa Tonokawa for sharing their clinical expertise, and Karen Iler Kirk for her editorial comments on an earlier version of this manuscript.

FOOTNOTES

[1]Nancy Tye-Murray and Cheryl Sobaski have produced an audiovisual instructional film entitled *Living with a family member who has a hearing loss: A guide for effective communication.* The film presents examples of repair strategies, inappropriate speaking behaviors, and clear speech. Copies of the film may be obtained by writing Nancy Tye-Murray.

[2]Danielle Kelsay is the co-developer of these materials.

REFERENCES

Abberton, E., Fourcin, A. J., Rosen, S., Walliker, J. R., Howard, D. M., Moore, B. C. J., Doucek, E. E., & Frampton, S. (1985). Speech perceptual and productive rehabilitation in electrocochlear stimulation. In R. A. Schindler & M. M. Merzenich (Eds.), *Cochlear implants* (pp.527–538). New York: Raven Press.

Ackehurst, S. (1989). *Broken silence,* Sydney, Australia: William Collins Pty Ltd.

Balkany, T., Gantz, B., & Nadol, J. (1988). Multichannel cochlear implants in partially ossified cochlea. *Annals of Otology, Rhinology, and Laryngology, 97,* 3–7.

Bergeron, F., Ferron, P., Gobeil, S., & Desgague, M. (1990). Multielectrode cochlear implantation in children: The Quebec experience. *Journal of Otolaryngology, 19,* 324–330.

Binnie, C.A. (1977). Attitude changes following speechreading training. *Scandinavian Audiology, 6,* 13–19.

Boothroyd, A., Hanin, L., & Waltzman, S. (1987). Development of speech perception skills in cochlear implantees. *Proceedings of Rehabilitation Engineering Society of America* (RESNA) *10th Annual Conference, San Jose, CA, 1987,* 428–430.

Brown, A. M., Dowell, R. C., Martin, L. F., & Mecklenburg, D.F. (1990). Training of communication skills in implanted deaf adults. In G. M. Clark, Y. C. Tong, & J. F. Patrick (Eds.), *Cochlear prostheses* (pp. 125–134), New York: Churchill Livingston.

Clark, G. M., Busby, P. A., Roberts, S. A., Dowell, R. C., Tong, Y. C., Blamey, P. J., Nienbuys, T. G., Mecklenburg, D. J., & Webb, R. L. (1987). Preliminary results for the Cochlear Corporation multi–electrode intracochlear implant on six prelingually deaf patients. *American Journal of Otology, 8,* 234–239.

Clark, G. M., Tong, Y. C., Patrick, J. F., Seligman, P. M., Crosby, P. A., Kuzma, J. A., and Money, P. K. (1984). A multichannel hearing prosthesis for profound to total hearing loss. *Journal of Medical Engineering Technology, 8,* 3–8.

Clark, G. M., Franz, B., Pyman, B., & Webb, R. (1991). Surgery for multichannel cochlear implantation. In H. Cooper (Ed.), *Cochlear implants: A practical guide* (pp. 169–200). San Diego: Singular Publishing Group, Inc.

Cook, B.O. (1991). Testing and rehabilitation of cochlear implant patients at the Department of Audiology, Sodersjukhuset, Stockholm. In H. Cooper (Ed.), *Cochlear implants: A practical guide* (pp. 240–250). San Diego: Singular Publishing Group, Inc.

Cooper, H. (1991a). Selection of candidates for cochlear implantation: an overview. In H. Cooper (Ed.), *Cochlear implants: A practical guide* (pp. 92–100). San Diego: Singular Publishing Group, Inc.

Cooper, H. (1991b). Training and rehabilitation for cochlear implant users. In H. Cooper (Ed.) *Cochlear implants: A practical guide* (pp. 219–239). San Diego, CA: Singular Publishing Group, Inc.

Craig, W. M. (1975). *Craig lipreading test* (1964). Pittsburgh: Western Pennsylvania School for the Deaf.

Davis, H. & Silverman, S. R. (1970). *Hearing and deafness.* New York: Holt, Rinehart & Winston.

De Filippo, C. L. (1991). Good talker/poor talker: What makes the difference? *CICI Contact, 6,* 30–32.

De Filippo, C. L., & Scott, B. L. (1978). A method for training and evaluating the reception of ongoing speech. *Journal of the Acoustical Society of America, 63,* 1186–1192.

Dodd, B., Plant, G., & Gregory, M. (1989). Teaching lip–reading: The efficacy of lessons on video. *British Journal of Audiology, 23,* 229–238.

Dorman, M. F., Dankowski, K., McCandless, G., Parkin, J. L., & Smith, L. (1990). Longitudinal changes in word recognition by patients who use the Ineraid cochlear implant. *Ear and Hearing, 11,* 455–459.

Dorman, M. F., Dove, H., Parkin, J., Zacharchuk, S., & Dankowski, K. (1991). Telephone use by patients fitted with the Ineraid cochlear implant. *Ear and Hearing, 12,* 368–369.

Downs, M. P. (1986). Psychosocial issues surrounding children receiving cochlear implants. *Seminars in Hearing, 7,* 383–406.

Eisenberg, L., & Berliner, K. (1983). Rehabilitative procedures for the cochlear implant patient. *Journal of the Academy of Rehabilitative Audiology, 16,* 104–113.

Erber, N. P. (1982). *Auditory training.* Washington DC: Alexander Graham Bell Association for the Deaf.

Erber, N. P. (1985). *Telephone communication and hearing impairment.* San Diego: College-Hill Press.

Evans, J. W. (1989). Thoughts on the psychosocial implications of cochlear implantation in children. In E. Owens & D. Kessler (Eds.), *Cochlear implants in young deaf children* (pp. 307–314). Boston: Little Brown.

Firszt, J. B., Novak, M. A., Reeder, R. M., & Proctor, L. A. (1991, November). *Cochlear implantation in children with severe cochlear deformities.* Paper presented at the American Speech-Language-Hearing Association, Atlanta, GA.

Firszt, J. B., Reeder, R. M., Zimmerman-Phillips, S., Tonokawa, L., & Proctor, L. A. (1991, June). *Rehabilitative plans and resulting performance of children using cochlear implants.* Paper presented at the Academy of Rehabilitative Audiology Summer Institutes XXV, Breckenridge, CO.

Fourcin, A. S., Rosen, S. M., Moore, B. C. J., Doucek, E. E., Clarke, G. P., Dodson, H., & Bannister, L. H. (1979). External electrical stimulation of the cochlear: Clinical psychophysical, speech-perceptual & histologic findings. *British Journal of Audiology, 13,* 85–107.

Fryauf-Bertschy, H. (1990, June). *Cochlear implantation of a blind child.* Paper presented at The Second International Cochlear Implant Symposium, Iowa City, IA.

Fryauf-Bertschy, H. (1992). Getting started at home. In N. Tye-Murray (Ed.), *Cochlear implants and children: A handbook for parents, teachers, and speech and hearing professionals* (pp. 1–24). Washington, DC: Alexander Graham Bell Association for the Deaf.

Fryauf-Bertschy, H., & Kirk, K. I. (1992). The child at school. In N. Tye-Murray (Ed.), *Cochlear implants and children: A handbook for parents, teachers, and speech and hearing professionals* (pp. 25–40). Washington, DC: Alexander Graham Bell Association for the Deaf.

Gagné, J. P., Parnes, L. S., La Rocque, M., Hassan, R., & Vidas, S. (1991). Effectiveness of an intensive speech-perception training program for adult cochlear implant recipients. *Annals of Otology, Rhinology, & Laryngology, 100,* 700–707.

Gantz, G. J., Woodworth, G. G., Knutson, J. F., Abbas, P. J., & Tyler, R. S. (in press). Multivariate predictors of success with cochlear implants. *Annals of Otology, Rhinology, and Laryngology.*

Gfeller, K., & Lansing, C. (1991). Melodic, rhythmic, and timbral perception of adult cochlear implant users. *Journal of Speech and Hearing Research, 34,* 916–920.

Graham, J. (1990). Cochlear implants for children? Conclusions. In M. Haggard & M. L. Page (Eds.), *Clinical developments in cochlear implants* (pp. 82–85). Southampton, England: Duphar Medical Relations.

Graham, J. (1991). Surgery for single-channel cochlear implantation. In H. Cooper (Ed.), *Cochlear implants: A practical guide* (pp. 155–168). San Diego: Singular Publishing Group, Inc.

Greenwald, A. B. (1984). *Lipreading made easy: Practice lessons.* Washington, DC: Alexander Graham Bell Association for the Deaf.

Heider, F., & Heider, G. M. (1940). An experimental investigation of lipreading. *Psychological Monographs, 52,* 124–133.

Jorgensen, S. (1991). Long-term follow-up for children with cochlear implants. *American Journal of Otology, 12* (Suppl.), 211–212.

Kessler, D. K. & Owens, E. (1989). Conclusions: Current considerations and future directions. In E. Owens & D. K. Kessler (Eds.), *Cochlear implants in young deaf children* (pp. 315–330). Boston: College-Hill Press.

Knutson, J. F., Schartz, H. A., Gantz, B. J., Tyler, R. S., Hinrichs, J. V., & Woodworth, G. (1991). Psychological change following 18 months of cochlear implant use. *Annals of Otolaryngology, Rhinology, and Laryngology, 100* (10), 877–882.

Lane, H. (1990). Cultural and infirmity models of deaf Americans. *Journal of the Academy of Rehabilitative Audiology, 23,* 11–26.

Lansing, C. R. (1990, November). *Longitudinal consonant recognition by adult multichannel cochlear implant users.* Paper presented at the American Speech-Language-Hearing Association Convention, Seattle, WA.

Lansing, C. R., & Davis, J. (1988). Early versus delayed speech perception training for adult cochlear implant users: Preliminary results. *Journal of the Academy of Rehabilitative Audiology, 21,* 21–42.

Lesner, S., Sandridge, S., & Kricos, P. (1987). Training influences on visual consonant and sentence recognition. *Ear and Hearing, 8,* 283–287.

Loeb, G. E. (1989). Neural prosthetic strategies for young children. In E. Owens & D. K. Kessler (Eds.), *Cochlear implants in young deaf children* (pp. 137–152). Boston: College-Hill Press.

Matthies, M. L. & Carney, A. E. (1988). A modified speech tracking procedure as a communicative performance measure. *Journal of Speech and Hearing Research, 31,* 394–404.

McKenna, L. (1991). The assessment of psychological variables in cochlear implant patients. In H. Cooper (Ed.) *Cochlear implants: A practical guide* (pp. 125–145). San Diego: Singular Publishing Group.

Mecklenburg, D. J., Blamey, P. J., Busby, P. A., Dowell, R. C., Roberts, S., & Rickards, F. W. (1990). Auditory (re)habilitation for implanted deaf children and teenagers. In G. J. Clark, Y. C. Tong, & J. F. Patrick (Eds.), *Cochlear prostheses* (pp. 207–222). New York: Churchill Livingston.

Miller, G. A., & Nicely, P. E. (1955). An analysis of perceptual confusions among some English consonants. *Journal of the Acoustical Society of America, 27,* 338–352.

Montgomery, A., & Demorest, M. (1988). Issues and developments in the evaluation of speechreading. *Volta Review, 90,* 119–148.

Moog, J. S., & Geers, A. E. (1991). Educational managements of children with cochlear implants. *American Annals of the Deaf, 136,* 69–76.

Moora, C. R., & Wallace, M. (1991). *Cochlear implant reimbursement guide.* Englewood, CO: Cochlear Corporation.

Nevins, M. E., Kretschmer, R. E., Chute, P. M., Hellman, S. E., & Parisier, S. C. (1991). Programs in action: The role of an educational consultant in a pediatric cochlear implant program. *The Volta Review, 93,* 197–206.

Owens, E., & Raggio, M. (1987). The UCSF tracking procedure for evaluation and training of speech reception by hearing-impaired adults. *Journal of Speech and Hearing Disorders, 52,* 120–128.

Picheny, M. A., Durlach, N. I., & Braida, L. D. (1986). Speaking clearly for the hard of hearing II: Acoustic characteristics of clear and conversational speech. *Journal of Speech and Hearing Research, 29,* 434–446.

Ramsden, R.T. (1990). Cochlear implants: patient selection. In M. Haggard & M. L. Page (Eds.), *Clinical developments in cochlear implants* (pp. 36–43). Southampton, England: Duphar Medical Relations.

Reeder, R. M., & Firszt, J. B. (1990, November). *A guide for optimizing auditory learning skills.* Paper presented at the American Speech-Language-Hearing Association, Seattle, WA.

Roberts, S. (1991). Speech-processor fitting for cochlear implants. In H. Cooper (Ed.), *Cochlear implants: A practical guide* (pp. 201–218). San Diego: Singular Publishing Group, Inc.

Robbins, A. (1990). Developing meaningful auditory integration in children with cochlear implants. *The Volta Review, 92,* 361–370.

Ross, M., & Lerman, J. (1971). *Word intelligibility by picture identification.* Pittsburgh, PA: Stanwix House.

Russell, R. L. (1987). *Read my lips: Speechreading instruction course no. 1.* Mustang, OK: Speechreading Laboratory, Inc.

Shallop, J. K., Dooley, G., Heller, J., Arndt, P., & Blamey, P. (1991, November). *BI-MODAL speech processor: Multichannel cochlear implant and hearing aid.* Paper presented at the American Speech-Language-Hearing Association, Atlanta, GA.

Sims, D. (1988). Video methods for speechreading instruction. *The Volta Review, 90,* 273–288.

Spivak, L. G., & Waltzman, S. B. (1990). Performance of cochlear implant patients as a function of time. *Journal of Speech and Hearing Research, 33,* 511–519.

Staller, S. J., Beiter, A. L., Brimacombe, J. A., Mecklenburg, D. J., & Arndt, P. (1991). Pediatric performance with the Nucleus 22-channel cochlear implant system. *American Journal of Otology, 12*(Suppl.), 126–136.

Staller, S. J., Dowell, R. C., Beiter, A. L., & Brimacombe, J. A. (1991). Perceptual abilities of children with the Nucleus 22-channel cochlear implant. *Ear and Hearing, 12*, 345–475.

Stark, R. E. (1986). Developmental aspects influencing implantation and rehabilitation of children. *Seminars in Hearing, 7*, 371–382.

Stout, G. G., & Windle, J. V. E. (1986). *The developmental approach to successful listening* (DASL). Houston: Stout & Windle.

Thielemeir, M. A., Tonokawa, L. L., Petersen, B., & Eisenburg, L. S. (1985). Audiological results in children with a cochlear implant. *Ear and Hearing, 6* (Suppl.), 275–355.

Tye-Murray, N. (1991). Repair strategy usage by hearing-impaired adults and changes following instruction. *Journal of Speech and Hearing Research, 23*, 921–928.

Tye-Murray, N. (1992a). Conversing with the implanted child. In N. Tye-Murray (Ed.), *Cochlear implants and children: A handbook for parents, teachers, and speech and hearing professionals* (pp. 60–78). Washington, DC: Alexander Graham Bell Association for the Deaf.

Tye-Murray, N. (1992b). Speech perception training: General guidelines. In N. Tye-Murray (Ed.), *Cochlear implants and children: A handbook for parents, teachers, and speech and hearing professionals* (pp. 79–90). Washington, DC: Alexander Graham Bell Association for the Deaf.

Tye-Murray, N. (1992c). Communication therapy. In N. Tye-Murray (Ed.), *Children with cochlear implants: A handbook for parents, teachers, and speech and hearing professionals* (pp. 136–168). Washington, DC: Alexander Graham Bell Association for the Deaf.

Tye-Murray, N. (1992d). Speechreading training. In N. Tye-Murray (Ed.), *Cochlear implants and children: A handbook for parents, teachers, and speech and hearing professionals* (pp. 115–135). Washington DC: Alexander Graham Bell Association for the Deaf.

Tye-Murray, N. (1992e). Laser videodisc applications in the aural rehabilitation setting: Good news for the severely and profoundly hearing-impaired patient. *The American Journal of Audiology: A Journal of Clinical Practice, 1*, 33–36.

Tye-Murray, N. (in press). *Communication training for hearing-impaired children and teenagers: Speechreading, listening, and using repair strategies.* Austin, TX: Pro-Ed.

Tye-Murray, N., & Schum, L. (in press). Conversation training for frequent communication partners. *Journal of the Academy of Rehabilitative Audiology.*

Tye-Murray, N., & Fryauf-Bertschy, H. (1992). Auditory training. In N. Tye-Murray (Ed.), *Cochlear implants and children: A handbook for parents, teachers, and speech and hearing professionals* (pp. 91–114). Washington, DC: Alexander Graham Bell Association for the Deaf.

Tye-Murray, N., & Kelsay, D. (in press). Communication therapy for parents of cochlear implant users. *Volta Review.*

Tye-Murray, N., Purdy, S. C., & Woodworth, G. (1992). The reported use of communication strategies by members of SHHH and its relationship to client, talker, and situational variables. *Journal of Speech and Hearing Research, 35*, 708–717.

Tye-Murray, N., & Tyler, R. S. (1988). A critique of continuous discourse tracking as a test procedure. *Journal of Speech and Hearing Disorders, 53*, 226–231.

Tye-Murray, N., Tyler, R. S., Woodworth, G., & Gantz, B. J. (1992). Performance over time with a multichannel cochlear implant. *Ear and Hearing, 13*, 200–209.

Tyler, R. S. (1988). Open set word recognition with the 3M Vienna single channel cochlear implant. *Archives of Otolaryngology, 114*, 1123–1126.

Tyler, R. S., & Fryauf-Bertschy, H. (1992). Hearing abilities of children with cochlear implants. In N. Tye-Murray (Ed.), *Cochlear implants and children: A handbook for parents, teachers, and speech and hearing professionals* (pp. 41–59). Washington, DC: Alexander Graham Bell Association for the Deaf.

Tyler, R. S., & Kelsay, D. (1990). Advantages and disadvantages reported by some of the better cochlear- implant patients. *American Journal of Otology, 11,* 282–289.

Tyler, R. S., Preece, J., & Tye-Murray, N. (1986). *The Iowa laser videodisc sentence test without context.* Iowa City, IA: University of Iowa Hospitals and Clinics.

Tyler, R. S., Tye-Murray, N., & Lansing, C. R. (1988). Electrical stimulation as an aid to speechreading. *Volta Review, 90,* 119–148.

Walden, B. E., Erdman, S. A., Montgomery, A. A., Schwartz, D. M., & Prosek, R. A. (1981). Some effects of training on speech recognition in hearing-impaired adults. *Journal of Speech and Hearing Research, 24,* 207–316.

Walden, B. E., Prosek, R. A., Montgomery, A. A., Scherr, C. K., & Jones, C. J. (1977). Effects of training on the visual recognition of consonants. *Journal of Speech and Hearing Research, 20,* 130–145.

Webb, R. L., Pyman, B. C., Franz, B. K., & Clark, G. M. (1990). The surgery of cochlear implantation. In G. J. Clark, Y. C. Tong, & J. F. Patrick (Eds.), *Cochlear Prostheses* (pp. 153–180). New York: Churchill Livingston Inc.

Woodworth, G. G. (submitted). *Misuse of Shearers' binomial test in audiology.* Manuscript submitted for publication.

Appendix 1

RELATIVE'S DAILY LOG OF COMMUNICATION ACTIVITIES

Date:_____

Instructions: Please answer the questions below in the appropriate column. All questions concern your family member who uses a cochlear implant.

1. How many times did you converse with your relative today (beyond a greeting)? Circle one response for each condition:

___ in a quiet place	Never	a few times	many times
___ in a noisy place	Never	a few times	many times
___ on the telephone	Never	a few times	many times
___ from another room	Never	a few times	many times
___ in a group of people	Never	a few times	many times
___ when only the two of us were present	Never	a few times	many times

2. On a scale of 1 to 10, where 1 = nothing and 10 = everything, how much of what you said today did your relative understand?

   ___ while watching you and listening
   ___ while listening only

3. Did your relative ever misunderstand your spoken message today (Yes or No)? _____

4. What did you do when your relative did not understand your message (check all that apply)?

   ___ started to talk more slowly
   ___ repeated my message word for word
   ___ said my message with different words
   ___ spoke one important word/identified the topic of conversation
   ___ elaborated my message by giving a little more information
   ___ simplified my message by using fewer words or more common place words
   ___ decided my message was not important enough to keep trying
   ___ wrote or spelled the message
   ___ used more gestures or sign language
   ___ other (describe) _____

(continued)

Appendix 1 *(continued)*

5. On a scale of 1 to 10, where 1 = never and 10 = always, how often did you attempt to establish eye contact with your relative before talking?

_____

6. Check all that apply:

_____ I encouraged my relative to practice speechreading me while I read the newspaper or a book aloud today.

_____ I identified at least one new environmental sound for my relative today.

_____ On at least one occasion today, I encouraged my relative to listen to my speech without watching my face.

Appendix 2

THE REPEATED SENTENCE FRAME TEST

The sentences are presented in random order, but are presented in sets of four here, with each set corresponding to one sentence frame. Key words are italicized. Whether the list is presented in audition-plus-vision or vision-only mode is noted in parentheses.

List A (Audition-plus-vision)

1. The *boat* is *fast*.
2. The *train* is *slow*.
3. The *plane* is *big*.
4. The *bike* is *small*.
5. A *lunchbox* is on the *bed*.
6. A *balloon* in on the *desk*.
7. A *baseball* is on the *chair*.
8. A *pencil* is on the *floor*.
9. The *snake* is looking at the *food*.
10. The *cat* is looking at the *moon*.
11. The *bear* is looking at the *tree*.
12. The *frog* is looking at the *bug*.
13. *Three stars* are in the sky.
14. *Ten birds* are in the sky.
15. *Six clouds* are in the sky.
16. *Eight kites* are in the sky.
17. The *silly* dog is *sleeping*.
18. The *funny* dog is *playing*.
19. The *ugly* dog is *sitting*.
20. The *pretty* dog is *eating*.
21. *Pick* up your *hat*.
22. *Put* on your *coat*.
23. *Put* on your *shoes*.
24. *Take* off your *boots*.

List B (Audition-plus-vision)

1. The *queen* is *nice*.
2. The *king* is *mean*.
3. The *nurse* is *fat*.
4. The *dog* is *bad*.

(continued)

Appendix 2 (*continued*)

5. Her *mom* is in the *bedroom.*
6. Her *friend* is in the *backyard.*
7. Her *dad* is in the *kitchen.*
8. Her *aunt* is in the *bathroom.*
9. *Grandma* is eating a *hotdog.*
10. *Mother* is eating a *cookie.*
11. *Grandpa* is eating a *pancake.*
12. *Father* is eating an *apple.*
13. The *birthday cake* and *plates* are on the table.
14. The *potatoes* and *forks* are on the table.
15. The *bananas* and *bowls* are on the table.
16. The *hamburgers* and *knives* are on the table.
17. I *want* the *soup.*
18. I *cook* the *eggs.*
19. I *need* the *meat.*
20. I *like* the *peas.*
21. Point to your *hair* and *nose.*
22. Point to your *arms* and *face.*
23. Point to your *hands* and *ears.*
24. Point to your *eyes* and *feet.*

List C (Vision-only)

1. The *pen* is in the *bowl.*
2. The *book* is in the *bag.*
3. The *key* is in the *jar.*
4. The *ball* is in the *room.*
5. The *football* is *outside* the box.
6. The *money* is *under* the box.
7. The *candy* is *inside* the box.
8. The *whistle* is *behind* the box.
9. *Drink* the *juice.*
10. *Buy* the *milk.*
11. *Stir* the *tea.*
12. *Pour* the *pop.*
13. The *lady* is washing the *shirts.*
14. The *teacher* is washing the *dress.*
15. The *farmer* is washing the *pants.*
16. The *woman* is washing the *dish.*
17. The *car* is *yellow.*
18. The *truck* is *blue.*

(*continued*)

Appendix 2 (*continued*)

19. The *kite* is *dirty*.
20. The *bike* is *little*.
21. The boy has a *pink* and *blue* bike.
22. The boy has a *white* and *green* bike.
23. The boy has a *brown* and *green* bike.
24. The boy has a *black* and *red* bike.

List D (Vision-only)

1. *Five boys* are in the water.
2. *Two ducks* are in the water.
3. *Four fish* are in the water.
4. *Nine boats* are in the water.
5. I see a *rabbit* and a *cow*.
6. I see a *turkey* and a *pig*.
7. I see a *turtle* and a *mouse*.
8. I see a *chicken* and a *horse*.
9. A cat is *running* in the *street*.
10. A cat is *waiting* in the *house*.
11. A cat is *walking* in the *grass*.
12. A cat is *standing* in the *yard*.
13. *Get* some *cake*.
14. *Take* some *pie*.
15. *Have* some *lunch*.
16. *Make* some *bread*.
17. The *cowboy* is *tall*.
18. The *mailman* is *mad*.
19. The *doctor* is *short*.
20. The *fireman* is *sad*.
21. A *boy* is *making* the paper airplane.
22. A *man* is *watching* the paper airplane.
23. A *clown* is *throwing* the paper airplane.
24. A *girl* is *making* the paper airplane.

CHAPTER 4

Speech Perception by Adults
MICHAEL F. DORMAN

Over a quarter of a century has passed since the publication of the first reports on patients fitted with cochlear implants (Doyle, Doyle, & Turnbull, 1964; Simmons, 1966). The first reports were not very encouraging—at best, speech signals were recognized as speech but were unintelligible. However, as the sophistication of signal processing increased and as the number of patients increased from a handful to hundreds, reports of patients with good, sometimes remarkably good, speech recognition abilities surfaced. Today, patients have achieved scores of 80% correct on single-syllable words and have achieved scores of 100% correct on tests of words in sentences. Many patients communicate with only minor difficulty, use the telephone, and have resumed careers interrupted by profound deafness. Cochlear implants have come a long way in a quarter of a century.

This chapter is organized into five sections. A description of some of the acoustic cues for speech recognition comes first. Cues in both the amplitude/time domain and the frequency domain are described. Reviews of speech recognition by patients with single-channel and multichannel implants follow. In this section, the performance of patients who use the Vienna single-channel implant and patients who use the Nucleus, Ineraid, and Research Triangle Institute multichannel implants are described in detail. A section on the recognition of nonspeech acoustic events—an important but often overlooked topic—comes next. In the penultimate section, data on the time course for reacquisition of speech and nonspeech recognition are reviewed. In the final section correlations among a variety of test and patient variables are described in an effort to account for differences in performance among patients.

ACOUSTIC CUES FOR SPEECH RECOGNITION

A necessary foundation for an appreciation of the speech recognition abilities of cochlear-implant patients is an understanding of visual and acoustic cues for speech perception (see Dodd & Campbell, 1987 and Pickett, 1980, respectively). We will discuss visual cues and their integration with auditory cues in a later section of this chapter. In this section, we will briefly review some of the acoustic cues for speech recognition in the context of cues that a cochlear prosthesis might make available to a patient fitted with a single channel or multichannel cochlear implant. Fortunately, a large amount of patient performance can be understood by reference to a small number of cues.

CUES AND FEATURES

The term "cue" refers to a specific aspect of an acoustic signal that has been demonstrated to be important for recognition of a phonetic segment, or for distinguishing between two phonetic segments. The term "feature" generally refers to *articulation*, and not to a particular acoustic cue. Thus, the feature "place of articulation" encompasses sounds with extremely different acoustic signatures. For example, the place cues for voiced stop-consonants reside in transient bursts and formant transitions of brief duration, but the place cues for fricatives reside in long duration fricative noises which differ greatly in frequency and in amplitude. This must be kept in mind when sorting through the results of studies that report on the reception of "features" by implant patients. Moreover, while some features are articulatory, others are acoustic. Thus, the "envelope" feature is defined by a set of amplitude profiles for consonants in intervocalic position. A feature-to-phoneme assignment matrix is shown in Table 4–1 (Wilson, Lawson & Finley, 1990).

MULTIPLE CUES FOR CONSONANTS AND VOWELS

One of the principal findings from the search for acoustic cues to consonant and vowel identity is that the articulation of a consonant or vowel produces multiple acoustic events and each event can have some value as a cue (e.g., Repp, 1982). Most generally, one cue, or set of cues, can be shown to be quite robust in guiding recognition while others (secondary cues) will be found to be effective only when other cues are altered in such a way as to be neutralized. The effectiveness of secondary cues in guiding recognition when primary cues are neutralized is particularly important to implant patients because primary cues, which are commonly in the frequency domain, may be altered, sometimes dramatically, by the characteristics of signal processors and by patients' damaged, peripheral auditory systems. Thus, for example, cues in the amplitude/time domain may provide information about speech features which normally are signaled by cues in the frequency domain.

VOWELS

For normal-hearing listeners, the principal cues to vowel identity are the frequencies of the first (F1) and second (F2) formants (see Figure 4–1). For some vowels, notably /ɝ/, the location of the third formant (F3) is also important. The range of frequencies covered by the first and second formants of men, women and children is approximately 270 Hz to 3200 Hz (Peterson & Barney, 1952). Secondary cues to vowel identity include vowel duration (House, 1961) and vowel intensity (Lehiste & Peterson, 1959). In English, vowels can differ in duration by more than 100 ms and can differ in intensity by 6 dB.

Table 4–1. *Assignment of consonant features*

Consonant	Voicing	Nasality	Frication	Duration	Place	Envelope
m	2	2	1	1	1	4
n	2	2	1	1	2	4
f	1	1	2	1	1	3
v	2	1	2	1	1	2
s	1	1	2	2	2	3
ʃ	1	1	2	2	3	3
ə	2	1	2	1	1	2
z	2	1	2	2	2	2
p	1	1	1	1	1	1
b	2	1	1	1	1	2
t	1	1	1	1	2	1
d	2	1	1	1	2	2
k	1	1	1	1	4	1
g	2	1	1	1	4	2
dʒ	2	1	2	1	3	2
l	2	1	1	1	2	4

Consider the potential information available to a multichannel implant patient about vowels with extreme formant frequencies in Figure 4–1, for example, /i/, /ɑ/ and /u/. The formant pattern of /i/ is distinctive because of the large separation of F1 and F2 and the high frequency of F2. Both /i/ and /u/ have low frequency F1s—which, most likely, accounts for the observation that the two vowels are often confused—but /u/ also has a low amplitude, low frequency F2. Thus, all of the auditory attributes of /u/ point to a very low frequency sound—one that is very distinct from /i/. Now consider /ɑ/. This vowel has a high F1 and low F2. The nearness of F1 and F2 in frequency space results in an increase in overall sound pressure level—/ɑ/ is 6 dB more intense than /i/ and 2 dB to 6 dB more intense than /u/. Moreover, /ɑ/ may be 80 ms longer than /i/ or /u/. Thus, there are cues in the frequency, time and intensity domains to guide implant patients to the identity of vowels.

ENVELOPE CUES FOR CONSONANT MANNER AND VOICING

If patients extract time/intensity (envelope) information from the signal with fidelity, then certain manner distinctions among consonants should be well marked (see, for example, Summerfield, 1985). As shown in Figure 4–2, in a vowel-consonant-vowel (vCv) environment, stop consonants

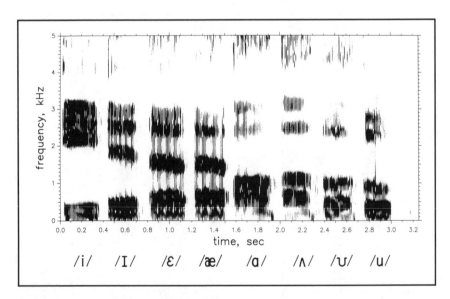

Figure 4–1. Spectrograms of steady-state vowels as spoken by a male informant. The vowels, in order, are those in "beet, bit, bet, bat, bought, but, put, boot."

(e.g., /dt/) are marked by a period of relative silence before signal onset and should not be confused with semivowels, nasals, or fricatives which lack the distinctive silent interval. By similar logic, the stop-initiated fricative, or affricate, in "a chin," should not be confused with the fricatives in "a sin" or "a fin."

Detailed envelope information could also contribute to the distinction between voiced and voiceless stop consonants (Rosen, 1989; Van Tassel, Soli, Kirby, & Widin 1987). As illustrated in Figure 4–2, in a vCv environment, voiced stops (e.g., /d/) are characterized by the presence of a low-amplitude, voicing signal during most of the period of stop closure. Voiceless stops (e.g., /t/) are characterized by a period of silence during

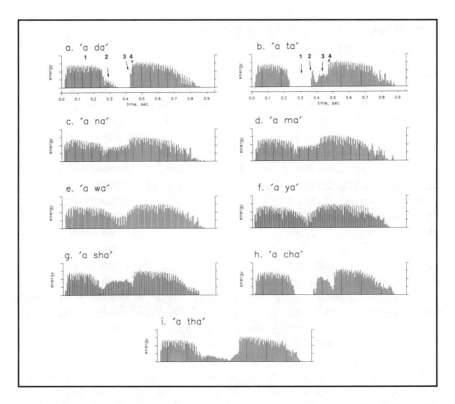

Figure 4–2. Amplitude envelopes for 9 consonants in intervocalic position. In the top left panel, event 1 marks the amplitude of the first vowel, event 2 marks the amplitude of voicing during the closure interval, event 3 marks the amplitude of the stop burst, and event 4 marks the onset of voicing for the consonant-vowel syllable. In the top right panel, event 1 marks the silent closure interval for the voiceless stop, event 2 marks the release burst, event 3 marks aspiration, and event 4 marks the onset of voicing.

closure. In other syllabic environments the voiced-voiceless distinction is marked by other envelope cues. For example, the duration of the interval between the release burst in F2/F3 and the onset of energy in F1, and the presence or absence of aspiration during that interval, signals the voicing contrast in syllable-initial position. Voiced stops are characterized by a short interval of 1–21 ms, and by the absence of aspiration. Voiceless stops are characterized by a longer interval of 40–80 ms and by the presence of aspiration.

As Figure 4–2 suggests, the semivowels /w r l y/ and the nasals /m n/ share a similar, though not identical, amplitude envelope in intervocalic position. Confusions among semivowels and nasals are not uncommon for implant patients with poor word understanding scores.

FREQUENCY AND ENVELOPE CUES FOR CONSONANT PLACE OF ARTICULATION

For stop consonants (/b d g p t k/), cues to place reside in the spectra of the release bursts and onsets and shapes of the formant transitions (Blumstein, Issacs, & Mertus, 1982; Liberman, Delattre, Cooper, & Gerstman, 1954). The stops /d t/ are characterized by energy at 3–4 kHz, /b p/ by energy near 1 kHz and /g k/ by energy between 1–3 kHz. The onset energy for /g k/ varies as a function of the following vowel. The voiced stop /g/ also has a potential cue in the amplitude envelope due to its relatively long voice-onset-time (Kewley-Port, 1983).

For semivowels (/w r l y/), place cues reside, most generally, in the onset frequencies and formant transitions of F2 and F3 (O'Connor, Gerstman, Liberman, Delattre, & Cooper, 1957). The lowest F2 onset belongs to /w/ (approximately 600 Hz.), while the highest belongs to /y/ (approximately 2100 Hz). Confusions between these two semivowels imply a lack of frequency resolution.

For nasal consonants, the cues to place reside in the nasal murmur and in the formant transitions to the vowel. The nasal murmurs for /m n ŋ/ are low in frequency (under 400 Hz) and are similar in frequency (Fujimura, 1962). Both the murmur and formant transitions are useful cues to nasal place of articulation (Repp, 1986).

For fricatives, place cues reside in the spectra of the noises (Heinz & Stevens, 1961), the formant transitions to the accompanying vowel (Harris, 1958) and in the time/amplitude waveform (Behrens & Blumstein, 1988). Most generally, the voiceless fricative /ʃ/ is characterized by a concentration of energy above 1.5 kHz and extending to above 4 kHz; /s/ is characterized by energy above 4.0 kHz; /f/ and /θ/ are both characterized by reasonably flat spectra (at least over the range of frequencies extracted by implant processors) with a small peak at

1.4–2.0 kHz. Envelope cues can aid greatly in sorting the voiceless fricatives into /s ʃ/, on the one hand, and /f θ/, on the other. The noises in "fin" and "thin" can be 15–20 dB less intense than the fricatives in "sin" and "shin" which, in turn, may be 5–10 dB less intense than an accompanying vowel.

WORD RECOGNITION

Acoustic cues and/or phonetic features need to be compared with a stored representation in memory if words are to be recognized. The process, or processes, by which recognition takes place is a matter of debate (see Pisoni & Luce, 1986 for a discussion). Nonetheless, an important concept from this literature is that of an "equivalence class." An equivalence class is a set of words having the same representation. Consider the features even a poor-performing implant patient might extract from the acoustic signal, for example, stress pattern, and broad phonetic categories such as [strong fricative], [high-front-vowel], [nasal], and [stop consonant]. Zue (1985) reports that if the 20,000 words in the Merriam Pocket Dictionary are coded in terms of six broad phonetic features, then the median class size (i.e., the number of words with the same feature representation) is 8 words and over one-third of the words are uniquely represented. In other words, word recognition can take place with some accuracy even when detailed acoustic or phonetic knowledge is absent. This works to the benefit of implant patients who may only be able to achieve a broad phonetic characterization of a signal.

CONNECTED DISCOURSE

Words in sentence context are more intelligible than words in isolation (e.g., Miller, Heise, & Lichten, 1951). The traditional interpretation of this finding has been that "higher level" sources of information, for example, syntax and semantics, interact with "lower level" information about prosody (pitch), rhythm and timing, and narrow the range of possible response alternatives for a listener (see, for example, Pisoni & Luce, 1986). For example, the word "homes" is more likely in the sentence context, "The real estate broker sold three _____ this week" than in the context, " Jim had two large _____." Postlingually deafened implant patients can be expected to have normal "higher level" sources of information about language, and can be expected to extract pitch and timing information with good fidelity. Thus, we may expect that highly predictable words in sentences will be recognized with greater accuracy than isolated words.

FREQUENTLY USED TESTS OF SPEECH RECOGNITION

As noted above, tests of consonant and vowel recognition, tests of isolated word recognition and tests of word recognition in sentences can probe different levels of speech processing. All can contribute to an understanding of patient, or signal processor, performance. Thus, if we are to understand *why* a patient does *what* she or he does, we need a battery of tests.

Most of the problems encountered in developing a test battery for cochlear-implant patients are similar to those encountered in the development of test batteries for other auditory disorders. Should the tests be open or closed set? What is the effect of repeated administration of the same test? Are multiple word lists of equal difficulty needed? Should only one token of a particular item be used, or should multiple tokens be used? Does performance on a test, or on the test battery, predict "real world" performance? Should all materials be recorded, or is there any role for "live voice" presentation of material? Is the material appropriate for patients with different levels of performance? Rosen et al. (1985) and Dowell, Brown, & Mecklenburg (1990) provide extensive discussions of these questions in the context of developing tests for cochlear-implant patients. In Chapter 5 of this text, Tyler discusses some of these issues with special reference to children.

The answer to the last question posed above—Is the material appropriate for patients with different levels of performance ?—has had, perhaps, the greatest influence on the development of a test battery for implant patients. Patients with very low levels of speech-recognition ability can be tested over a period of years with the same "easy" closed-set materials from a single speaker (e.g., four-choice spondee words) and not be limited by a ceiling effect on performance. Materials in audiovisual format may be appropriate for other patients with low levels of sound-only performance. At the other extreme, some patients achieve 100% scores on closed-set tests and on open-set tests with "easy" words. For these patients, open-set materials with "difficult" single-syllable words and with words in "difficult" sentences are necessary to document changes in speech recognition ability.

In response to the need for standardized test materials for implant patients, Owens, Kessler, & Schubert (1981) developed the Minimum Auditory Capabilities (MAC) battery. The MAC battery includes both open- and closed-set materials, assesses the identification of speech and nonspeech signals, and can be used to assess vowel, consonant, isolated word, and word-in-sentence recognition. The battery also includes an assessment of speech-reading. The battery has been found to be useful in documenting changes in speech and nonspeech recognition ability for a wide range of patients and, thus, is widely used by clinicians.

The MAC battery has only one test of audiovisual speech recognition and does not assess speech recognition in noise. Moreover, the audiovisual tests must be administered in person. This produces the unwelcome circumstance of "live voice" and "live face" presentation of material and the probability of changes in patient performance as a function of changes in test administrators. In response to these considerations, Tyler and colleagues at the University of Iowa developed a test battery for cochlear-implant patients (Tyler, Preece, & Lowder, 1983) which has been recorded on laser videodisc (Tyler, Preece, & Tye-Murray, 1986). The battery contains a wide variety of test materials in audio, visual, and audiovisual format. This battery, like the MAC battery, has been shown to be effective in assessing changes in performance for patients with a wide range of speech recognition abilities and is used widely.

SPEECH PERCEPTION WITH SINGLE CHANNEL PROSTHESES

Single-channel prostheses are of interest on several accounts. From the point of view of a patient, single-channel devices are appealing because they should cost less and be easier to maintain than multichannel devices. These considerations will be very important as implant technology becomes available to worldwide markets. Equally important, from the point of view of many patients, is the consideration that all of the electronics can be packaged in a behind-the-ear processor (Hochmair-Desoyer, 1991). In this regard, cochlear-implant patients are like other hearing-impaired patients—the more invisible the device, the better.

From the point of view of clinicians and researchers, single-channel prostheses are of interest on several grounds. One is that they may be the prosthesis of choice for patients with ossified cochleas and in whom only a single, short electrode can be inserted. Indeed, single-channel *extracochlear* prosthesis may the best choice for patients whose cochlea are completely ossified. A second reason for interest in single-channel prostheses is that some single-channel patients perform remarkably well, and we would like to know why. In this regard, the performance of single-channel patients can be used as a baseline against which to measure the performance of patients with mulitichannel devices.

The general absence of open-set speech understanding with the original House, single-channel implant (e.g., Gantz et al., 1988; Tye-Murray & Tyler, 1989) was not surprising given the poor frequency resolution and poor detail in the time/intensity waveform (Edgerton, Doyle, Brimacombe, Danley, & Fretz, 1983). However, a quite different result has been found for patients who use the Vienna single-channel implant. Some patients who use this device have shown remarkably good speech understanding (Hochmair-Desoyer, Hochmair, & Stiglbrunner, 1985). Other patients using single-channel, extracochlear devices have also shown good speech understanding (Tyler, 1988b). To gain an appreciation of why the speech-recognition abilities of these patients are of interest, consider the following.

The most obvious limitation imposed by a single electrode on the encoding of speech is the absence of place coding of frequency. Further, rate, or temporal, encoding of frequency by single fibers is constrained by the neural refractory period—resulting in an upper limit of about 1 kHz on frequency resolution (see Abbas, Chapter 7). Thus, on a single channel, information from the frequency domain should be limited to two critical aspects of speech: vocal pitch, or the fundamental frequency of the voice, and the frequency of the first formant. As noted in the section on acoustic cues, the presence of the fundamental frequency in a signal indicates the presence of voiced sounds. Changes in pitch provide information about sentence prosody. An accurate indication of F1 can provide information about consonant manner and voicing and about vowel identity.

If time/intensity information and the limited frequency information described above were available to a patient, then the voicing status of a consonant might be recognized (e.g., patients could discriminate between the sets /b d g/ and /p t k/), the manner of consonant production might be recognized (e.g., patients could discriminate among the sets /s ʃ θ f/, /b d g p t k/, and /w r l y/) and vowels that differ greatly in F1 frequency might be recognized (e.g., patients could discriminate between /i u/ and /a æ/). For languages in which vowel duration is distinctive, long and short vowels should not be confused. Finally, for tone languages in which pitch plays a phonemic role, at least some distinctions in tones should be distinguished. The data on speech recognition by patients who use the Vienna single-channel implant indicates that some patients can extract most of the information just described.

VOWEL RECOGNITION

Figure 4–3 (left) illustrates the formant frequencies of German vowels used in a recognition experiment. Note the small difference in first-formant frequency for the vowels in the set /i y u/ and for the vowels in the set /e ø o/. In contrast, both /ɛ/ and /ɑ/ have distinctive F1s. Figure 4–3 (right) shows the results of a recognition task from a typical patient (von Wallenberg, Hochmair-Desoyer, & Hochmair, 1990). The recognition data mirror the distinctiveness of the F1 frequencies, that is,/ɛ/ and /ɑ/ are recognized essentially without error, some confusions occur between the sets /i y u/ and /e ø o/, and many confusions occur within the vowel sets. Note that /i/ is identified most often as /u/, indicating the the F2 of /i/ is not used as a cue. Most generally, signals which differ principally in F2 frequency are not well identified (see Hochmair-Desoyer et al., 1985 for summary data on vowel identification; see also Rosen & Ball, 1986; Tyler, Tye-Murray, Moore, & McCabe, 1989b).

The best patients, however, appear to extract more information from the auditory representation of a vowel than information about F1. Consider the performance of the patient in Figure 4–4. Recognition of vowels with similar F1s but different F2s, that is, recognition within the sets /i y u/ and /e ø o/, is well above chance. Either this patient is better able to exploit the small differences in F1 within the vowel sets, or uses other information—signal duration, signal level, or F2—for identification. The results of an experiment with filtered speech suggests the added information comes from frequencies above 900 Hz. As the frequency of a low pass filter in the patients' signal processor was reduced successively from full bandwidth to 900 Hz, and then to 300 Hz, percent correct vowel recognition fell from 78% correct, to 58% correct, and then to 41% correct (Hochmair & Hochmair-Desoyer, 1985). The 20% reduction in percent correct with a reduction in bandwidth from 5000–900 Hz indicates that information from F2 and F3 contributes to vowel recognition. The nature of the manner in which F2/F3 aids in vowel recognition is,

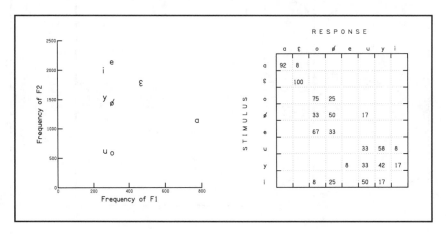

Figure 4–3. The formant frequencies for 8 German vowels are shown in the left panel. The identification of the 8 vowels by a patient who uses the Vienna single-channel implant is shown in the right panel. (Adapted from von Wallenberg et al., 1990.)

however, unclear. It seems unlikely that neurons code the frequency of F2 and F3 by discharge rate. The addition of F2 and F3 to the signal alters the waveform so, perhaps, timbre or loudness differences distinguish some of the vowels.

CONSONANT RECOGNITION

Consonant recognition scores for a select group of six patients who evidence some open-set word understanding are shown in Figure 4–5 (see Hochmair-Desoyer et al., 1985 for summary data). We have suggested that manner and voicing, which have cues in the time/intensity waveform, might be relatively well identified. The results shown in Figure 4–5 confirm that they are. For example, the stop consonants /b d g/ are rarely confused with nasals and semivowels. Note, also, that the voiced stop consonants /b d g/ are rarely confused with the voiceless stops /p t k/.

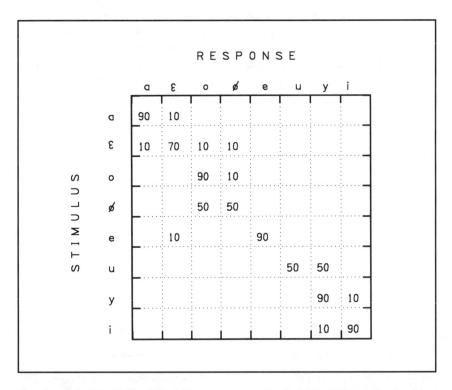

Figure 4–4. Vowel identification by a patient fitted with a Vienna single-channel implant who evidences better than average identification. (Adapted from Hochmair & Hochmair-Desoyer, 1985.)

It is surprising to see that place of articulation is relatively well identified, at least in some manner categories. For example, /l/ and /r/ are not confused and /b p/, /d t/ and /g k/ are not often confused.

Experiments with filtered speech suggest that information above 1 kHz is important for recognition of some place contrasts. For example, for one patient a wide-band condition allowed a score of 56% correct while a low-pass filter at 900 Hz allowed a score of only 33% correct. For consonants, as for vowels, we are left with the puzzle of how information above 1 kHz is encoded by means of a single electrode.

WORD AND SENTENCE RECOGNITION

Gantz et al. (1988) and Rosen and Ball (1986) report no open-set speech intelligibility for four and three patients, respectively. However, as shown in Figure 4–6, Hochmair-Desoyer et al. (1985) and von Wallenberg, Hochmair-Desoyer, & Hochmair (1985) report, for a sample of 22

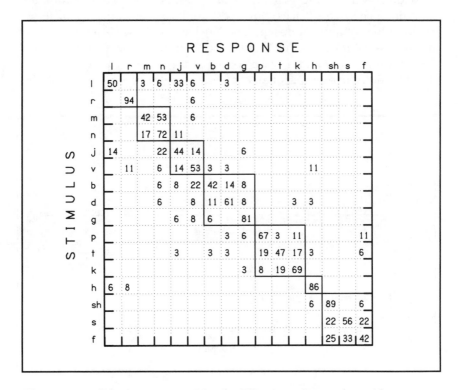

STIMULUS	l	r	m	n	j	v	b	d	g	p	t	k	h	sh	s	f
l	50		3	6	33	6		3								
r		94				6										
m			42	53		6										
n		17	72	11												
j	14				22	44	14			6						
v		11		6	14	53	3	3				11				
b				6	8	22	42	14	8							
d				6		8	11	61	8		3	3				
g				6	8	6		81								
p						3	6			67	3	11			11	
t				3		3	3			19	47	17	3		6	
k							3			8	19	69				
h	6	8											86			
sh													6	89	6	
s														22	56	22
f														25	33	42

Figure 4–5. Consonant recognition by Vienna patients who evidence some sound-alone sentence recognition. The solid lines bracket manner and voicing categories. (Adapted from Hochmair-Desoyer et al., 1985.)

patients, a mean score of 30% for one-syllable word identification (range = 0–90%), and a mean score of 45% for words in sentences (range= 0–98%). Tyler (1988a) tested nine of the better patients with single syllable words and reported a mean score of 37% with a standard deviation of 17%. For words in sentences the mean score was 54% with a standard deviation of 28%. As we will see in the following sections, these scores from "better" patients are quite comparable with the scores from patients who use multichannel devices.

MULTICHANNEL DEVICES

In this section, we describe the speech recognition abilities of patients fitted with two commercially available prostheses, the Nucleus device (Clark et al., 1981) and the Ineraid device (Eddington, 1980), and one research prosthesis, the CIS device from Research Triangle Institute (see Wilson, Chapter 2). Both the Nucleus device and the Ineraid device are in widespread use and provide about the same level of speech understanding. The two devices, however, are based on radically different philosophies of implant design. The Nucleus processor is an example of a "speech-feature extracting" signal processor (the frequencies of F1 and F2/F3 are tracked) and a place coding strategy for frequency analysis. The Ineraid is an example of an analogue signal processor and a rate *and*

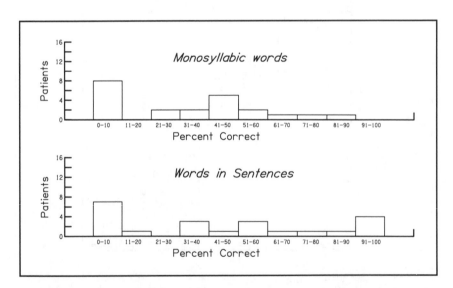

Figure 4–6. Distribution of scores for monosyllabic word recognition and the recognition of words in sentences for patients who use the Vienna implant. (Adapted from Hochmair-Desoyer et al., 1985 and von Wallenberg et al., 1985.)

place coding strategy for frequency analysis. The Nucleus device uses a 22-electrode array and stimulates the electrodes in a nonsimultaneous manner. Signals are transmitted from the signal processor to the electrodes via a receiver implanted in the temporal bone. In contrast, the Ineraid device uses only four electrodes and stimulates the electrodes simultaneously. Signals are transmitted from the processor to the electrodes via a percutaneous carbon pedestal implanted in the temporal bone. The CIS processor is presently a nonwearable, laboratory device which holds promise for improving the speech recognition abilities of patients currently fitted with other devices (e.g., the Ineraid). This processor digitizes analogue signals, generates very brief pulses, and outputs the pulses to multiple channels in a nonsimultaneous fashion. Current interaction among channels is minimized by nonsimultaneous stimulation of electrodes and by a stimulation order which alternates between apical and basal electrodes. The increase in the number of channels and the reduction in channel interaction results in better transmission of both frequency and time/amplitude information when compared to the Ineraid.

NUCLEUS DEVICES

The Nucleus device has gone through a number of improvements since its debut. The original configuration mapped the frequency of a combination of F2 and F3 along the whole electrode array (Tong, Clark, Seligman, and Patrick, 1980). Energy in the F2/F3 region was chosen as the mapping variable because place of articulation is signaled, most generally, by the frequencies of F2 and F3. F0 was, and continues to be, mapped by pulse rate at each electrode site. A second configuration (introduced in 1985) mapped F1 with five apical electrodes and mapped F2 with the remaining electrodes (see Blamey, Dowell, Brown, Clark, & Seligman, 1987). A third revision (introduced in 1989) added to the 1985 version a mapping of three relatively high frequency bands of energy to three electrodes in the base (see Skinner et al., 1991). And, in a fourth version, the device assesses the energy in 16 band-pass filters and stimulates electrodes according to the 6 channels which have the highest root mean square (RMS) energy (McKay, McDermott, Vandali, & Clark, 1991).

The evolution of the Nucleus device illustrates in an elegant fashion the improvement in coding capacity of signal processors, changes in thought about the perceptual capabilities of implant patients and an appreciation of the information necessary to code not only speech but also environmental sounds. The first processor—the F0/F2 processor—may be seen as an example of the "keep it simple" approach to implants. The design of the most recent processor, the spectral maxima processor, is consistent with the view that patients can make use of more than a few pieces of information and that relatively rich descriptions of auditory spectra are necessary if very high levels of *both* speech and non-speech recognition are to be achieved.

F0/F2 Versus F0/F1/F2

We should expect that recognition scores for consonants, vowels and words would increase when F1 frequency and energy are added to the information about F2/F3. Tye-Murray, Lowder, & Tyler (1990) report a 22% increase in NU-6 word recognition (from 29% correct to 51% correct) and a 33% increase in word recognition in sentence context (from 31% to 64% correct) (see also Dowell et al., 1987 and Dowell, Seligman, Blamey, & Clark, 1990). The increase in word recognition stems from improved recognition of both consonants and vowels. Blamey et al. (1987) reported that two patients, who were tested with both coding strategies, increased vowel recognition scores by 12–25% (in the latter case from 69–94% correct) and increased consonant recognition scores by 18–20% (in the later case from 53–73% correct). In contrast, Tye-Murray et al. (1990) reported no significant increase for hearing-alone consonant recognition for five patients tested with both strategies. However, Tye-Murray et al. (1990) did find a significant improvement in vision-plus-hearing conditions for the F0/F1/F2 strategy when compared to the F0/F2 strategy. In both Blamey et al. (1987) and Tye-Murray et al. (1990), feature analyses indicated increased scores for voicing and amplitude envelope. The increase in accuracy for the identification of voicing is reasonable given the addition of the voice-onset-time cue, that is, the timing of energy onset in F2 and F1. The addition of F1 energy would lead also to a better indication in the waveform of the consonant amplitude envelope.

Vowel Recognition

Figure 4–7 shows the confusion matrix for a nine vowel stimulus set for a small number of patients fitted with the F0/F1/F2 processor (Skinner et al., 1991). Overall accuracy was 62%. Note, by reference to Figure 4–1, that the error responses tended to be the vowels with the most similar F1 and F2/F3 frequencies. This is, of course, as it should be if (a) the processor accurately extracts F1 and F2/F3, (b) if there are a sufficient number of electrodes to discretely map F1 and F2/F3 along the cochlea, and (c) if the electrodes produce pitch sensations that are tonotopically organized. For other data on vowel recognition see Blamey and Clark, 1990; Tyler et al., 1989b; Tyler, Tye-Murray, & Otto, 1989).

Consonant Recognition

Figure 4–8 shows the confusion matrix for a 13 consonant test set (/iCi/) for 10 of the better performing patients fitted with the F0/F1/F2 processor (Tyler & Moore, in press). Manner and voicing are relatively well recognized. Error responses for voiced sounds are almost always another voiced sound. As we would expect, error rates are highest for place of articulation and vary somewhat with manner.

Word Recognition Scores with the F0/F1/F2 Processor

Dowell et al. (1987) report mean scores of 26% for spondee recognition, 35% for CID sentence recognition and 12% for monosyllabic word recognition for a sample of 9 patients. Similar monosyllabic word recognition scores were reported by Gantz et al. (1988) and Tye-Murray & Tyler (1989) for small samples. For a sample of "better" performing patients, Tyler et al. (1989a) report word scores of 11% correct

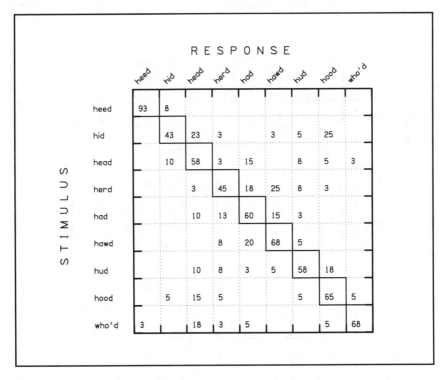

Figure 4–7. Vowel recognition by patients who use the FO/F1/F2 version of the Nucleus implant. (Adapted from Skinner et al., 1991.)

(with a range of 3–20%) and sentence scores of 30% correct (with a range of 18–51%).

The distribution of NU-6 and CID sentence scores for a relatively large sample of patients in the United States (n = 100) who had used their processors for at least a year are shown in Figure 4–9 (data provided by J. Brimacombe). The range of NU-6 scores was 0–60% correct with a mean of 12% correct. The range of CID sentence scores was 0–98% correct with a mean of 38% correct. Note that the mean scores for this large sample are encouragingly similar to the mean scores for the smaller samples cited in the previous paragraph.

F0/F1/F2 Versus Multipeak Processor

The "multipeak" processor adds coding of energy in three bands—2.0–2.8 kHz, 2.8–4.0 kHz and 4.0–6.0 kHz—to the coding of F1 and F2/F3. Energy in the three bands is directed to three basal electrodes

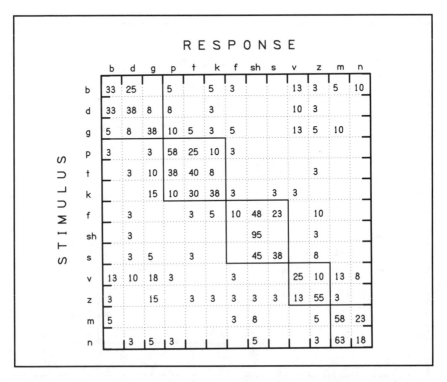

Figure 4–8. Consonant recognition by patients who use the F0/F1/F2 version of the Nucleus implant. (Adapted from Tyler & Moore, in press.)

with the obvious tonotopic relation to the bands. With this coding scheme we might expect that the spectra of stop consonant bursts and of fricatives would be better resolved than in the F0/F1/F2 coding scheme. There is little reason to suspect that vowel recognition would improve.

Skinner et al. (1991) report no difference in percent correct for either vowels or consonants for patients tested with both the F0/F1/F2 and "multipeak" processor. However, the multipeak processor allowed significantly better monosyllabic word recognition (NU-6) scores: 29% correct versus 14% correct. It appears that the vowel and consonant tests were not sufficiently sensitive to detect the improved resolution of some segmental features.

Spectral Maxima Processor

As noted above, this processor passes a speech signal through a 16-channel filter bank and then activates electrodes in accordance with the 6 channels that have the most energy. This scheme should provide better

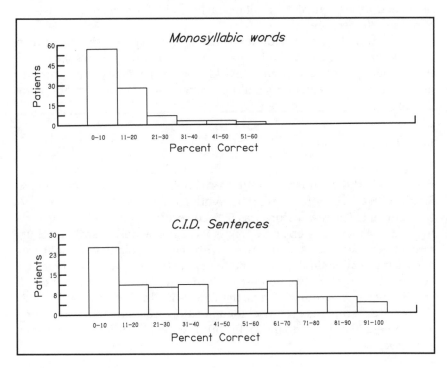

Figure 4–9. Distribution of scores for monosyllabic word recognition and the recognition of words in the CID sentences by 100 patients who use the F0/F1/F2 version of the Nucleus implant.

resolution of the amplitude envelope of a signal and should provide a better indication of the distribution of energy as a function of frequency. Accordingly, McKay et al. (1991) report better performance for two patients with the spectral maxima processor than with the F0/F1/F2 processor. In the test context of a consonant-vowel-consonant word list, one patient increased word, vowel, and consonant scores from 9–21% correct, from 37–49% correct and from 23–43% correct, respectively. Another patient's scores changed from 1–16% words correct, from 32–51% vowels correct, and from 16–39% consonants correct.

INERAID DEVICE

Signal processing by the Ineraid device is relatively simple. The energy in four bandpass filters is detected and current proportional to that energy is delivered to four monopolar electrodes (Eddington, 1980). The center frequencies for the filters are at .5, 1, 2, and 3.4 kHz. In contrast to the Nucleus device, the Ineraid provides analog stimulation, not pulsatile, and directs current simultaneously to the four electrodes instead of nonsimultaneously.

The Ineraid should provide information about speech similar to that of the Vienna single-channel device and should add some resolution of the frequency spectrum from 1 to 4 kHz. Most generally, then, resolution of place of articulation should be better with this device than with the single-channel device.

Vowel Recognition

Vowel recognition for a sample of patients with good word-understanding scores is shown in Figure 4–10 (Dorman, Dankowski, McCandless, & Smith, 1989a). The stimuli were 12 synthetic vowels in /b/-vowel-/t/ environment. The mean score was 60% correct (range = 49–79% correct). In most instances, the error responses were not widely distributed but, rather, were the one or two vowels with the most similar formant frequencies. Recall a similar outcome for patients fitted with the Nucleus F0/F1/F2 processor. The poorest performance was for vowels with F1 and F2 in close proximity, that is, the vowels in "but, bought, and bout." For other experiments on vowel identification see Dorman, Dankowski, McCandless, Parkin, and Smith, (1991a); Tyler et al. (1989b), and Tyler et al. (1989c).

Coding Formant-Frequency with a Small Number of Electrodes

The best Ineraid patients achieved scores of 80% correct on the difficult (12 synthetic vowels) test of vowel identification used by Dorman et al.

(1989a) and have achieved scores of 100% correct on smaller (8 vowels), naturally produced vowel sets (Wilson et al., 1990). These results imply better frequency resolution than we might have expected given only four channels of stimulation. The mechanism responsible for frequency resolution is not well understood. One possibility, in terms of coding F1, is that frequency is coded by neurons firing to the period of F1. Another, more likely, possibility is that the distribution of energy among channels codes frequency. On this view, changes in the balance of channel energy provide continuously changing frequency percepts. To see how this might occur, consider the signal levels in channels 1 and 2 of the Ineraid when a low frequency F1 is presented. The root mean square (RMS) energy in channel 1 will be high and the RMS energy in channel 2 will be low. As F1 frequency increases, the energy in channel 1 will stay the same, or decrease slightly, but the energy in channel 2 will increase. Indeed, as F1 moves up in frequency the balance of energy in channels 1 and 2 will change continuously and tip toward channel 2. **If changes in**

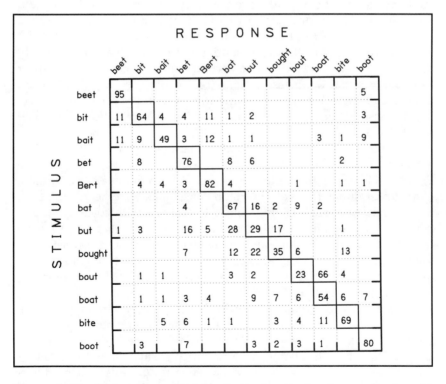

STIMULUS \ RESPONSE	beet	bit	bait	bet	Bert	bat	but	bought	bout	boat	bite	boot
beet	95											5
bit	11	64	4	4	11	1	2					3
bait	11	9	49	3	12	1	1			3	1	9
bet		8		76		8	6			2		
Bert		4	4	3	82	4		1			1	1
bat				4		67	16	2	9	2		
but	1	3		16	5	28	29	17			1	
bought				7		12	22	35	6		13	
bout		1	1			3	2		23	66	4	
boat		1	1	3	4		9	7	6	54	6	7
bite			5	6	1	1		3	4	11	69	
boot		3		7			3	2	3	1		80

Figure 4–10. Vowel recognition by "better" patients who use the Ineraid implant. (Reprinted from Dorman et al., 1989a.)

the balance of energy between channel 1 and channel 2 produce continuous changes in pitch, then a mechanism exists for coding F1. Data from Townshend, Cotter, Compernolle, and White (1987) confirm the existence of such a mechanism. Townshend and colleagues report, for two patients, that when two electrodes are stimulated simultaneously, and the balance of current is varied on the two electrodes, then pitch varies from lower to higher as current balance is tipped toward the more basal electrode (see also Shannon, Chapter 8).

Consonant Recognition

Consonant recognition for seven patients with average scores are shown in Figure 4–11, left panel (Dorman et al., 1990c). Manner and voicing were well recognized. Manner errors for nasals were other voiced signals. The identification of place varied with manner. Neither stop nor nasal place of articulation was well identified. The intense fricative "sh" was well identified as was the affricate "ch."

Contrast the errors made by the patients just described with the errors made by three patients with excellent scores (Figure 4–11, top panel). Recognition of stop consonant place of articulation was much improved as was discrimination between the intense fricatives "s" and "sh." Recognition of nasal place and semivowel place remained relatively poor. The increased identification accuracy for stop consonants and for /s/ suggests that the better patients received more information from middle and high frequencies than patients with poorer performance. Similar observations have been made by Tye-Murray and Tyler (1989) and Tyler (1990).

It is instructive to compare the performance of the patients described above with that of a patient with very poor consonant recognition (see Figure 4–11, right panel). Envelope cues seem to dominate recognition. Note, for example, that voiceless stop consonants were heard predominately as the affricate "ch"—a phone which shares with voiceless stops a period of silence in the amplitude envelope. Note also that /w l y/ were heard as /m/ or /n/ which are signals that share the characteristic of a high-amplitude voiced signal in intervocalic position. Note, finally, that the two intense fricatives "s" and "sh" were not confused with signals of lower signal amplitude.

For patients with average to excellent speech understanding, errors in the recognition of voicing were rare. To further explore perception of the voicing contrast, Dorman et al. (1991a) created synthetic versions of "ga" and "ka," in which the voice-onset-time varied in small steps, for classification by Ineraid patients. At issue was whether the patients evidenced normal resolution of the temporal cues which underlie the identification of

voicing. Four of the six patients exhibited normal classification of the stimuli, that is, normal phonetic boundaries and a normal slope to the identification function (see also Dorman, Hannley, McCandless, & Smith, 1988).

Word and Sentence Recognition

The distribution of scores for 50 patients on tests of spondee recognition,
monosyllabic word recognition and the recognition of words in sentences

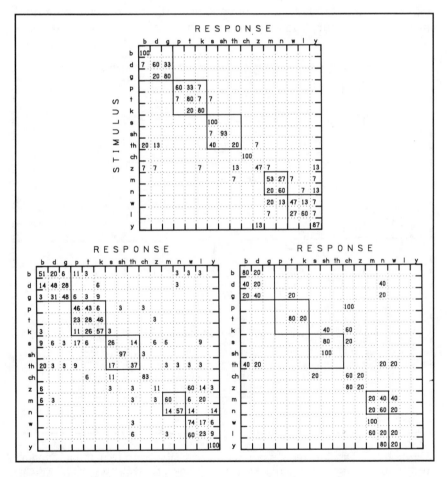

Figure 4–11. Consonant identification by patients who use the Ineraid implant.
The performance of patients with excellent scores are shown in the top panel, the
performance of patients with average scores are shown in the left panel, and the
performance of a patient with poor performance is shown in the right panel.
(Adapted from Dorman et al., 1990c.)

are shown in Figure 4–12 (Dorman, Hannley, Dankowski, Smith, & McCandless, 1989b). For monosyllabic words, the median score was 14% correct with a range of 0–60% correct. For spondee words, the median score was 44% correct with a range of 0–100% correct. For the CID sentences, the median score was 45% correct with a range of 0–100% correct.

Perhaps the most surprising aspect of the Ineraid device has been its success in providing speech understanding when measured against the performance of patients fitted with the F0/F1/F2 version of the Nucleus processor. It would be reasonable to suppose that the more channels the better, and that bipolar, nonsimultaneous, pulsatile stimulation would provide more accurate information than monopolar, simultaneous, ana-

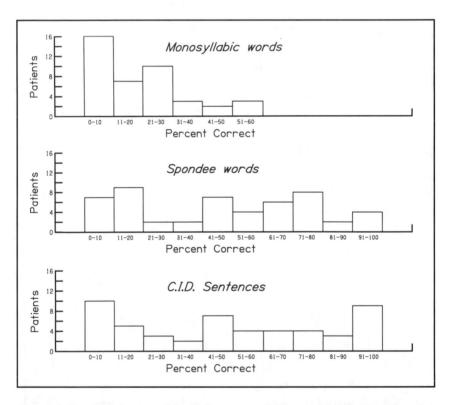

Figure 4–12. Distribution of scores for monosyllabic word recognition, spondee recognition and the recognition of words in the CID sentences by 50 patients who use the Ineraid implant. (Reprinted from Dorman et al., 1989b. Word recognition by 50 patients fitted with the Symbion multichannel cochlear implant. *Ear and Hearing, 10,* 44–49, with permission.)

logue stimulation. However, Gantz et al. (1988) and Tye-Murray & Tyler (1989) report no difference in word scores for a randomized sample of patients fitted with the Ineraid and the Nucleus processors. A similar conclusion can be drawn from a comparison of the scores for the large samples of Nucleus and Ineraid patients shown in Figures 4–9 and 4–12. Tyler et al. (1989a) report no difference in word and phoneme recognition scores for groups of the best performing Ineraid and Nucleus patients.

THE RESEARCH TRIANGLE INSTITUTE DEVICE

The "supersampler" is a research device under development at Research Triangle Institute under the auspices of the Neural Prosthetics Program of the National Institute of Health (Wilson et al., 1990; Wilson, Lawson, and Finnley, 1991). The hallmarks of the "continuous interleaved sampling (CIS)" processor are (a) the use of brief, nonsimultaneous pulses for stimulation, (b) a rapid rate of stimulation, and (c) stimulation of at least six electrodes. Access to six electrodes, in contrast to the four used by the Ineraid, increases the probability of frequency resolution by means of cochlear place of stimulation. The use of brief, nonsimultaneous pulses reduces current spread in the cochlea and thus might improve the discriminability of multiple sites of stimulation. The use of a rapid rate of stimulation allows the amplitude waveform of signals to be accurately represented.

The CIS strategy has been tested extensively only with patients who use the Ineraid prosthesis. The percutaneous pedestal of the Ineraid (and the absence of implanted electronics) allows easy access to the implanted electrodes. The speech-recognition scores reported below, and shown in Figure 4–13, were obtained for seven patients who had less than 1 hour experience with the processor. For comparison, the patients' performance with their Ineraid processors is also shown. Performance with the Ineraid processor is coded by the initials CA (compressed analogue processor).

Vowel Recognition

The stimuli were eight vowels in /h/-vowel-/d/ environment. The patients averaged 95% correct with the compressed analogue processor. The patients averaged 93% correct with the CIS processor. This outcome illustrates a problem many in the field of cochlear implants thought they might never face—levels of performance so high, on stimulus sets of reasonable size, that differences between processors could not be assessed.

Consonant Recognition

The stimuli were 16 consonants in an /a/-consonant-/a/ environment. The patients averaged 66% correct with the compressed analogue processor. The patients averaged 82% correct with the CIS processor. Performance was significantly better with the CIS processor. Feature analyses indicated that the features of nasality, frication, place, and envelope were transmitted better by the CIS processor. The improvement in transmission this set of features suggests that both frequency resolution and resolution of envelope cues is enhanced by the CIS strategy.

Word and Sentence Recognition

With the CIS strategy, scores improved by 18% for spondee words (from 76–94%), improved by 18% for words from the NU-6 list (from 43–61%), and improved by 38% for words from the Speech Perception in Noise (SPIN) test (50–88%) (Wilson et al., 1991). Two patients achieved NU-6 scores of 80% correct. This score is within the range of scores obtained by individuals with mild-to-moderate, sensorineural hearing impairment (Bess & Townsend, 1977).

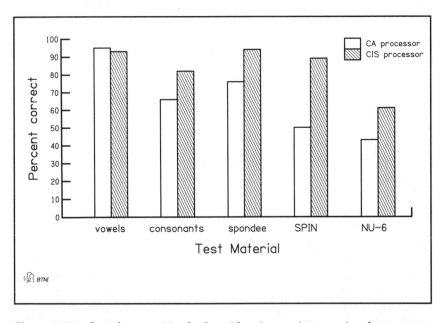

Figure 4–13. Speech recognition by Ineraid patients using two signal processors: the Ineraid processor (CA) and the CIS processor from Research Triangle Institute.

A version of the CIS strategy has been implemented in the Clarion prosthesis manufactured by MiniMed Technologies. Patients were first implanted with this device in 1991. No data are available on patient performance. It is expected that the CIS strategy will be implemented in future revisions of the Ineraid prosthesis.

TELEPHONE USE

Reports of telephone use by implant patients have been controversial. The controversy stems from a confusion between telephone use qua telephone use and telephone use as a measure of speech understanding. Consider the situation in which the implantee initiates a telephone call. In this circumstance she or he can constrain the conversation in a such a manner that only a small number of words are possible responses. Thus, a patient would not have to have a large vocabulary of understandable words to use the telephone successfully—so telephone use is not a good measure of speech understanding. But that is not to imply that a telephone can not be used functionally by implantees. It most certainly can. In fact, in light of the speech understanding skills of the best performing patients, we should expect that a small number of patients could use the telephone for more than brief, highly constrained interactions.

To obtain an objective indication of telephone use among patients, Dorman, Dove, Parkin, Zacharchuk, & Dankowski (1991b) sent a questionnaire on telephone use to a large number of Ineraid patients. Since Nucleus patients have been found to have, on average, the same scores as Ineraid patients on tests of speech identification (Gantz et al., 1988; Tye-Murray & Tyler, 1989), the incidence of telephone use should be similar (see, for example, Brimacombe quoted in Cohen, Waltzman, & Shapiro, 1989). The results of the survey indicated that about half of the sample initiated calls and two thirds answered the telephone. Of the 66% who answered the telephone, 48% indicated that they could understand a familiar caller and familiar topic most of the time. Thus, about one third of the sample claimed to understand a familiar speaker and a familiar topic most, not all, of the time. As the speaker and message uncertainty increased, the number of patients who claimed to understand a caller decreased to a lower limit of only 5% who claimed to understand an unfamiliar caller and an unfamiliar topic.

AUDIOVISUAL SPEECH RECOGNITION

Most speech understanding occurs in the context of being able to see and hear a speaker. If we wish to assess the ability of implant patients to understand speech in realistic communication settings, then we should include tests of audiovisual speech perception.

Before we describe the results for implant patients on tests of audiovisual speech recognition, we should consider the interaction of visual and auditory information in speech recognition. To gain an appreciation of the power of combined auditory and visual information, consider that seeing the face of a talker can be equivalent to improving the signal-to-noise ratio by 15 dB (Sumby & Pollack, 1954). For normal-hearing individuals listening in a noise background, at – 9 dB signal-to-noise ratio only 10% of words in sentences are reported. With a 15 dB improvement in signal-noise-ratio, intelligibility is 90%. Thus, as Summerfield (1987) has noted, seeing the face of a speaker can transform performance from a failure to understand to one of complete understanding.

Summerfield (1987) points out that when the auditory signal is degraded, as it is in the case of the signal provided by cochlear implants, then visual information can both supplement and complement auditory information. In one role, visual information can direct a listeners attention to the speech signal rather than background noise. Seeing *who* the speaker is, that is, whether the speaker is male or female, can direct the listener to a likely set of harmonics in the incoming signal. Seeing *when* the speaker moves his or her articulators can alert the listener to which part of the incoming acoustic information is related to speech.

In a second role, visual information can add to impoverished auditory information about both vowels and consonants. The information in the optical signal which allows "lipreading" of vowels and consonants is reasonably well documented (for a recent discussion see Summerfield, 1985). For consonants, visual information provides a great deal of information about place of articulation, which is the feature of the speech signal that is transmitted the least well by cochlear implants. For vowels, the visabilty of the teeth, indicating a high front vowel, lip rounding, and jaw opening can assist in recognition.

The results of a consonant identification test in a vision-alone condition and in a vision-plus-implant condition for patients using the Nucleus F0/F1/F2 processor are shown in Figure 4–14 (Tye-Murray et al., 1990). Note that in the vision-alone condition, place of articulation is recognized the best. Adding the signal provided by the implant did not add significantly to the information about place of articulation available to the patient. However, transmission of the other speech features was greatly improved. As a consequence, the mean score increased from 39% correct for the vision-alone condition to 73% for the vision-plus-audition condition.

The results of a word identification task in sentence context for patients who use the Ineraid are shown in Figure 4–15 (redrawn from Gantz et al., 1988). The lipreading scores varied from 0–90% correct with a mean score of 55% correct. In the implant-alone condition the range of scores was 0–95% correct with a mean score of 33% correct. In the combined implant-plus-vision condition the mean score was 91% correct. Note, in particular, the "superadditivity" of auditory and visual information for patients 5, 6, and 10. For these patients the scores for the vision-plus-implant condition are greater than a simple addition of the scores for the vision-alone and implant-alone conditions (see Massaro, 1987, and Summerfield, 1987 for models of how visual and auditory information are combined in phonetic perception). "Superadditivity" is common in studies of combined auditory and visual perception of speech and can work to the great advantage of implant patients.

RECOGNITION OF NONSPEECH ACOUSTIC EVENTS

ENVIRONMENTAL SOUND RECOGNITION

The detection and recognition of environmental sounds is an extremely important aspect of using a cochlear implant. When Ineraid patients

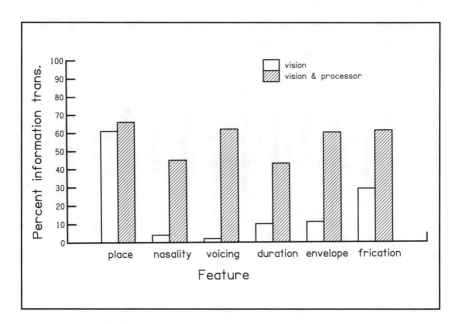

Figure 4–14. Feature transmission for Nucleus patients in a vision-alone condition and in a vision-plus-processor condition. (Adapted from Tye-Murray et al., 1990.)

were asked to partition their satisfaction with the device into portions appropriate to understanding speech, recognizing environmental sounds and listening to music, the patients as a group allotted almost as much satisfaction to recognizing environmental sounds as they allotted to understanding speech (Dorman, unpublished; also see Tyler & Kelsay, 1990).

The importance of nonspeech recognition may be difficult to appreciate for those of us who have heard all our lives. Consider the following diary entry.

[On the seventh day of implant use] I was startled to realize that I recognized someone was coming down a corridor at a 90 degree angle to the one I was walking in, and I had recognized what it was before I turned the corner. Only if you have had as many collisions and near misses as I have had at corridor corners can you have any appreciation for this event !

And, on a more profound topic:

I will never be able to overlook the total simplicity, but incredible value, of being able to hear the friendly "pat on the back" of human hands as people greet and hug one another.

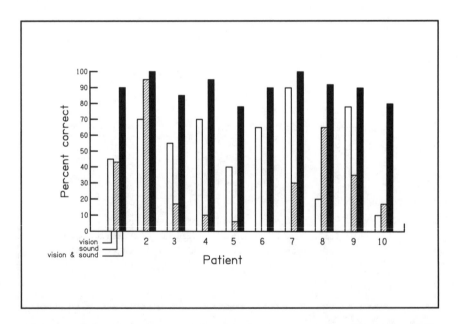

Figure 4–15. Percent correct word recognition for Ineraid patients in vision-alone, implant-alone, and in implant-plus-vision conditions. (Adapted from Gantz et al., 1988.)

On a test of environmental sound recognition, Gantz et al. (1988) report scores of 54% correct for Ineraid patients, 43% correct for Nucleus patients and 38% correct for patients with the Vienna device. Tyler et al. (1989a) assessed environmental sound recognition for samples of the better patients who used the three devices and reported scores of 83% correct for Ineraid patients, 58% correct for Nucleus patients (F0/F1/F2 processor) and 41% correct for Vienna, single-channel patients.

Ineraid patients appear to be significantly better at nonspeech recognition than patients fitted with other devices. The improvement in scores relative to single-channel devices is due, no doubt, to increased information about the frequency composition of the signals. The poorer group mean score for patients who use the F0/F1/F2 processor is due, one supposes, to the specificity of the processor for extracting information about speech. We should expect that the spectral maxima processor, described above, will provide a large increase in scores for nonspeech recognition relative to scores obtained with the F0/F1/F2 processor.

MUSIC APPRECIATION

Gfeller and Lansing (1991) indicate that Ineraid patients report a greater variety of musical instruments to sound pleasant than Nucleus patients. A survey of Ineraid patients revealed that 47% listened to music more than occasionally, 22% listened occasionally and 31% did not listen at all (McCandless, unpublished). In an objective test of musical ability with 16 patients, 91% were able to identify which third of the keyboard was being played. However, most were unable to determine the direction of a scale. The patients were also tested on open- and closed-set identification of five familiar melodies and five musical instruments (voice, violin, piano, flute, and horn). The majority were unable to recognize any of the melodies in an open-set format (see also Gfeller & Lansing, 1991). One patient, however, identified three of the five melodies. In closed-set format, 9 of the 16 patients were able to identify three of the five melodies. In the test of musical instrument identification, the majority of patients correctly identified only one or two instruments. However, in closed-set format, 75% of the patients were able to identify four or five of the instruments (Dorman, Basham, McCandless and Dove, 1991c; McCandless, unpublished).

As noted above, a small number of patients listen to music more than occasionally. The following was written by an individual who was a piano instructor before she lost her hearing and who, today, continues to teach with the aid of her implant.

> I hear the keyboard in complete form, but a few notes have a nuance all their own. The G, A, and B above middle C are softer than notes below

middle C. But the volume returns for notes above these. Indeed, G, A, and B in the second and third octaves above middle C are the loudest notes on the keyboard. My students discovered this quickly. If I point a finger at one of them for not practicing, they sometimes jokingly reach up and sharply strike one of these notes to give me a good jolt. Some instruments have taken on a new sound quality. For instance, brass instruments, when played loudly, can produce a "splatter" of tone. However, the sound of horns improves after the initial attack and becomes much more melodious as a piece continues. Most string and reed instruments sound pure at all volume levels. The violin, viola, and flute are particularly pleasant through the implant. Small group recitals are more enjoyable than large group concerts. A full band or orchestra seems to produce more sound than can be processed. I constantly try to piece it together, so sometimes a band concert can wear me out.

THE REACQUISITION OF WORD AND SOUND RECOGNITION

The reacquisition of speech recognition takes time and the rate of reacquisition varies across patients. Consider the following descriptions of speech recognition on the first day of implant use.

Patient 1: My first impressions with the processor were really very disappointing after the ease with which we seemed to go through the tonal check with the individual electrodes. The [speech] sounds were totally indistinguishable.

Patient 2: On the first test following hookup, I got 55% correct on the [spondee] word test.

The rate at which reacquisition takes place is of interest on two broad accounts. On one account, information about the time course of reacquisition is essential for proper counseling of patients about likely levels of performance at different times following implantation. This information is necessary also to plan and evaluate rehabilitation strategies (see Tye-Murray, Chapter 3).

On another account, information about the time course of reacquisition can provide a window on the fidelity of electrically evoked auditory representations of speech and on the plasticity of central neural mechanisms responsible for word recognition. The most likely outcome, given that patients undoubtedly differ in the magnitude of damage to their peripheral auditory system, and may differ in rate of accommodation to a distorted representation of speech, is that the rate of reacquisition of word recognition will be relatively slow and will vary among patients. However, two other outcomes would be of particular interest. If all patients require a long period, perhaps a year or more, to achieve a high level of word recognition, then we might suppose that the auditory representation of speech is always greatly degraded and that a great deal of accommodation by central mechanisms is necessary for word recognition. Consider now the possibility that patients can identify words soon after fitting with the prosthesis, for example, within a month. This outcome would suggest that it is possible to provide a nontrivial auditory representation of speech and that a great deal of central accommodation is not always necessary for word recognition.

WORD RECOGNITION

The results from several studies indicate that, on average, the largest gains in word intelligibility come within the first nine months of implant use (e.g., Dorman, Dankowski, McCandless, Parkin, and Smith, 1990a; Spivak & Waltzman, 1990; Tye-Murray, Tyler, Woodworth, & Gantz, in press). Representative data from Dorman et al. (1990a) are shown in Table 4–2. Three aspects of this data set are of particular interest. First, note that at 1 month performance ranges from nil to extraordinarily good. Thus, an extremely long period of accommodation to the device is not a necessary condition for a relatively high level of word recognition. Second, note that some patients with high asymptotic scores evidenced high scores at 1 month, while others gradually improved over a 2-year period. Thus, "star" patients do not always present as "star" patients early in the postsurgery period. Third, note that some patients make relatively large gains in word recognition after 1 year of implant use. This outcome is of particular interest because it indicates that central mechanisms of signal decoding can continue to improve over a period of years. The practical significance of this outcome is that patients can be advised that a plateau, or a very small gain over a period of 6 months to 1 year, need not herald asymptotic performance in word recognition.

One fascinating aspect of the reacquisition of word recognition is an all-too-brief "window in time" during which speech can be startlingly clear. Consider the following description penned by a patient who had used his Ineraid for eight months.

> I was with my wife, mother, and sister in a doctor's office. I was sitting next to my mother on one side of the waiting room. My wife and sister were sitting next to a wall at the end of the room. I usually can't understand in such a situation, as I have to speechread to understand. I was reading a book when at once it dawned on me that I had heard and understood what my mother had said to my wife. It was just as clear as anything! I quit reading and just quietly sat there listening without looking at them. I clearly understood their conversation for 2 or 3 minutes. I heard

the nurse call them to go to see the doctor. When they came back, we immediately left ... **and the ability to hear that way [i.e., understand speech by hearing alone] had left me.**

Our understanding of this phenomenon is best described in the last sentence of the diary entry just cited: "There is a lot they still don't understand about how these implants work."

FEATURE RECOGNITION

Any increase in isolated word recognition must be based on increased recognition of the constituent parts of words—consonants and vowels. Tye-Murray et al. (1992) report that most features of consonants—voicing, place, nasality, frication, envelope and duration—are better received at 9 months than at 1 month. Patients who use the Ineraid device show

Table 4–2. *Percent correct spondee recognition as a function of time since device activation*

	Months postfitting			
Patient	1	6–9	12–15	22–28
1	0	4	4	0
2	0	16	16	32
3	0	28	24	52
4	2	16	16	18
5	2	10	32	28
6	4	16	32	16
7	4	44	50	56
8	6	22	20	64
9	8	24	24	56
10	8	40	52	76
11	10	22	12	28
12	10	36	30	64
13	10	72	58	88
14	12	42	58	38
15	16	8	48	48
16	24	48	44	32
17	24	56	68	82
18	28	52	64	84
19	30	52	60	52
20	32	72	72	64
21	32	52	70	86
22	36	84	84	96
23	44	76	76	78
24	80	100	100	100
25	84	72	100	92

the largest improvement for the frication feature. Patients who use the Nucleus device show the largest improvement for the voicing feature. Only Ineraid patients evidenced gains in feature recognition between 9 and 18 months and only for the features of frication and duration, both of which code the presence of fricative energy.

ENVIRONMENTAL SOUND RECOGNITION

During the first days of implant use many patients comment on the variety of environmental sounds they hear and on the change in the nature of the sounds over a short period of time. This was recorded by one patient in the following manner.

> [While in my motel room on the second night of implant use] the slow closing of the room door changed from a all-the-same noise to a faint "click-thump" of the latch hitting the strike plate and the door hitting the frame. It seemed very faint [and] it startled me to recognize it.

The recognition of sounds commonly requires activity on the part of the patient. Consider the following report.

> The door closing sound is well-set now. When I left the men's room and walked down the hall a little way and turned the corner, I heard the very distinctive "ka-thump"! It was kind of exciting! And so was the urinal! Yesterday I heard only the handle "clicking" when I flushed it— today I heard the "whoosh" sound before the water drained down inside. After the water was through flowing, the last bit make a very low pitched "gurgle-sloop" as it went down the hollow drain pipe. Needless to say, I flushed the toilet almost as many times as I "vroomed, vroomed" my car engine last Saturday! The staff now have their own little jokes about me going around tapping, knocking, humming, flushing, banging, rattling, and grabbing everything in sight!

After a period of implant use, the sounds which the implantee wished so much to hear before implantation, can even become annoying. Each summer one patient returns to our clinic to have the gain on his high-frequency channels turned down so that the cicadas in his back yard "won't drive me crazy."

Tye-Murray et al. (1992) report limited improvement on the Iowa Environmental Sounds Test during the first 9 months of implant use. Scores improved only after 18 months of implant use. However, in a review of patients in the Utah sample for whom scores were obtained on the Environmental Sounds Recognition Test of the MAC battery at 1, 3, 6, and 12 months postfitting, we find a significant ($p < .01$)

improvement in identification at 1 year postfitting. This outcome is consistent with the increase in word identification scores shown in the first 9 months of implant use.

IN THE FUTURE WHO SHOULD BE IMPLANTED?

Most adult patients who are currently fitted with cochlear implants were deafened after the acquisition of language and obtain little or no open-set speech understanding with a hearing aid. When looking toward the future, we should ask (a) would patients who were deafened before the onset of language acquisition benefit from a cochlear implant, and (b) would patients who obtain some open-set speech understanding with a hearing aid benefit from an implant?

Too little data have been published to answer the first question without reservation. Tong, Busby, & Clark (1988) report poor consonant and vowel recognition for three patients fitted with the Nucleus device (see also Busby, Roberts, Tong, & Clark, 1991). Chouard, Fugain, & Lacombe (1983) report a small gain in word understanding for 3 of 10 prelingually deafened patients when lip reading-plus-implant was compared to lip reading alone. Slightly more optimistic results were reported by Burian (1984) who reported that about half of the prelingually deafened patients in the Vienna sample achieved some vowel, consonant and sentence recognition. The general absence of speech understanding is to be expected given that these patients do not have an auditory memory for speech sounds against which to compare the information provided by a prosthesis. It remains to be determined whether sound awareness and minimal discrimination provide enough information to sustain device use by this population.

The answer to the second question is "yes." At issue is the level of speech understanding with a hearing aid that *would not* be improved by the addition of an implant. Recall that the best patients with the CIS processor achieved scores of 80% correct on the NU-6 word list. This a level of speech understanding better than that obtained by many patients who use hearing aids.

Two groups of patients who have some open-set speech understanding by means of a hearing aid have been fitted with the Nucleus prosthesis. The patients in one group have less than 10% sentence recognition when assisted by a hearing aid. Patients in the other group have up to 25% sentence recognition when aided monaurally and up to 30% sentence recognition when aided binaurally. Brimacombe, Arndt, Staller, & Beiter (1991) report that 69% of the 16 patients in the first group evidenced significantly improved sentence understanding with the implant. The scores ranged from 0–97% correct. In the binaural condition of hearing aid plus implant, 75% of the patients evidenced improved sentence understanding. The range of scores was 3–99% correct. One half of the patients (8) showed better performance in the implant plus hearing aid condition than in the implant-alone condition.

Only two patients in the group with up to 30% sentence understanding when aided binaurally have been tested postoperatively. Brimacombe et al. (1991) report a 30% correct preoperative score for binaural aids, a 75% correct postoperative score for implant alone and an 82% correct score for implant plus hearing aid.

The results described above indicate that patients with some residual speech understanding by means of a hearing aid may achieve much higher levels of speech understanding when fitted with a cochlear implant. It is quite likely that in the near future many patients will use *both* a cochlear implant and a hearing aid.

COCHLEAR NUCLEUS IMPLANT

An intracochlear implant is not an option for some patients because the auditory nerve has been damaged in the course of removal of an acoustic tumor. For these patients restoration of hearing must depend on stimulation above the level of the auditory nerve. The cochlear nucleus is a logical place for such stimulation.

Twenty-two patients who lost hearing bilaterally due to the removal of acoustic tumors have been fitted with a cochlear nucleus implant at the House Ear Institute. The mesh electrode lies over the dorsal cochlear nucleus but stimulates, most likely, a large area of neural tissue. Most generally, this single-channel, analogue system works as well, or poorly, as the House, single-channel system implanted in the cochlea. However, one patient fitted with a research processor developed at Research Triangle Institute has shown spectacular results. The processor used a train of short-duration pulses whose amplitudes were modulated with the envelope of the speech signal. The patient's scores increased from 2% correct to 40% correct for spondee words, from 11% correct to 25% correct for CID sentences and from 2% correct to 12% correct for NU-6 words (Shannon, Zeng, & Wygonski, in press). Consonant recognition improved from 45% correct to 60% correct on the Iowa Medial Consonant Test. Vowel recogntion did not improve. These scores are similar to the average scores for patients using the multichannel Nucleus and Ineraid devices.

ACCOUNTING FOR DIFFERENCES AMONG PATIENTS

For a given type of implant, scores on tests of speech recognition can range from 0 to nearly 100% correct. Contrast the reports of two patients.

First patient: I can understand most of what is being said to me with my implant. Speech sounds like it should; I use the telephone ... and [I] sometimes listen to music.

Second patient: I can hear ... from across the room. But I can't understand anything that's said.

We would like to understand the factors responsible for these differences. Understanding can take place at different levels of analysis. We can ask, for example, whether personality factors, such as willingness to accept responsibly for one's own health care, are correlated with performance on tests of speech understanding. At another level, we can ask whether the age of onset of deafness, or the duration of profound deafness, is correlated with performance. At yet another level, we can ask whether frequency resolution, temporal resolution, or dynamic range is correlated with performance on tests of speech understanding. And, at yet another level, we can ask whether evoked-potential measures of auditory nerve function are related to performance. And finally, we can count the number of ganglion cells, axons, and dendrites in the auditory periphery of patients who have come to autopsy.

FIBER AND CELL BODY COUNTS

Direct measurement of the peripheral auditory mechanism of implant patients has been limited, most generally, to patients fitted with the House single-channel implant (Linthicum & Anderson, 1991). Few dendrites were found in the cochlea of these patients—which suggests that the excitable neural elements were cell bodies or axons in the spiral ganglion. Linthicum and Anderson (1991) report no correlation between the number of surviving ganglion cells and performance on the monosyllable-trochee-spondee word test. The absence of a significant correlation is not unexpected given a single place of stimulation and the limited speech recognition abilities of the patients. We would expect a very different outcome for patients with multichannel prostheses. In this instance we would expect that the number of cell bodies and, perhaps more important, the **distribution** of cells bodies would be correlated with performance.

AUDITORY NERVE REFRACTORY STATE AND SPEECH UNDERSTANDING

There is a relatively high correlation between speech intelligibility and the auditory nerve's rate of recovery from the refractory state (see Abbas, Chapter 7). Brown, Abbas, and Gantz (1990) stimulated and recorded the whole-nerve action potential from the intracochlear electrodes in 11 Ineraid patients. Recovery from the refractory state was measured by assessing the amplitude of the electrically elicited response to the second of two clicks as a function of the interval between the clicks. The correlation between the rate of recovery from the refractory state and speech understanding was .76 for the Iowa Sentence Test and .84 for the NU-6 word test. That is to say, the faster the recovery, the better the score on tests of speech understanding. As the authors note, if patients rely heavily on time/amplitude cues for speech understanding, then it is not surprising that the patients with fast recovery rates from stimulation perform better than patients with slow recovery rates.

PSYCHOACOUSTIC MEASURES

As we should expect, psychoacoustic measures of temporal resolution and of frequency resolution are related to speech understanding (see Shannon, Chapter 8). Patients with very poor temporal resolution, as measured by gap detection and temporal difference limens, tend to evidence very poor speech understanding. However, patients with good temporal resolution can evidence either good or poor speech understanding (Hochmair,-Desoyer, Hochmair, & Stiglbrunner, 1985; Tyler et al., 1989a).

There is also a relationship between the range of pure-tone signals that can be scaled in frequency and speech intelligibility, at least for patients who use the Ineraid. Dorman et al. (1990b) report much larger pitch ranges for patients with excellent speech understanding than for patients with very poor speech understanding. In this experiment, the best patients could scale pitch over a range of 2–3 kHz while the poorest could scale pitch over a range of less than 1 kHz.

Some reports with small patient samples suggest that electrical thresholds may be related to speech understanding (Eddington, 1990), but other reports suggest no relationship (Dankowski, McCandless, & Dorman, 1990).

RESIDUAL HEARING

There has been a suspicion that the best performing implant patients are those with "residual hearing" of some sort. Tye-Murray, Gantz, Kuk, and Tyler (1988) comment that patients with thresholds of 85 dB or less at a number of frequencies were better at word recognition than other patients. Tyler (1988b) noted that the best patient with the Banfai device (Banfai, Hortmann, Karczag, Kubik, & Wustrow, 1984), whose scores compared favorably with those of some of the better multichannel implant patients, had the most residual hearing when tested before implantation. However, a review of 40 patients in the Utah sample revealed no significant correlation between preimplant audiogram and postimplant speech understanding (McCandless, 1990).

DURATION OF DEAFNESS

The duration of profound deafness is related to speech recognition ability (Dorman et al, 1989b; Dowell, Mecklenburg, & Clark, 1986; Gantz et al., 1988; Tyler, 1991), but the correlation is only moderate—in the neighborhood of .40 to .50. Thus, many patients with recent onset of deafness evidence poor identification, while some patients with deafness of long duration, even 20 years, evidence some speech understanding.

ETIOLOGY OF DEAFNESS

The etiology of deafness has not yet been shown to affect speech understanding (e.g., Dorman et al., 1989b). However, sample sizes are small, and the most common etiology is "unknown." Note, under the category of etiology, that meningitis is a common disease of childhood. In this instance, etiology and duration of profound deafness are confounded. In the sample studied by Dorman et al. (1989a) meningitic patients with long periods of deafness performed particularly poorly on tests of speech understanding. However, recent data from younger meningitic patients with short periods of deafness indicate high levels of performance. Thus, meningitis, per se, does not seem to be a significant factor in poor speech understanding.

GRADUAL VERSUS ABRUPT HEARING LOSS

It would be reasonable to suspect that the rate at which a patient loses his or her hearing might be related to speech recognition performance. Patients with a slow deterioration of hearing have a longer period to adapt to a distorted speech signal than patients who lose their hearing suddenly. However, the correlation between rate of hearing loss and speech identification is not significant (Gantz et al., 1988).

PSYCHOLOGICAL VARIABLES

The psychological health and well-being of implant patients has been assessed with a large number of test instruments. Of the many variables examined, only "willingness to participate in one's own health care" was correlated significantly with speech understanding (Gantz et al., 1988; Knutson, et al., 1991). At the time of preimplant assessment, an important finding was that patients who have just lost their hearing feel more isolated than any other population for whom test data exist. The previous record-holding group was college freshmen.

CONCLUSION

As we noted at the beginning of this chapter, it has taken nearly 25 years of diligent work by research groups in many countries to achieve the success that cochlear implants currently enjoy. From the point of view of the patient, and sometimes the researcher, progress has been slow, even frustratingly slow. However, every once in a while we have the opportunity to be a part of an event like the following, which makes the long hours spent in the laboratory more than just worthwhile.

It was late on a Friday afternoon on a warm summer day. Three researchers and a patient had spent a very long and very tiring 2 weeks testing new signal processors for cochlear implants. The speech-perception experiments had been completed and a processor had been identified which produced a large gain in intelligibility. As the researchers were switching off pieces of equipment, the patient asked if he could listen to his favorite song from before he lost his hearing through the best of the new signal processors. As unneeded pieces of equipment were being shut off, the patient put his head in his hands and listened intently to the tape. When the song was over, he looked up. Tears were streaming down his face. In a voice choked with emotion, he said that he had almost forgotten how good the song sounded ... and wondered if the new signal processor could be put in a box for him to take home.

ACKNOWLEDGMENTS

The following individuals graciously provided material for this chapter: J. Brimacombe of Cochlear Corporation; I. Hochmair-Desoyer of the University of Innsbruck; D. Lawson and B. Wilson of Research Triangle Institute; P. Blamey of the Austrialian Bionic Ear Institute; and R. Tyler of the University of Iowa. I thank our patients for permission to quote from their diaries. Preparation of this manuscript was supported by grant DC-00654 from the National Institute on Deafness and Other Communication Disorders.

REFERENCES

Banfai, P., Hortmann, G., Karczag, A., Kubik, S., & Wustrow, F. (1984). Results with eight-channel cochlear implants. *Advances in Audiology, 2,* 1–18.

Behrens, S., & Blumstein, S. (1988). On the role of the amplitude of the fricative noise in the perception of place of articulation in voiceless fricative consonants. *Journal of the Acoustical Society of America, 84,* 861–867.

Bess, F., & Townsend, T. (1977). Word discrimination for listeners with flat sensorineural hearing losses. *Journal of Speech and Hearing Disorders, 42,* 232–237.

Blamey, P., & Clark, G. (1990). Place coding of vowel formants for cochlear implant patients. *Journal of the Acoustical Society of America, 88,* 667–673.

Blamey, P., Dowell, R., Brown, A., Clark, G., & Seligman, P. (1987). Vowel and consonant recognition of cochlear implant patients using formant-estimating speech processors. *Journal of the Acoustical Society of America, 82,* 48–57.

Blumstein, S., Issacs, E., & Mertus, J. (1982). The role of gross spectral shape as a perceptual cue to place of articulation in initial stop consonants. *Journal of the Acoustical Society of America, 72,* 43–50.

Brimacombe, J., Arndt, P, Staller, S., & Beiter, A. (1991, May). *The use of a multichannel cochlear implant in severely-to-profoundly hearing-impaired adults.* Paper presented at the 1991 Conference on Implantable Auditory Prostheses, Pacific Grove, CA.

Brown, C., Abbas, P., & Gantz, B. (1990). Electrically-evoked whole-nerve action potentials: Data from human cochlear implant users. *Journal of the Acoustical Society of America, 88,* 1385–1391.

Burian, K. (1984). Clinical results. *Acta Otolaryngologia,* (Suppl. 411), 217–220.

Busby, P., Roberts, S., Tong, Y., & Clark, G. (1991). Results of speech perception and speech production training for three prelingually deaf patients using a multiple-electrode cochlear implant. *British Journal of Audiology, 25,* 291–302.

Clark, G., Tong, Y., Dowell, R., Martin, L., Seligman, P., Busby, P., & Patrick, J. (1981). A multiple channel cochlear implant: An evaluation using nonsense syllables. *Annals of Otology, Rhinology and Laryngology, 90,* 227–230.

Chouard, C., Fugain, C., & Lacombe, H. (1983). Long term results for the multichannel cochlear implant. In C. Parkins and S. Anderson (Eds.), *Cochlear prostheses: An international symposium. Annals of the New York Academy of Sciences, 405,* 311–322.

Cohen, N., Waltzman, S., & Shapiro, W. (1989). Telephone speech comprehension with use of the Nucleus cochlear implant. *Annals of Otology, Rhinology and Laryngology, 98,* 8–11.

Dankowski, K., McCandless, G., & Dorman, M. (1990). *Relationship between electrical and acoustical dynamic range and measures of speech discrimination.* Paper presented at the Second International Cochlear Implant Symposium, Iowa City, IA.

Dodd, B., & Campbell, R. (1987). *Hearing by eye: The psychology of lip-reading.* Hillsdale, NJ: Lawrence-Erlbaum Associates.

Dorman, M. (1990). *Survey of implant patients.* Unpublished manuscript.

Dorman. M., Basham, K., McCandless, G., & Dove, H. (1991c). Speech understanding and music appreciation with the Ineraid cochlear implant. *The Hearing Journal,* June, 34–37.

Dorman, M., Dankowski, K., McCandless, G., Parkin, J., & Smith, L. (1990a). Longitudinal changes in word recognition by patients who use the Ineraid cochlear implant. *Ear and Hearing, 11,* 455–459.

Dorman, M., Dankowski, K., McCandless, G., Parkin, J., & Smith, L. (1991a). Vowel and consonant recognition with the aid of a multichannel cochlear implant. *Quarterly Journal of Experimental Psychology, 43A*(3), 585–601.

Dorman, M., Dankowski, K., McCandless, G., & Smith, L. (1989a). Identification of synthetic vowels by patients using the Symbion multichannel cochlear implant. *Ear and Hearing, 10,* 40–43.

Dorman, M., Dove, H., Parkin, J., Zacharchuk, S., & Dankowski, K. (1991b). Telephone use by patients fitted with the Ineraid cochlear implant. *Ear and Hearing, 12,* 368–369.

Dorman, M., Hannley, M., Dankowski, K., Smith, L., & McCandless, G. (1989b). Word recognition by 50 patients fitted with the Symbion multichannel cochlear implant. *Ear and Hearing, 10,* 44–49.

Dorman, M., Hannley, M., McCandless, G., & Smith, L. (1988). Acoustic/phonetic categorization with the Symbionmultichannel cochlear implant. *Journal of the Acoustical Society of America, 84,* 501–510.

Dorman, M., Smith, L., McCandless, G., Dunnavant, G., Parkin, J., & Dankowski, K. (1990b). Pitch scaling and speech understanding by patients who use the Ineraid cochlear implant. *Ear and Hearing, 11,* 310–315.

Dorman, M. F., Soli, S., Dankowski, K., Smith, L., McCandless, G., & Parkin, J. (1990c). Acoustic cues for consonant identification by patients who use the Ineraid cochlear implant. *Journal of the Acoustical Society of America, 88,* 2074–2079.

Dowell, R., Brown, A., & Mecklenburg, D. (1990). Clinical assessment of implanted deaf adults. In G. Clark, Y. Tong, & J. Patrick (Eds.), *Cochlear Prostheses* (pp. 193–206), Edinburgh: Churchill Livingstone.

Dowell, R., Mecklenburg, D., & Clark, G. (1986). Speech recognition for 40 patients receiving multi-channel cochlear implants. *Acta Otolaryngologia, 12,* 1054–1059.

Dowell, R., Seligman, P., Blamey, P., & Clark, G. (1987). Speech perception using a two formant 22-electrode cochlear prosthesis in quiet and in noise. *Acta Otolaryngologica, 104,* 439–446.

Doyle, J., Doyle, J., & Turnbull, F. (1964). Electrical stimulation of the eighth cranial nerve. *Archives of Otolaryngology, 80,* 388–391.

Eddington D. (1980). Speech discrimination in deaf subjects with cochlear implants. *Journal of the Acoustical Society of America, 68*(3), 885–891.

Eddington, D. (1990). *Psychophysical correlates of speech reception in subjects using multichannel cochlear implants.* Paper presented at the Second International Cochlear Implant Symposium, Iowa City, IA.

Edgerton, B., Doyle, K., Brimacombe, J., Danley, M., & Fretz, R. (1983). The effects of signal processing by the House-Urban single-channel stimulator on auditory perception abilities of patients with cochlear implants. In C. Parkins and S. Anderson (Eds.), Cochlear prostheses: An international symposium. *Annals of the New York Academy of Sciences, 405,* 311–322.

Fujimura, O. (1962). Analysis of nasal consonants. *Journal of the Acoustical Society of America, 34,* 1865–1875.

Gantz, B., Tyler, R., Knutson, J., Woodworth, G., Abbas, P., McCabe, B., Hinrichs, J., Tye-Murray, N., Lansing, C., Kuk, F., & Brown, C.(1988). Evaluation of five different cochlear implant designs: Audiologic assessment and predictors of performance. *Laryngoscope, 98,* 1100–1106.

Gfeller, K., & Lansing, C. (1991). Melodic, rhythmic and timbral perception of adult cochlear implant users. *Journal of Speech and Hearing Research, 34,* 916–920.

Harris, K. (1958). Cues for the discrimination of American English fricatives in spoken syllables. *Language and Speech, 1*, 1–7.

Heinz, J., & Stevens, K. (1961). On the properties of voiceless fricative consonants. *Journal of the Acoustical Society of America, 33*, 589–596.

Hochmair, E., & Hochmair-Desoyer, I. (1985). Aspects of sound signal processing using the Vienna intra- and extracochlear implants. In R. A. Schindler and M. M. Merzenich (Eds.), *Cochlear Implants* (pp.101–110). New York: Raven Press.

Hochmair-Desoyer, I. (1991). *Advances with different speech-processors for analog and combined analog and pulsatile (CAP) strategies.* Paper presented at the International Symposium on Neural and Artifical Control of Hearing and Balance, Rheinfelden, Switzerland.

Hochmair-Desoyer, I., Hochmair, K., & Burian, K. (1985). The Viennaextra- and intracochlear prosthesis: Speech-coding and speech understanding. In E. Myers (Ed.), *New dimensions in otorhinolaryngology-head and neck surgery.* Elsevier Science Publishers.

Hochmair-Desoyer, I., Hochmair, E., & Stiglbrunner, H. (1985). Psychoacoustic temporal processing and speech understanding in cochlear implant patients. In R. A. Schindler and M. M. Merzenich (Eds.), *Cochlear Implants* (pp. 291–304). New York: Raven Press.

House, A. (1961). On vowel duration in English. *Journal of the Acoustical Society of America, 33*, 1174–1178.

Kewley-Port, D. (1983). Time-varying features as correlates of place of articulation in stop consonants. *Journal of the Acoustical Society of America, 73*, 322–335.

Knutson, J., Schartz, H., Gantz, B., Tyler, R., Hinrichs, J., & Woodworth, G. (1991). Psychological change following 18–months of cochlear implant use. *Annals of Otology, Rhinology and Laryngology, 100* (11), 877–882.

Lehiste, I., & Peterson, G. (1959). Vowel amplitude and phonemic stress in American English. *Journal of the Acoustical Society of America, 31*, 428–435.

Liberman, A.M., Delattre, P.Cooper, F., & Gerstman, L.(1954). The role of consonant-vowel transitions in the perception of the stop and nasal consonants. *Psychological Monographs, 68*(8, Whole No. 379), 1–13.

Linthicum, F., & Anderson, W. (1991). Cochlear implantation of totally deaf ears: Histologic evaluation of candidacy. *Acta Otolaryngologia, 111*, 327–331.

Massaro, D. (1987). Speech perception by ear and eye. In B. Dodd & R. Campbell (Eds.), *Hearing by eye: The psychology of lip-reading* (pp. 53–85). London: Lawrence Erlbaum.

McCandless, G. (1990). *Factors which affect function with the Ineraid multichannel cochlear implant.* Paper presented at the Second International Cochlear Implant Symposium, Iowa City, IA.

McCandless, G. (1990). *Music perception by Ineraid patients.* Unpublished manuscript.

McKay, C., McDermott, H., Vandali, A., & Clark, G. (1991). Preliminary results with a six spectal maxima sound processor for the University of Melbourne/Nucleus multiple-electrode cochlear implant. *Journal of the Otolaryngological Society of Australia, 6*, 354–359.

Miller, G., Heise, G., & Lichten, W. (1951). The intelligibility of speech as a function of the context of the test materials. *Journal of Experimental Psychology, 41*, 329–335.

O'Connor, J., Gerstman, L., Liberman, A., Delattre, P., & Cooper, F. (1957). Acoustic cues for the perception of initial /wjrl/ in English. *Word, 13*, 24–43.

Owens, E., Kessler, D., & Schubert, E. (1981). The minimal auditory capabilities (MAC) battery. *Hearing Aid Journal, 34*, 9–34.

Peterson, G., & Barney, H. (1952). Control methods used in a study of vowels. Journal of the *Acoustical Society of America, 24,* 175–184.

Pickett, M. (1980). *The sounds of speech.* Austin, TX: Pro-Ed.

Pisoni, D., & Luce, P. (1986). Speech perception: Research,theory and the principal issues. In E. Schwab & H. Nusbaum (Eds.), Pattern recognition by humans and machines (pp. 1–42). Orlando, FL: Academic Press.

Repp, B. (1982). Phonetic trading relations and context effects: New experimental evidence for a speech mode of perception. *Psychological Bulletin, 92,* 81–110.

Repp, B. (1986). Perception of the [m]–[n] distinction in CV syllables *Journal of the Acoustical Society of America, 79,* 1987–1999.

Rosen, S., (1989). Temporal information in speech and its relevance for cochlear implants. In B. Fraysse and N. Cochard (Eds.), *Cochlear implant: Acquisitions and controversies* (pp. 3–26). Basel, Switzerland: Cochlear AG.

Rosen, S. & Ball, V. (1986). Speech perception with the Vienna extra cochlear single-channel implant: A comparison of two approaches to speech coding. *British Journal of Audiology, 20,* 61–83.

Rosen, S., Fourcin, A., Abberton, E., Walliker, S., Howard, D., Moore, B., Douek, E., & Frampton, S. (1985). Assessing assessment. In R. A. Schindler and M. M. Merzenich (Eds.), *Cochlear implants* (pp. 479–498). New York: Raven Press.

Shannon, R., Zeng, F-G., & Wygonski, J. (in press). Speech recognition using only temporal cues. In M. E. Schouten (Ed.), *Audition, speech and language.* Berlin: Mouton-DeGruyter.

Simmons, B. (1966). Electrical stimulation of the auditory nerve in man. *Archives of Otolaryngology, 84,* 2–54.

Skinner, M., Holden, L., Holden, T., Dowell, R., Seligman, Brimacombe, J., & Beiter, A. (1991). Performance of postlinguistically deaf adults with the wearable speech processor (WSP III) and mini speech processor (MSP) of the Nucleus multi-channel cochlear implant. *Ear and Hearing, 12,* 3–22.

Spivak, L., & Waltzman, S. (1990). Performance of cochlear implant patients as a function of time. *Journal of Speech and Hearing Research, 33,* 511–519.

Sumby, W., & Pollack, I. (1954). Visual contribution to speech intelligibility in noise. *Journal of the Acoustical Society of America, 26,* 212–215.

Summerfield, A. Q. (1985). Speech-processing alternatives for electrical auditory stimulation. In R. A. Schindler & M. M. Merzenich (Eds.), *Cochlear implants* (pp.195–222). New York: Raven Press.

Summerfield, A. Q. (1987). Lip-reading and speech perception: Theoretial perspectives. In B. Dodd & R. Campbell (Eds.), *Hearing by eye: The psychology of lip-reading* (pp. 3–52). London: Lawrence Erlbaum.

Tong, Y, Busby, P., & Clark, G. (1988). Perceptual studies on cochlear implant patients with early onset of profound hearing impairment prior to normal development of auditory, speech and language skills. *Journal of the Acoustical Society of America, 84,* 951–962.

Tong, Y., Clark, G., Seligman, P., & Patrick, J. (1980). Speech processing for a multiple-electrode cochlear implant hearing prosthesis. *Journal of the Acoustical Society of America, 68,* 1897–1899.

Townshend, B., Cotter, N., Compernolle, D., & White, R. (1987). Pitch perception by cochlear implant subjects. *Journal of the Acoustical Society of America, 82,* 106–115.

Tye-Murray, N., Gantz, B., Kuk, F., & Tyler, R. (1988). Word recognition performance of patients using three different cochlear implant designs. In P. Banfai (Ed.), *Cochlear implant: Current situation* (pp. 605–612). Duren, West Germany.

Tye-Murray, N., Gantz, B., Kuk, F., & Tyler, R. (1988).*(continued)* Proceedings of the International Cochlear Implant Symposium, Cologne, West Germany, 1987.

Tye-Murray, N., Lowder, M., & Tyler, R. (1990). Comparison of the F0F2 and F0F1F2 processing strategies for the Cochlear Corporation cochlear implant. *Ear and Hearing, 11,* 195–200.

Tye-Murray, N., & Tyler, R. (1989). Auditory consonant and word recognition skills of cochlear implant users. *Ear and Hearing, 10,* 292–298.

Tye-Murray, N., Tyler, R., Woodworth, G., & Gantz, B. (in press). Performance over time with a Nucleus or Ineraid cochlear implant. *Ear and Hearing.*

Tyler, R. (1988a). Open-set word recognition with the 3M/Vienna single-channel cochlear implant. *Archives of Otolaryngology, Head and Neck Surgery, 114,* 1123–1126.

Tyler, R. (1988b). Open-set word recognition with the Duren/Cologne extra-cochlear implant. *Laryngoscope, 98,* 999–1002.

Tyler, R. (1990). What should be implemented in future cochlear implants? *Acta Otolaryngologia* (Suppl. 469), 268–275.

Tyler, R. (1991). What can we learn about hearing aids from cochlear implants. *Ear and Hearing, 6* (Suppl.), 177–186.

Tyler, R., & Kelsay, D. (1990). Advantages and disadvantages reported by some of the better cochlear-implant patients. *The American Journal of Otology, 11,* 282–89.

Tyler, R., & Moore, B. (in press). Consonant recognition by some of the better cochlear-implant patients. *Journal of the Acoustical Society of America.*

Tyler, R., Moore, B., & Kuk, F. (1989a). Performance of some of the better-cochlear-implant patients. *Journal of Speech and Hearing Research, 32,* 887–911.

Tyler, R., Preece, J., & Lowder, M. (1983). Iowa Cochlear Implant Tests. Iowa City: Department of Otolaryngology–Head and Neck Surgery, The University of Iowa.

Tyler, R., Preece, J., & Tye-Murray, N. (1986). The Iowa Phoneme and Sentence Tests (Laser Videodisc). Iowa City: Department of Otolaryngology – Head and Neck Surgery, The University of Iowa.

Tyler, R., Tye-Murray, N., Moore, B., & McCabe, B. (1989b). Synthetic two-formant vowel perception by some of the better cochlear-implant patients. *Audiology, 28,* 301–315.

Tyler, R., Tye-Murray, N., & Otto, S. (1989). The recognition of vowels differing by a single formant by cochlear-implant subjects. *Journal of the Acoustical Society of America, 86,* 2107–2112.

Van Tassel, D., Soli, S., Kirby, V., & Widin, G. (1987). Speech waveform envelope cues for consonant recognition. *Journal of the Acoustical Society of America, 82,* 1152–1161.

von Wallenberg, E., Hochmair-Desoyer, I., & Hochmair, E. (1985). Speech processing for cochlear implants. *Proceedings of the Seventh Annual Conference on the IEEE Engineering in Medicine and Biology Society,* 1114–1118.

von Wallenberg, E., Hochmair, E., & Hochmair-Desoyer, I. (1990). Initial results with simultaneous analogue and pulsatile stimulation of the cochlea. *Acta Otolaryngologia,* (Suppl. 469), 140–149.

Wilson, B., Lawson, D., & Finley, C. (1990). Speech processors for auditory prostheses. *Fourth Quarterly Progress Report on NIH Project N01-DC-9-2401,* 4–24.

Wilson, B., Lawson, D., Finley, C., Eddington, D., & Rabinowitz, W. (1991). Better speech recognition with cochlear implants. *Nature, 352,* 236–238.

Zue, V. (1985). The use of speech knowledge in automatic speech recogition. *Proceedings of the IEEE, 73,* 1602–1615.

CHAPTER 5

Speech Perception by Children
RICHARD S. TYLER

The provision of cochlear implants has enormous potential rewards for profoundly hearing-impaired children. Conceivably, the exposure to sound via electrical stimulation could change the entire life of a young deaf child. Enhanced sound perception could dramatically influence speech production, language, and cognitive development. Cochlear-implant use could change the way a child communicates with parents, siblings, and friends. It may change the educational opportunities available and the manner in which the deaf function in society when they become adults.

Providing cochlear implants to children represents a challenging task because testing and fitting young children can be difficult and uncertain. Furthermore, we are only beginning to quantify the performance of children using cochlear implants to demarcate their potential abilities and limitations. Many profoundly hearing-impaired children benefit substantially from hearing aids. Providing these children with cochlear implants may not improve their speech-perception performance; cochlear implants may even decrease performance in some children. Furthermore, there are some hearing-impaired children who successfully use sign language and may not need or want the sound sensations provided by a cochlear implant (see Boothroyd, Chapter 1; Lane, 1990; Tyler, 1992).

There is much to learn about the potential uses of cochlear implants in children. This chapter begins by reviewing some of the important issues in measuring speech perception in children, including a discussion of many tests used to evaluate speech-perception performance in children.

This is followed by a review of the results from numerous studies of speech perception in children with cochlear implants. We then discuss several issues related to cochlear implants in children, including educational placement, predicting performance, cochlear implants for children with multiple handicaps, and the implications of these results for selection criteria.

CONSIDERATIONS FOR TESTING SPEECH PERCEPTION IN CHILDREN

There are several important issues that should first be considered to understand, design, and evaluate speech-perception tests for children. Dorman (see Chapter 4) has reviewed the speech features and their coding by cochlear-implant type. His discussion is applicable to understanding speech perception in children. There are additional concerns that arise when testing young children, which are highlighted in the present section.

SPEECH SHOULD BE THE STIMULUS TO EVALUATE SPEECH PERCEPTION

If our goal is to measure and understand speech-perception abilities, then we should use speech as the signal (Boothroyd, 1991). Speech is a complex acoustical signal that changes rapidly. We are not yet able to fully understand speech-perception ability by studying responses to isolated nonspeech segments. Particularly for young children, speech is a more meaningful stimuli, and is therefore more likely to capture and hold their attention when extensive testing is required.

However, there are some applications where the use of nonspeech stimuli may be helpful, such as in removing the effects of vocabulary, or producing a simple test for young prelingually deaf children. Psychoacoustical tests have been partially successful in examining the underlying factors in speech perception in hearing-impaired adults (e.g., Dreschler & Plomp, 1985; Lutman & Clark, 1986; Stelmachowicz, Jesteadt, Gorga, & Mott, 1985; Tyler, Summerfield, Wood, & Fernandes, 1982). Utilizing synthetic speech-like stimuli in psychoacoustical paradigms can contribute to our understanding of fundamental speech-perception abilities (e.g., Dorman, Dankowski, McCandless, & Smith, 1989: Kirk, 1990). Shannon (see Chapter 8) and Dorman (see Chapter 4) discuss some applications of nonspeech stimuli in cochlear-implant testing.

For the present, however, the speech-perception abilities of children will be most easily interpretable, and generalizable, if natural speech is used as the stimulus.

FOCUS ON SENSORY RECEPTION

Figure 5–1 schematically shows how cochlear implants intervene primarily on the perception of sound. If there is a successful transmission of meaningful sound by the cochlear implant, then there may be changes in the secondary areas of speech production, language skills, and cognition. The secondary areas can all be influenced by many variables; the ability to hear is only one of these variables. For example, it may be possible to teach some totally deaf children to talk intelligibly (see Tobey, Chapter 6). Language development will be affected by the quality and duration of exposure to language, family, and school environment (and

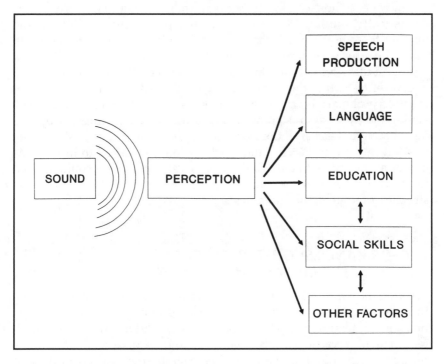

Figure 5–1. A schematic representation showing that the primary effect of the cochlear implant is on speech perception, with secondary effects on many other areas. These secondary areas can be influenced by many other variables that are difficult to isolate and control. (Adapted from Tyler et al., 1986.)

all are difficult to quantify). While these other areas are of utmost importance to the overall understanding of the impact of cochlear implants, the specific effects of the cochlear implant on these secondary areas is often difficult to isolate. Thus, the influence of the cochlear implant is best studied by using speech-perception measures (Boothroyd, 1991; Tyler, Berliner, Demorest, Hirshorn, Luxford, & Mangham, 1986).

TESTS SHOULD BE WITHIN THE LANGUAGE AND VOCABULARY LEVEL OF THE CHILD

Speech-perception tests should not be influenced by factors unrelated to perceptual abilities, particularly, limitations imposed by the child's vocabulary and language. It is necessary to ensure that the test words are within the vocabulary of the child. For example, if the test item is "horse," but the child does not know what a horse is, then the child might repeat "house" simply because that is a familiar word that is acoustically similar. This error does not reflect the inability of the implant to code the word "horse" or the child's ability to recognize it. Thus, the error is not a reflection of speech-perception abilities. Rather it is a vocabulary limitation. This problem can occur in both open-set and closed-set tests. It is the responsibility of the audiologist to ensure that the test vocabulary is within the child's vocabulary. This can be done by having the child say or sign the words when shown pictures, or by asking a parent or teacher. If the words are not known, then they should not be used in the test. Parents and teachers could be asked to include the objects and words into the child's activities so that the test could be used in the future. Similar comments can be made about the grammatical structure of sentence or phrase tests.

PERFORMANCE SHOULD REFLECT CONVERSATIONAL SPEECH

Tests should represent the true performance of the child in natural situations because this is the ultimate communication environment that the implant is designed to effect (Boothroyd, 1991). This is a difficult requirement, because it is also necessary to develop tests that are independent of confounding variables, like cognition, memory, vocabulary, and grammar.

Conversational speech in natural situations is influenced by many factors, including the following; the child's knowledge of the topic, familiarity with the talker, vocabulary, ability to control the conversation, and the speaking rate of the talker. These factors are not related to the information provided by the implant, and therefore, tests should be used that limit their effect on the results.

It is possible to devise tests using speech stimuli that have little bearing on conversational speech. For example, you could determine if a child can discriminate the words "toe" and "baseball." However, because these words can be distinguished based on duration only, the test's ability to reflect conversational speech understanding is probably very limited.

Tests using a series of single sentences have high face validity because we typically communicate in sentences. However, there are some additional considerations. First, unlike word tests, the results of sentence tests can be influenced by the child's knowledge of grammar. Second, contextual information within the sentence can provide clues about the words (e.g., a sentence that contains the word "ski" is likely to also contain the word "snow"). Third, the presence of one word can influence the way an adjacent word is produced (coarticulation). Fourth, speech is presented at a rapid rate (Bilger, 1983). The ability of a person to follow the incomplete speech signal presented by the cochlear implant may be influenced by talker rate. Consider how difficult it can be to understand someone talking very quickly in a familiar foreign language. Fifth, there may be characteristics of the cochlear implant (or hearing aid) speech processor, such as automatic gain control circuits, that will alter the acoustic signal differently for sentences and isolated words. Thus, sentence testing is important in an evaluation provided that the grammar and vocabulary are appropriate to the child.

Paragraphs can also be used for testing speech perception, but, in addition to the effects of grammar, they can be influenced by the child's familiarity with the topic. The ability to remember what was said may also be a factor. This could provide an artificial advantage for one child over another or reflect changes not related to speech perception per se.

Continuous discourse tracking (De Filippo & Scott, 1978) has many confounding factors when used as a test. For example, it is difficult to control the sender and receiver strategies (the strategies used at low and high tracking rates can be particularly different), even when comparing across conditions in the same subject (De Filippo, 1988; Tye-Murray & Tyler, 1988). Different passages will likely not be equally difficult, even within the same book. Live-voice testing with familiar talker often precludes any comparisons across centers. Thus, in its present form, we do not recommend its application as a test. However, it can be a viable training procedure (Owens & Raggio, 1987; see Tye-Murray, Chapter 3). Thus, tests should relate to conversational speech. This does not imply, however, that all tests must be of sentence length or longer.

TESTS SHOULD PROVIDE ANALYTICAL INFORMATION ABOUT WHAT SPEECH FEATURES ARE PERCEIVED

Although it is important to obtain global measures of speech recognition, it is also desirable to determine detailed information about which speech features are being perceived (see Dorman, Chapter 4). Analytical information about speech features perceived and misperceived can suggest new processor designs, adjustments in the processor for an individual, and rehabilitation strategies (see Tye-Murray, Chapter 3). Tests of this type include stimuli that differ primarily by one or two phonetic features. There are powerful statistical tools for the evaluation of the error patterns on these tests, giving a detailed analysis of the kind of features perceived (see Dorman, Chapter 4; Miller & Nicely, 1955; Wang & Bilger, 1973).

TEST-RETEST RELIABILITY SHOULD BE SUFFICIENTLY SMALL SO THAT THE TEST CAN BE USED TO MEASURE CLINICAL DIFFERENCES

For any test to be useful, it must be reliable enough to measure significant differences (Boothroyd, 1991). The reliability of a test is partly related to the number of items on the test; a test with more items has more reliability than the same test with fewer items (Thornton & Raffin, 1978). This creates problems when it is necessary to test a young child with a short attention span. For this reason, many tests have been designed with a small number of test items, 20 or less. However, this is usually insufficient to evaluate differences between tests, particularly if chance performance on the test is 25% (a four-choice test) or 50% (a two-choice test) correct. It will be difficult to measure significant changes in a test with a small number of items and a high chance score. In situations like this it may be inappropriate to use the test altogether. Sometimes the test can be repeated two or three times and the scores added. However, in this case the test items will not be independent, and the use of the binomial theorem is no longer valid to test critical differences. The reliability of any test should be known before it can be used for clinical and research issues.

EQUIVALENT LISTS ARE DIFFICULT TO FIND

It is often important to compare the performance among two or more presentations of the same test. This occurs when it is of interest to determine if a child's performance has changed compared with an earlier test date, or it may be of interest to compare the performance of the test in two or more modalities (e.g., vision-only compared to audition-plus-vision), or using two or more different signal processors. Finally, it is often of interest to compare the performance among many individuals on the same test.

There are at least four different ways that the "equivalency" of multiple presentations of a test have been approached. First, and perhaps the most common, is to use different lists made up of different items. These lists have gone through some re-arrangement of the items across lists to make them "equivalent." However, the entire notion of equivalent lists is tenuous. Often, the equivalency may be based on averages and have little bearing on individuals, or it may be based on one modality, such as lipreading, and be unequal in another modality. In the extreme, each individual's hearing aid, cochlear implant, or auditory system filters the signal differently, and it is likely impossible for two lists to have the exact same difficulty level for large numbers of individuals. Thus, it is unlikely that different test lists that use different items can be truly equally difficult.

A second approach is to use different lists which contain the same closed set of response items and the same stimuli in different orders. This guarantees that the lists are equivalent and is a powerful advantage of closed-set tests.

A third approach, used for open-set testing, is to use a single list of items and to repeat the items in each test (usually presenting them in different random order). Although this also guarantees the lists are equivalent, it creates another problem. It is possible (and often likely) that some of the test items may be learned and remembered. Performance on a later test may be influenced by the child's memory (and overall score) for items on an earlier test. This is particularly a problem for sentence material because the message conveyed by the sentence is more likely to be remembered than when the test is composed of individual words. The learning of test items can be reduced by using a large number of items and by increasing the time between test replications, but it may not prevent the problem altogether.

The fourth approach is similar to the first in that different lists of open-set items are used. However, in this approach it is acknowledged that the lists are not equally difficult. The test-retest variability is measured for different lists, and this statistic is used to evaluate differences among scores.

Thus, it is important to critically evaluate supporting data for tests that claim to have "equivalent" lists, particularly open-set tests. An understanding of the equivalency of lists is needed to determine if the two scores from different lists represent real differences or not.

TESTS SHOULD BE WITHIN THE COGNITIVE, MOTORIC, AND ATTENTIONAL CAPABILITIES OF THE CHILD

Children must understand what is required of them, the response must be within their physical abilities, and the test should measure perceptual abilities, not their concentration (Boothroyd, 1991). Children who do not fulfill these requirements should not be tested. Test sessions lasting more than 10 or 15 minutes may tax the attentional capabilities of some children. Many do not have the memory capabilities to listen and respond to a 4- or 6-item sentence. Some young or multiply handicapped children will not be able to understand that they must point to an object or select from among 6 to 12 choices. Others may not be able to point to a picture. Some children are not motivated to select the correct answer. They may not be interested in the task, may have something else on their mind, or simply not care about the results. These children should not be tested. They may require an additional visit, more feedback, encouragement, reinforcers, or more training on the task.

If a child performs poorly on a speech-perception test, it should be because the child has difficulty understanding speech. If a child cannot perform the test, then the child should not receive any score on the test ("could not test"). It is equally important that a child who cannot understand any test items because of perceptual limitations should be evaluated and given a score, even if the score represents chance performance. **Not reporting the test score suggests that the child could not be tested, and this will inappropriately inflate group average results.**

It is the responsibility of the audiologist to rule out these factors before testing a child. One approach is to test the child using the visual modality. Using the same test procedure, present a visual stimulus (or using sign plus audiovisual speech) in the same spatial and temporal relationships as the auditory test. For example, show the child a ball and then have him or her select the picture of the ball on the six-choice picture set. To limit the influence of memory, the **ideal** response should occur shortly after the stimulus. It may be that some children will not be able to perform some tests.

We must be certain that we are testing speech-perception abilities. If factors like attention, memory, or motoric limitations influence the results, then we could misrepresent the child's perceptual abilities.

CHILDREN SHOULD NOT BE TRAINED ON THE TEST MATERIALS

If the child has been trained on or is overly familiar with the specific test items, the results obtained may overestimate the child's true speech-perception abilities. It is inappropriate to train the child on the same items on which he or she will be tested. Although children may learn the auditory patterns of the small set of test items, this may not be representative of their overall speech-perception ability. This also places trained children at an unfair advantage over untrained children (or children trained less well).

Similar complications can also occur when the child is very familiar with the test items. The child can be so familiar with the words "ball" and "hot dog" that only minimal auditory clues are needed for the child to guess the correct answer. This is particularly a problem when the number of test items is small, and the child can anticipate some of the test items. If the particular item was not so familiar, then that item would not have been identified.

Audiologists should not train the child on the test items. Correct/incorrect feedback should not be provided on test items, and tests should be administered sparingly. Training is important (see Tye-Murray, Chapter 3), but training on the test items confounds the interpretation of the results.

RECORDED TEST MATERIALS ARE PREFERRED

Recorded test materials are preferable over live-voice materials for a number of reasons. The acoustical characteristics of the recorded stimuli can be measured and analyzed. There is less opportunity for bias introduced by the talker unintentionally slowing down or talking more clearly or loudly. The same test conditions can be exactly repeated to the child at another time, or to another child. In live-voice testing, the talker is often familiar to the child, and this may inflate performance. The talker could mispronounce the word.

With computer-digitized speech, interactive compact disks and laser videodiscs, it is possible to present the stimulus when the child is ready for it and provide computer games to make the test fun and interesting for young (and older) children, thereby increasing the number of children for whom recorded test materials are appropriate.

It is also true that some children are difficult to test with recorded material and will respond more consistently to a tester in live-voice conditions. Live-voice data are acceptable and are better than no data at all, provided that the data are truly representative of the child's performance and are repeatable. However, misleading **data that are inflated or unrepresentative are worse than no data.** When using live-voice testing, monitor the level of the voice and, if possible, use an unfamiliar talker. Using the same talker across different children and across different test sessions for the same child at a particular center would reduce differences introduced by different talkers.

Whenever possible, recorded test materials should be used. If live-voice tests are used, the test conditions should be reported explicitly. This includes the familiarity of the tester to the child, talker gender, rate of talking (words or phonemes per minute) and perhaps voice fundamental frequency.

PERFORMANCE CATEGORIES AND COMPOSITE SCORES DISCARD INFORMATION

Although it can sometimes be helpful to summarize performance on a test by assigning a qualitative label, this practice discards information. For example, we often summarize a particular type of audiogram as representing a "moderate hearing loss." Similarly, the performance on several tests can often be summarized by a single number or response-category label. Children who obtain some open-set word recognition are sometimes referred to as "open-set responders" or "stars." This approach is often helpful in summarizing performance and providing a general idea of what the real-life consequences might be for that particular level of performance.

However, this simplification or reduction in the data by its very nature discards information, and such categorizations should be used cautiously. Although the reduction of the audiogram to "mild, moderate, and severe" is sometimes useful, most would agree that it is more informative to examine the entire audiogram.

Geers and Moog (1987) categorized the speech-perception abilities of hearing-impaired children into four groups: (1) no pattern perception, (2) pattern perception, (3) inconsistent word recognition, and (4) consistent word recognition, to predict which children would develop spoken language skills. Recently, the scale has been applied to children with cochlear implants. Such a generalization is useful because it provides a simple tool to discuss the global performance of patients and to relate speech-perception test scores to practical consequences. Others have added new categories in an attempt to increase the sensitivity of the four-category scale.

However, such simplification, by definition, ignores information and relinquishes the resolution achieved by the tests. For example, performance could improve within a category, but this would not be reflected in the category assignments. When determining how well one implant compares to another, or how performance changes over time, or comparing performance across children, it will be more effective to utilize all the information provided by test scores.

It is often useful to summarize performance with a single metric. This is best achieved by submitting all the test scores to a factor analysis. A single score is obtained that represents the weighted average of all the other test scores. Thus, all the information is utilized. Henderson, Fisher, Cohen, Waltzman, and Weber, (1991) have applied a factor analysis to the results obtained from adult cochlear-implant patients.

It can be useful to provide a summary or categorization score, but caution should be used in relinquishing information. In general, it will be best to report performance for each test.

INDIVIDUAL SCORES SHOULD BE REPORTED

Variability across children with cochlear implants is enormous. Most clinical and research questions about children's speech-perception abilities focus on whether an individual has shown improvement with the implant, compared to preimplant scores. Reporting average scores across individuals does not specify the most critical information. It can also be misleading to report the percentage of children scoring above chance pre- and postoperatively; it fails to indicate the magnitude of the pre- and postoperative differences. Furthermore, some children may have scored above chance preoperatively, but failed to show a significant increase postoperatively. What is important is the absolute levels of performance for each child. Results from large groups of children can be reported by stating how many benefited from the implant and by how much, or how many showed a statistically significant increase, for example. The best approach is to show individual data in scattergrams or bar graphs.

DO NOT REPEAT TEST ITEMS THAT ARE MISHEARD

To compare performance across time or across children, it is important that the test conditions be as similar as possible. Repeating the test stimuli creates two problems. First, if some children receive repetitions and others do not, it provides an unfair advantage for the former group. Second, even if all children receive the same number of repetitions, there may be individual differences, unrelated to the information provided by the cochlear implant, that confound the results. For example, some children may be able to make better use of integrating phonetic information in reconstructing the entire word on the second presentation than other children. This skill may be important in everyday communication, but it is a confounding factor in the measurement of the effect of the cochlear implant on speech perception. It may be possible to repeat a test item that the child wasn't attending to at the end of a test. Audiologists need to ensure that the child is engaged attentively during the test.

A VARIETY OF TESTS ARE NEEDED TO MEASURE SPEECH PERCEPTION

Speech perception involves a multitude of skills, and no one test is likely to fulfill all the requirements. In addition, a wide range of performance levels across children is common. Some tests will be too easy for some children, and others will be too difficult. Tests of pattern and spectral perception focus on different cues. Word and sentence level materials are needed. Analytic tests which often utilize nonsense syllables are very powerful for understanding which features are perceived. Finally, it is important to include **audiovisual** tests, since most conversational situations include visual information.

THE AGE AT ONSET AND DURATION OF PROFOUND DEAFNESS

One of the most important factors in speech perception in children with cochlear implants is their exposure to speech in the first 2 to 3 years of life (see Boothroyd, Chapter 1). Therefore, it is important that we define and clarify a few related issues before describing speech-perception performance.

During this early period the child is exposed to hundreds of thousands, perhaps millions, of speech utterances that begin to form templates of these meaningful acoustical signals in the brain. Eventually, children have a very good notion of what a particular word, for example, "table," is supposed to sound like, whether spoken by a male or female adult or another child.

First, children can be born with a profound hearing loss (congenital) and never develop a speech memory. Second, children can lose their hearing after only a limited exposure to speech (prelingual-noncongenital). Third, children may lose their hearing after the speech memory has been firmly established (postlingual). Finally, there are many cases where the onset of deafness cannot be precisely determined but the deafness likely began between 1 to 3 years of age (perilingual) (see Table 5–1).

It should be appreciated that the exact years to distinguish these groups are not clear. There exists great interchild variability in the amount of speech memory children develop for a given amount of exposure to spoken language. Some children may develop useful speech memory if deafened at 1 year, others may have a poor speech memory if deafened at 3 years. In addition, many have some hearing initially which progressively deteriorates, and the amount of residual hearing and progression varies enormously. In practice, it is not possible to determine precisely how much exposure to speech most children have experienced.

Table 5–1. *Categorization of deafness based on age at onset of profound deafness. The particular age of 2 years was chosen somewhat arbitrarily to reflect the approximate age at which sufficient exposure to verbal language has occurred that the child might be expected to achieve some memory for speech*

	Prelingual		Perilingual	Postlingual
	Congenital	Noncongenital		
Age at onset of profound deafness	born deaf	< 2 years but not born deaf	uncertain but probably between 1 and 3 years	> 2 years

The duration of profound deafness also plays a critical role in performance. Children who have been deaf for many years may forget some of the speech sounds they once heard. In congenitally deaf children, the receptivity of the nervous system may decrease over time. The effect of the duration of profound deafness should be examined separately for each of the groups discussed above.

The most important issue is the amount of auditory memory for speech that is available to the child. The labels of prelingual, postlingual, or perilingual may not be as important as simply reporting their age at onset and length of deafness. If there is uncertainty about the onset of deafness in some children, this should be stated. It is unwise to group prelingual and postlingual deafened children when reporting results. It will always be necessary to know to which group of children one is referring to when examining the effects of cochlear implants. Boothroyd (see Chapter 1) discusses this important issue in more detail.

SPEECH PERCEPTION TESTS FOR CHILDREN

There are many speech-perception tests available for children and several new ones are being developed. The purpose of this section is to provide an overview of some of these tests. We cannot review all tests, but we can discuss some of the common, unique, or informative tests. We pay particular attention to tests for which there are data on children with cochlear implants. Some of the tests have significant shortcomings and should not be used for speech-perception evaluation.

The descriptions of these tests can be referred to when reading the discussion of the performance of children with cochlear implants provided in the next section. Table 5–2 to Table 5–8 summarize the important characteristics of some of the tests. Although the tests are grouped according to their primary category of use, some of the tests can be used to assess several different levels of perception.

ENVELOPE AND STRESS PERCEPTION

Discrimination After Training (DAT)

This test (Thielemeir, 1984) consists of 12 levels of increasing difficulty, ranging from the detection of a voice to the recognition of speech in a four-choice closed set. A small set of words is used at each level. The first eight levels focus on time-envelope cues, and the other levels include some items that also differ based on spectral cues. Unfortunately, the test protocol includes training on the test materials and therefore it is difficult to interpret the results.

Monosyllable-Trochee-Spondee Test (MTS)

The Monosyllable-Trochee-Spondee test (Erber & Alencewicz; 1976) utilizes 12 pictures of nouns (Figure 5–2). They are divided equally into three syllable stress patterns of one-syllable words, two-syllable words with equal stress (spondees), and two-syllable words with unequal stress (trochees). A "stress" and "word" score is obtained. The stress score depends on whether the word selected comes from the correct syllable-stress category (monosyllable vs. spondee vs. trochee). The word score is determined by the number of words identified correctly. Because the recognition of stress category can be an easy task and can focus the child's attention to a row of four words within the same stress category, the chance score on the word score should be one out of four (25%) correct.

The primary advantage of this test is that the items are within the vocabulary level of many deaf children. Because stress perception depends on envelope cues, it should be relatively easy compared to tests that rely on spectral differences. The test provides a measure of performance for children who do not perceive spectral cues very well. However, with only 12 test items and the test's frequent use, it is possible that the items will be recognized by only minimal cues. Furthermore, this small set of words is sometimes used in auditory training. Therefore, it may overestimate the actual perceptual abilities of some children.

Table 5–2. *Description of some of the important characteristics of tests that focus on envelope and stress perception. The age given in this and in subsequent tables is the approximate minimal age of a child before they are ready for the test*

Test Name	Type	Stimulus Materials	Response Format	Chance Percent	No. of Items	Minimal Age (in years)
Glendonald Auditory Screening Procedure	Stress	Mono, spondee, trochee, 3-syllables	4-choice	25	24	4
	Word	3 words in each stress category	3-choice	33	24	4
	Sentences	10 sentences	open set	0	10	6
Monosyllable-Trochee-Spondee Test	Stress	Monosyllabic, spondee, trochee	3-choice	33	24	4
	Word	4 words in each stress category	4-choice if get stress correct	25	24	4

Table 5–3. *Description of some of the important characteristics of the Sound Effects Recognition Test, used for the evaluation of environmental-sound perception*

Test Name	Type	Stimulus Materials	Response Format	Chance Percent	No. of Items	Minimal Age (in years)
Sound Effects Recognition Test	Everyday sounds	Recordings of everyday sounds	4-choice	25	10 (can give 20 or 30)	5

Table 5–4. Description of some of the important characteristics of tests that focus on closed-set word recognition

Test Name	Type	Stimulus Materials	Response Format	Chance Percent	No. of Items	Minimal Age (in years)
Auditory Numbers Test	Word	Number 1 to 5	5-choice	20	5	3
Early Speech Perception Standard Version	Pattern Perception	12 words monosyllables	4-choice	25	24	6
	Spondee Identification	Spondee trochees and 3-syllable words	12-choice	8	24	6
	Monosyllabic Word Identification	12 monosyllables	12-choice	8	24	6
Low-Verbal Version	Pattern Perception	4 toys, monosyllable spondee trochee 3-syllable words	4-choice	25	12	2
	Spondee Identification	4 spondees	4-choice	25	12	2

Test Name	Type	Stimulus Materials	Response Format	Chance Percent	No. of Items	Minimal Age (in years)
Monosyllable Identification	Word	4 monosyllables	4-choice	25	12	2
Northwestern University Children's Perception of Speech	Word	Single-syllable words 4 lists of 50	4-choice	25	50	6
Word Intelligibility by Picture Identification	Word	1-syllable words 4 lists of 20	6-choice	17	25	6

Table 5-5. *Description of some of the important characteristics of the Phonetically Balanced-Kindergarten open-set word recognition test*

Test Name	Type	Stimulus Materials	Response Format	Chance Percent	No. of Items	Minimal Age (in years)
Phonetically Balanced Kindergarten Test	Word 4 lists	1-syllable words 8 lists	open	0	50	6

Table 5-6. *Description of some of the important characteristics of tests that focus on sentence perception*

Test Name	Type	Stimulus Materials	Response Format	Chance Percent	No. of Items	Minimal Age (in years)
Bamford-Kowal-Bench	Sentence	21 list of 16 sentences	open	0	16	6
Matrix	Sentence	Level A; four 2 × 3 matrixes	2-choice	50	60	5
		Level B; two 4 × 4 matrixes	4-choice	25	120	6

Table 5-7. *Description of some of the important characteristics of tests that focus on vowel and consonant feature perception*

Test Name	Type	Stimulus Materials	Response Format	Chance Percent	No. of Items	Minimal Age (in years)
Audiovisual Feature Test	Syllable audiovisual	b, c, d, p, t, v, z, key me, knee	10-choice	10	60	5
Change/No Change	Nonsense syllables	9 feature lists	2-choice	50	15	4
Children's Vowel Test	Word audiovisual	5 sets of four monosyllabic words, each differing by a medial vowel	4-choice	25	40	5

Test Name	Type	Stimulus Materials	Response Format	Chance Percent	No. of Items	Minimal Age
Speech Pattern Contrast	Word Phrase	10 subtests 2 suprasegmental 8 segmental	4-choice	25	12	10
Three Interval Forced Choice Test of Speech Pattern Contrasts	Features	10 subtests 2 suprasegmental 8 segmental	3-choice	33	24	6

Table 5-8. *Description of some of the important characteristics of the Craig Lipreading Inventory, used to test audiovisual perception. The Audiovisual Feature Test, the Children's Visual Perception Test, the Word Intelligibility with Picture Identification test, and the Bamford-Kowal-Bench sentences can also be presented audiovisually*

Test Name	Type	Stimulus Materials	Response Format	Chance Percent	No. of Items	Minimal Age (in years)
Craig Lipreading Inventory	Word	1- and 2-syllable; words	4-choice	25	33	6
	Sentences	pictures of brief statements	4-choice	25	24	7

Glendonald Auditory Screening Procedure (GASP).

The word-test version of this (Erber, 1982) can be considered an extension of the MTS test. Compared to the MTS, the GASP contains an extra syllabic category (there is a three-syllable option on the GASP but not on the MTS). However, the inclusion of an extra group is done at the expense of one alternative within each group. Thus, the chance score for the GASP within a category is 1 in 3 (33%), whereas it is 1 in 4 (25%) for the MTS. One must be careful to make sure that the child has not overlearned the 12 test items, which contain words such as "ball, table, toothbrush, and elephant."

The sentence test contains 10 questions (e.g., "What is your name?" "When is your birthday?"), and is scored correct only if the child responds to the question appropriately. This subjective scoring technique could result in some errors due to tester biases in some situations. In an extension of this test, Plant (1983) added an extra polysyllabic category.

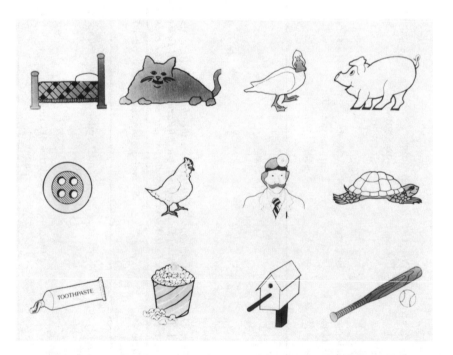

Figure 5–2. The test items on the Monosyllabic-Trochee-Spondee Test (MTS) developed by Erber and Alencewicz (1976). The task is "Point to ... chicken," for example. (Reprinted from Erber, N., & Alencewicz, C. (1976). Audiologic evaluation of deaf children. *Journal of Speech and Hearing Disorders, 41*, 256–267, with permission.)

Test of Auditory Comprehension (TAC)

This test was developed to measure a wide range of auditory comprehension abilities. Subtests 1, 2, and 3 examine a child's ability to discriminate suprasegmentals using speech and nonspeech stimuli (Trammell, et al., 1981). Subtest 1 is a noise-versus-voice test (e.g., horn or drum versus. male or female voice). Subtest 2 tests linguistic (voice), human-nonlinguistic (coughing, sneezing) versus environmental (drum, dog barking) items. Subtest 3 examines common phrases that differ in stress, rhythm, and intonation (e.g., "wash your hands," and "where are your shoes?"). The remaining subtests are highly dependent on language and cognitive skills and should not be used for speech-perception tests.

The **Early Speech Perception** test (see below) also includes stress-perception subtests.

ENVIRONMENTAL SOUND PERCEPTION

Sound Effects Recognition Test (SERT)

This is the only widely used environmental sound test for children (Finitzo-Hieber, Matkin, Cherow-Skalka, & Gerling, 1977) (Figure 5–3). Although there are only 10 items on each of three lists, two or three lists can be administered. Not all of the sounds and pictures are familiar to all children, particularly those less than 6 years of age. Some of the sounds may be inappropriate. For example, there is a picture of a child playing in a pool, and children do not use their cochlear implants in the water! The authors report that normally hearing 3-year-olds score about 83% correct, and 5-year-olds score about 97% correct. It is necessary to ensure that the children know the sounds and can associate them with the picture. However this is sometimes very difficult to ascertain, even when the child can identify what the picture represents. An audiotape is available.

CLOSED-SET WORD RECOGNITION

Auditory Numbers Test (ANT)

This test (Erber, 1980) was intended to distinguish between those children who hear envelope cues from those who hear spectral cues. The stimulus materials are the numbers "one to five." The child must be able to count to five. The tester familiarizes the child with the numbers by counting pictures of "ants" on cards, 1, 1 2 (for two), 1 2 3 (for three), and so on. During the test, either the sequence of numbers is presented (such as 1 2 3) or a single number is presented (such as 3). Only the single-number presentations are the test stimuli. Selecting the correct single number signifies spectral recognition. Always pointing to the number 1 suggests envelope perception.

Having only five test items limits the generalization to everyday speech. It is possible that a child may hear a distorted version of something that sounds like a number other than the test number, but because he or she was taught that a single-syllable presentation represented 1, he might be biased to select number 1 instead of the closest approximation to what was actually heard.

Erber (1980) suggested an alternative procedure, where the number is repeated (e.g., 4, 4) and could also be used as the test stimulus. Perhaps each number could be repeated five times (e.g., 4, 4, 4, 4, 4) to distinguish more clearly between spectral and envelope cues, or be taught that single-number presentations might also be the entire set of test stimuli.

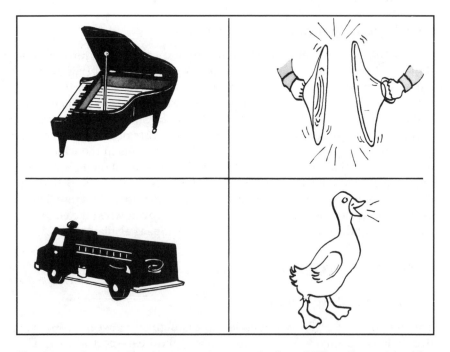

Figure 5–3. An example of some test items on the Sound Effects Recognition Test developed by Finitzo-Hieber, Matkin, Cherow-Skalka, and Gerling (1977). The child hears an environmental sound and must point to the picture that represents something that could have produced the sound. (Reprinted from Finitzo-Hieber, T., Matkin, N. D., Cherow-Skalka, E., & Gerling, I. J. (1977). *Sound Effects Recognition Test*. St. Louis, MO: Auditec, with permission.)

Auditory Perception of Alphabet Letters (APAL)

This test (Ross & Randolph, 1990) requires the recognition of the letters of the alphabet. The child hears a letter and must select among the 26 alphabet letters (a, b, c, d, etc.). Response errors are categorized based on phonetic dissimilarity. Knowledge of the names of all the alphabet letters is required, which would limit the test to many hearing-impaired children approximately 5 years of age and older.

Body Parts

A number of clinics use body parts (nose, eyes, teeth, ears, hands, toes, knees, mouth) as stimuli for live-voice testing for very young children ("point to your nose," for example). Although no formal test exists to our knowledge, the approach may be the only one that can be administered to some children. The strategy could be used when nothing else is possible. The body parts should be distinguished based on whether the words contain one or two syllables so that information provided by gross envelope cues are controlled. As with all tests, it is necessary to ensure that the child knows the stimuli before and to report the actual words used. Comparisons across tests are only valid if the same stimuli are used. We suggest using "hair, eyes, ears, nose, mouth" as an abbreviated set for 2- to 3-year-olds, because they are usually learned at an early age and are all single-syllable words.

Early Speech Perception Tests (ESP)

This test was developed to provide a similar format of testing for children above and below 6 years of age. The words chosen for this test (Moog & Geers, 1990) are known by most hearing-impaired children 6 years of age and older. The "Low-Verbal" version is for children who do not have the vocabulary for the "Standard" version, and it can be used on some children who are 2 to 3 years old.

The **Standard** version has three tests (see Figure 5–4). The **Pattern Perception Test** is similar to the word-categorization subtest of the GASP (Erber, 1982). The **Spondee Identification Test** contains a closed set of 12 familiar (and acoustically different) spondees. The **Monosyllabic Identification Test** contains 12 monosyllables, all starting with "b."

The **Low-Verbal** version (Figure 5–5) contains three tests that parallel those in the Standard version but uses toys instead of pictures. In the **Low-Verbal Pattern Perception Test**, the examiner must select four objects, one from each of the stress-pattern categories. In the **Low-Verbal Spondee Identification Test**, four of six two-syllable words are selected for testing. In the **Low-Verbal Word Identification Test**, four of six mono-syllabic words are selected.

The Low-Verbal version is one of the only tests available for 2-year-old children, and is therefore an important contribution. However, with only four test items it is not clear how the test results generalize to realistic speech-perception abilities. It is also advisable to record and report which test items were selected, as the items are probably not equally difficult. We try to use "french fries, popcorn, airplane, hot dog," and "ball, book, bird, boat" for our test stimuli, to be consistent across children and over time. An audio cassette and a computer program are available.

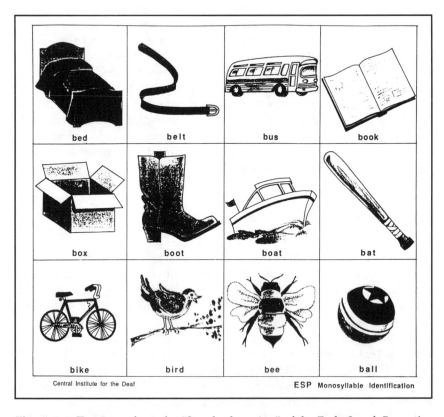

Figure 5–4. Test items from the "Standard version" of the *Early Speech Perception Test* developed by Moog and Geers (1990). (Reprinted from Moog, J. S., & Geers, A. E. (1990). *Early Speech Perception Test*. St. Louis, MO: Central Institute for the Deaf, with permission.)

Northwestern University Children's Perception of Speech (NU-CHIPS)

This four-choice picture-pointing test (Figure 5–6) uses the most frequently occurring phonemes in English (Elliott & Katz, 1980). The foils were selected to be phonemically similar to the test item. Hearing-impaired children with receptive language abilities of at least 2.6 years (measured by the Peabody Picture Vocabulary Test; Dunn, 1965) should be familiar with the words and pictures of the test. Another advantage is that the test has been widely used. A tape recording of the test is available.

Toy Discrimination Test

This test was designed for children with "a mental age of two" (McCormick, 1977, p. 71), and uses actual toys, not pictures. The toys are placed in front of the child, and the child must select one of the toys in response to the test stimulus. There are phonetic similarities among some of the items (e.g., plate

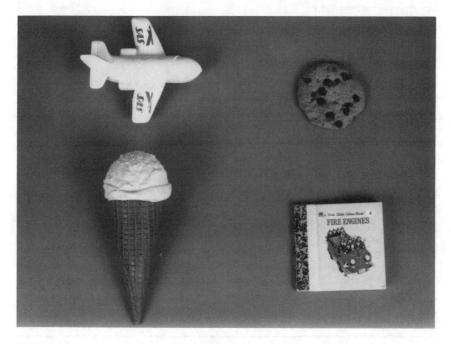

Figure 5–5. Examples of the test items from the "Low-Verbal" version of the Early Speech Perception Test developed by Moog and Geers (1990). (Reprinted from Moog, J. S., & Geers, A. E. (1990). *Early Speech Perception Test.* St. Louis, MO: Central Institute for the Deaf, with permission.)

and plane; sheep, key, and tree). It is suggested that a subset of the items can be selected depending on the vocabulary of the child. If this were the case, a record of the test items used should be maintained.

Word Intelligibility by Picture Identification (WIPI)

This six-choice picture-pointing test (Ross & Lerman, 1971) is one of the most widely used (Figure 5–7). Many of the foils share phonetic similarities with test items. The test is recommended for children ages five to six with a moderate hearing loss and to ages seven or eight for those with severe hearing loss. At the University of Iowa, we use a "reduced-set WIPI," eliminating some of the less-familiar items so that a subset can be administered to younger children. A few of the pictures are somewhat

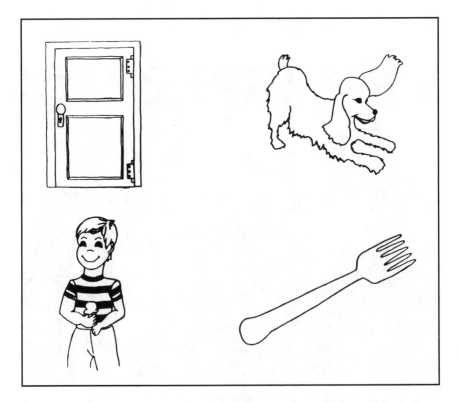

Figure 5–6. An example of a response set for the NU-CHIPS (Elliott & Katz, 1980). The task is "Show me ... dog," for example. (Reprinted from Elliott, K., & Katz, D. (1980). *Development of a new children's test of speech discrimination*. St. Louis, MO: Auditec, with permission.)

dated. The test is often administered audiovisually, although the lists are probably not equally difficult. Audiotape recordings are available.

OPEN-SET WORD RECOGNITION

Phonetically Balanced Kindergarten Test (PBK)

This widely used open-set word recognition test (Haskins, 1949) has four lists of 50 words. It can be scored based on the number of phonemes or number of words identified correctly. It is one of the few open-set word-recognition tests developed for children. Although the test was produced in 1949, only a few of the items are beyond the vocabulary of most of today's 6-year-old hearing-impaired children. At the University of Iowa, we utilize a 20-word subset that can be administered to many 3-year-olds. A tape recording is available.

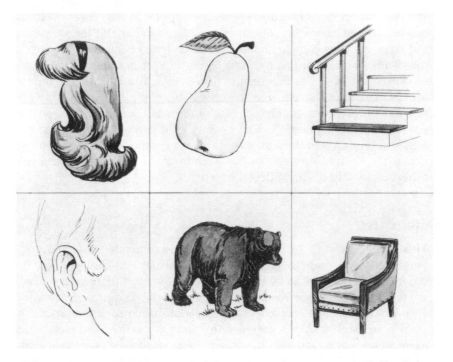

Figure 5–7. An example of a response set for the Word Intelligibility by Picture Identification (WIPI). (Reprinted from Ross, M., & Lerman, J., 1971. *Word Intelligibility by Picture Identification*. Pittsburgh: Stanwix House, Inc., with permission.)

SENTENCE PERCEPTION

Bamford-Kowal-Bench Sentences (BKB)

This test (Bench & Bamford, 1979) was developed in the United Kingdom, based on vocabulary and grammar produced by 8- to 16-year-old hearing-impaired children. The child is presented with a single sentence and must repeat as many words from the sentence as possible. The sentences are all simple statements. The number of keywords correctly identified is scored, although sometimes all the words (excluding articles) are scored. Some of the words are peculiar to British English. Tyler, Preece, and Tye-Murray (1986) adapted 100 sentences for use in the United States. This test is available on laser videodisc. Others in the United States and Australia have also produced modified recordings of the original BKB sentences.

Common Phrases Test

This test attempts to measure speech perception in a setting where the child has some contextual information (Osberger et al., 1991a). Before the test begins, a pretest topic familiarization is done by showing the child a card with 10 different pictures and telling him or her that the following sentences will be about the pictures. The card is removed before the test begins. The child is required to repeat short, highly predictable and familiar phrases. For statements, the entire sentence must be repeated. For questions, the question must be answered precisely. The test is presented in audition and audition-plus-vision conditions. A disadvantage is that the ability to remember the topic from the pretest pictures could differ across children and affect the results.

Matrix Test

This sentence test (Tyler & Holstad, 1987) was intended for children as young as 4 to 6 years of age. A closed-set format was chosen to control the learning effects associated with repeated presentations and to make the test independent of vocabulary, language, and cognitive maturation. Figure 5–8 shows the two different levels of difficulty of materials. The child is presented with a sentence that is composed of one word from each column, and responds by either repeating the sentence or pointing to the words. The test can be too easy for some children who perform well with their cochlear implant.

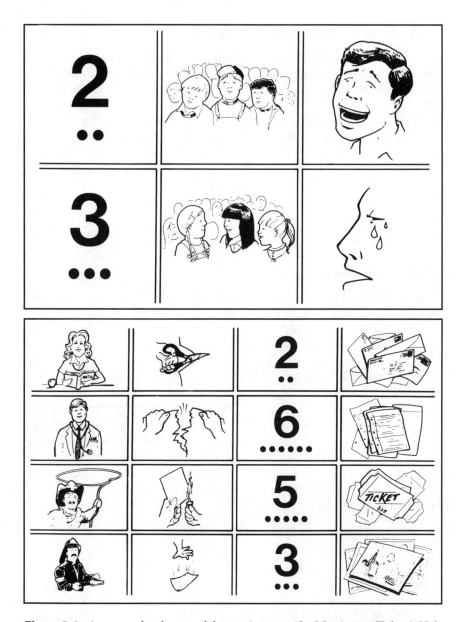

Figure 5–8. An example of some of the test items on the Matrix test (Tyler & Holstad, 1987). The top shows Level A, and the bottom shows Level B. The task is "Show me … two children cry," or "Show me … The cowboy drops three letters." (Reprinted from Tyler, R. S., & Holstad, B. (1987). *A closed-set speech perception test for hearing-impaired children.* Iowa City: University of Iowa, with permission.)

Pediatric Speech Intelligibility Sentence Test

This is a four-choice closed-set sentence test (Jerger, Lewis, Hawkins, & Jerger, 1980). The sentences and vocabulary were carefully obtained from the production of 3- to 9-year-old hearing-impaired children (see also Jerger, Jerger, & Lewis, 1981). Format I sentences are of the noun-verb-object type, preceded by "show me" (e.g., "Show me a rabbit painting an egg"). Format II omits the "show me" (e.g., "A rabbit is painting an egg"). Each format has two five-sentence lists and a card containing five pictures, one of which the child must select. The sentences are appropriate for many young children.

The **Glendonald Auditory Screening Procedure** (see above) also contains sentence material.

VOWEL AND CONSONANT FEATURE PERCEPTION

Audiovisual Feature Test

This test (Tyler, Fryauf-Bertschy, & Kelsay, 1991) was developed to examine speech-feature perception in young children. Figure 5–9 presents a sample response form used to administer the test. The stimulus materials include seven alphabet letters (see also Ross & Randolph, 1990, who developed a test using all alphabet letters) and three words that are recognized by many 4- to 5-year-old deaf children. One advantage of the test is its ability to provide information about speech features; for example, nasality, place of articulation, and manner. The closed-set format means that the test can be repeated without the items being learned from test to test. Therefore, multiple presentations in different audiovisual modalities are possible. One difficulty is the test is lengthy, although it can be given in several sessions. Using the same response form and a limited stimulus set can result in a test that is not very interesting for some children. It is also necessary to ensure that the children consider all the alternatives.

Change/No Change Test

This test contains nonsense syllables produced by a male talker. The stimuli examine one characteristic in each of seven subtests (Osberger et al., 1991b): syllable length, intonation, fundamental frequency, talker gender, vowel height, vowel place, and consonant manner. The stimuli are presented in a series, such as "ba ba ba ba ba ba ba ba" or "ba ba ba ba ba pa pa pa pa pa." After each presentation, the child must decide whether the stimuli in that series "changed" or "did not change."

The main advantage of the test is that it examines speech features in young children. One disadvantage of the test is that chance performance is 50%. Another is that only 15 trials are used for each feature, so that discovering a significant difference between two presentations for a particular feature requires a large difference.

Childrens Vowel Perception Test

This test (Tyler, Fryauf-Bertschy, & Kelsay, 1991) was designed to measure vowel recognition in young children. There are five sets of pictures, each with four items. Within each group of four, the items (e.g., hit, hat, hot, hurt) differ by only the medial vowel. Figure 5–10 presents a sample response form used to administer the test, which can be given audiovisually. The test may be easy for some children who perform well with their implant.

Indiana Minimal Pairs

This test (Osberger et al., 1991a) contains pairs of pictured words that differ in one speech feature. The child is shown a pair, hears a word, and

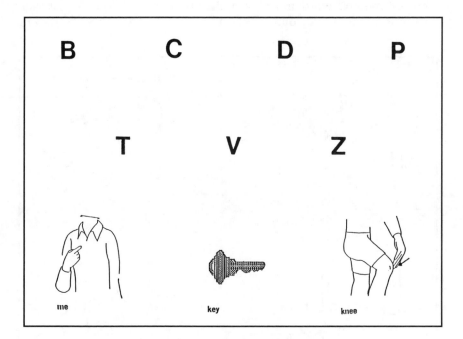

Figure 5–9. Response items of the Audiovisual Feature Test. Each item is of the form consonant-/i/. The task is "Show me the 'Vee' ...," for example. (Reprinted from Tyler, R. S., Fryauf-Bertschy, H., & Kelsay, D. 1991. *Audiovisual Feature Test for Young Children.* Iowa City: University of Iowa, with permission.)

must select among the two items. The advantage of the test is that it is one of the few tests available to test feature perception in young deaf children. One of the disadvantages of the test is that chance performance is 50%, so many items must be presented to determine a significant difference, particularly when the individual features are of interest.

Phonetic Task Evaluation

This speech-feature test (Mecklenburg, Shallop, & Ling, 1987) examines pitch, manner, place, voicing, and vowel perception. In the discrimination version, the child reports whether two items are the same or different. The identification task has six alternatives. The discrimination and identification tasks require different skills, and the results from each should be reported separately. The test requires a substantial amount of time to administer. An audiotape is available.

Speech Pattern Contrast Test (SPAC)

This test requires word and phrase identification in a closed set of four response items (Boothroyd, 1984). The suprasegmental contrasts are

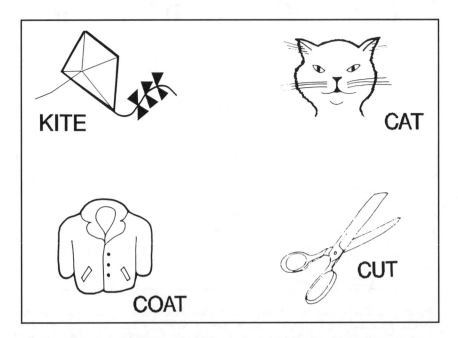

Figure 5–10. The four-choice vowel test, developed at the University of Iowa. Each set of four pictures differs by only the medial vowel. (Reprinted from Tyler, R. S., Fryauf-Bertschy, H., & Kelsay, D. [unpublished], with permission.)

vowel height and place, initial and final consonant voicing, continuance, and place. Suprasegmental contrasts include word stress and pitch rise/fall. Advantages include the use of meaningful stimuli. The 12 items in each subtest can be repeated to increase reliability. The main disadvantage is that the required vocabulary and reading level is high. Boothroyd (1991) suggests that this restricts the test to children older than 10 years. The test is available on audiotapes and laser videodisc.

A similar test was developed for younger children, called the **Imitative SPAC (IMSPAC)** (Boothroyd, 1991). For this test the child is asked to orally imitate a normal-hearing talker. These utterances are recorded, edited, and used as test stimuli in a listening test for a group of normal subjects. The normal-hearing subjects listen to the child's production, for example, "see," and must select the correct production among four choices, for example, "dee, zee, see, tee." Limitations imposed by speech production skills are quantified by using any appropriate combination of inputs, including audition, lipreading, fingerspelling, text, or sign. Although the editing of the tapes requires considerable time, Boothroyd believes the task is appropriate for postlingually deafened children who were deafened as young as 2 years old.

Three-Interval Forced-Choice Test of Speech Pattern Contrast Perception (THRIFT)

This test was designed to obtain speech feature information from 5- to 6-year-old children (Boothroyd, 1986). It utilizes similar feature contrasts to those used in the SPAC, except in a three-interval forced-choice format. For example, the child hears "dee zee zee" and must select the first one as different. Boothroyd reports that the oddity paradigm is unsuitable for children less than 5 years of age, but the monotonous nature of the task makes it difficult for some 7-year-olds. A "Minithrift" version is available (Boothroyd, 1991) using fewer test items and can be given when less time is available for testing. Both versions are recorded on audiotape and laser videodisc.

The **Auditory Perception of Alphabet Letters** (see above) test also provides some information about phonetic perception.

AUDIOVISUAL ENHANCEMENT

Craig Lipreading Inventory

This test contains both a word and a sentence test (Craig, 1964). Both are four-choice closed-set tests, and utilize pictures. The sentence material contains straightforward relational sentences (e.g., "a drum is on a chair"). Children must have the appropriate language concepts for the sentence test. One potential advantage could be achieved if the same stimuli were presented in all modalities. The test would then be equally difficult for all presentations. Because it is a closed-set format, the effects of learning the stimuli are not a concern. An audiovisual tape recording of this test is available.

Hoosier Auditory Visual Enhancement Test (HAVE)

This test is a three-choice, closed-set picture test (Osberger et al., 1991a). Two of the three items in the set are homophenous (that is, they are visually similar). The test is presented in an audiovisual condition only, but is scored for "visual" correctness (either of the two homophenous words would be considered correct), or "word correctness." However, since the test is not given in vision alone, it is difficult to determine the actual contribution of lipreading to the audiovisual score. The test appears easy for many children with cochlear implants, so ceiling effects may be a problem.

The **Word Intelligibility by Pictures Index** and the **Audiovisual Feature Test** were also designed to be given audiovisually. The **Bamford-Kowal-Bench** sentence test is also frequently administered audiovisually.

SPEECH-PERCEPTION ABILITIES

We focus on five different areas of speech perception in children with cochlear implants; envelope and stress perception, environmental sound perception, closed-set word recognition, open-set word recognition, sentence recognition, vowel and consonant recognition, and audiovisual enhancement. No attempt is made to cite all published work, only to provide a broad basis for an understanding of the abilities and limitations of speech perception in this population.

ENVELOPE AND STRESS PERCEPTION

The ability to recognize the stress or envelope patterns of words is one of the easier speech-perception tasks, requiring only perception of time-intensity information (see Dorman, Chapter 4). Its perception can be useful for syllabic demarcation and to identify an emphasized word in a sentence. Sometimes it can be used to recognize the talker identity, distinguish a statement or question, and distinguish a stern or humorous voice. It can also be a useful supplement to lipreading. Stress and envelope perception do not provide in and of themselves sufficient information to communicate effectively.

The Cochlear Corporation has coordinated a study of children from several centers (Staller et al., 1991b) using the Nucleus multichannel cochlear implant (Clark, Tong, & Patrick, 1990; see Wilson, Chapter 2). On the MTS stress test, 83 children (age at onset unspecified) averaged 64% correct (*sd* = 24) after 12 months of use.

Figure 5–11 shows the results from these children on the MTS stress test for children with congenital, prelingual-noncongenital, postlingual with more than 2 years of deafness before receiving their implant, and postlingual with 2 years or less of profound deafness before receiving their implant. Children who became deaf after 2 years of age were called postlingually deafened. Although the postlingually deafened children clearly show higher scores than the other groups, the distributions of the other three populations are similar. Each group has children that perform well and do not perform above chance. The congenital group has 10 of 43 (23%) who did not score significantly above chance, indicating they are not able to utilize stress cues.

Figure 5–12 compares the preimplant and 12-month postimplant results. Fourteen of the 56 (25%) children did not perform significantly above chance after 12 months of implant use. Twenty-three of the 56 children (41%) showed a statistically significant increase in their 12-month score compared to their preimplant score.

Osberger et al. (1991a) compared performance in 11 children using the House single-channel cochlear implant (Danley & Fretz, 1982) with that of 11 children using the Nucleus multichannel implant. The children in both groups were mostly prelingual. On the MTS stress test, children with the House cochlear implant averaged 52% correct (*sd* = 25) and children with the Nucleus implant averaged 74% correct (*sd* = 14).

On the Change/No Change test, the average score of 11 children with the House implant was 66% (*sd* = 25) on syllable duration, 51% (*sd* = 10) on intonation, 61% (*sd* = 21) on fundamental frequency, and 58% (*sd* = 14) on gender recognition (Osberger et al., 1991a). With a chance score of 50% on the test, it appears that most of these children could not perceive these characteristics. The 11 Nucleus children scored 94% (*sd* = 9), 64% (*sd* = 21), 79% (*sd* = 18), and 79% correct (*sd* = 21), respectively, on the same four tests. A statistical advantage for children with the Nucleus patients was found for the syllable-duration and talker-gender test. Similar scores were reported by Osberger et al. (1991b) for a larger group of Nucleus subjects.

On a test requiring the identification of the number of syllables in a word (designed for adults; Tyler, Preece, & Lowder, 1983), Staller et al. (1991a) observed that 16 children with the Nucleus implant averaged

54% correct (*sd* = 19.5). Staller et al. (1991b) reported that 65 children averaged 63.9% correct (*sd* = 20.3) on a test requiring them to identify a talker as being male or female (a test designed for adults; Tyler, Preece, & Lowder, 1983).

It is notable that many children perform poorly on these tasks of envelope-stress perception. About one-quarter of the children do not score above chance on the MTS stress test. Some of the distinctions, for example between spondees and trochees, require amplitude or voicing fundamental-frequency discrimination of which they are incapable. Many children apparently cannot tell whether a voice is produced by a male or female talker. These results were largely obtained after only 12 months of implant use, and it is likely that performance will improve for most of these children.

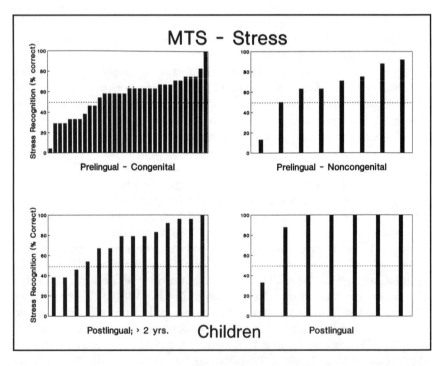

Figure 5–11. Results on the Monosyllable-Trochee-Spondee (MTS) stress test obtained from children using the Nucleus cochlear implant after 12-months of use (Data from Staller et al., 1991b). The "postlingual; >2 yrs." group represent postlingually deafened children who were implanted 2 years or more after becoming profoundly deaf. Data above the dashed line represent a significant difference from chance (one-tailed test) at the 95% confidence level, using the binomial model and 0 variance associated with chance (Thornton & Raffin, 1978).

ENVIRONMENTAL SOUND RECOGNITION

One important contribution of the cochlear implant is that it can provide children the opportunity to perceive everyday sounds. These sounds provide valuable information about the environment in which they live. This includes an awareness of when they are being called, when the telephone or doorbell ring, recognition of musical instruments, and so forth (see Bilger & Hopkinson, 1977; Tyler, Moore, & Kuk, 1989).

Staller (1991b) reported that 57 out of 58 children detected the presence of environmental sounds presented at 70 dB SPL. Thirty of 58 (52%) children scored above chance on the Sound Effects Recognition Test.

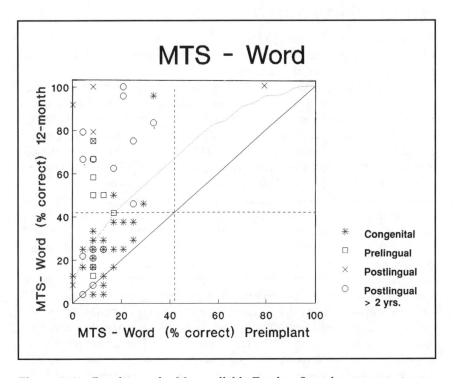

Figure 5–12. Results on the Monosyllable-Trochee-Spondee stress test comparing preimplant and 12-month, postoperative performance for children using the Nucleus cochlear implant. Data to the right of the vertical dashed line represent preoperative data that are significantly different from chance. Data above the horizontal dashed line represent 12-month data that are significantly different from chance. Data above the curved, dotted line represent a significant increase in 12-month postoperative performance compared to preimplant performance (two-tailed test) at the 95% confidence level, using the binomial model (Thornton & Raffin, 1978). (Data provided by Staller from Staller et al., 1991b.)

Osberger et al. (1991b) reported that 24 children (prelingual and postlingual combined) with the Nucleus implant averaged 52% correct (sd = 23) on the Sound Effects Recognition Test (chance is 25%). About 50% of the children scored above 40% correct.

Thus it appears that about one-half of the children with the Nucleus cochlear implant can recognize some environmental sounds without visual cues. It is likely that most obtain useful additional visual and contextual cues. Learning to associate the sounds perceived through the cochlear implant while interacting with the environment will likely improve performance in most of these children.

CLOSED-SET WORD RECOGNITION

Testing word recognition in children, in a closed-set format, offers the advantage that all the alternatives are available to the child. Cognitive and vocabulary factors are minimized.

Geers and Moog (1989) studied 12 of the better-scoring children (presumably chosen from over two hundred) with the House implant (see also Moog & Geers, 1991). Scores on the Standard Version of their Early Speech Perception tests ranged from 17/24 to 24/24 correct (chance performance is 6/24) on Pattern Perception, from 10/24 to 24/24 correct (chance performance is 2/24) on Spondee Identification, and from 12/24 to 21/24 correct (chance performance is 2/24) on Monosyllable Identification.

Geers and Moog (1991) reported on four children with the Nucleus cochlear implant ages 2 to 10 years (see also Moog & Geers, 1991). They were matched to two other groups, one with hearing aids and one with tactile aids. The variables on which they were matched included age, general speech-perception ability, pretrial language, intelligence, the percentage of speech sounds that they produced that were intelligible, and family support. All became deaf before age 4. Children with cochlear implants typically outperformed children from the other two groups. A 2-year-old scored 95% correct pattern recognition and 60% correct word recognition on the Low-verbal tests. Two of the other three implanted children also showed significant improvements on the Early Speech Perception pattern and word tests, when their preimplant hearing-aid performance was compared with their 12-month cochlear implant performance.

Several groups have evaluated performance on the MTS word test. Eighty-four (prelingual and postlingual) children with the Nucleus implant averaged 39% correct (sd = 29) after 1 year of implant use (Staller et al., 1991b) (chance performance is 25% correct). The individual results for different implant groups are shown in Figure 5–13 (see also Staller et al., 1991a). Clearly the congenitally deaf children performed poorly on this test, and 6 of the 7 postlingual deafened children performed very well. The distributions of the prelingual-noncongenital group and the postlingual-deafened group who were implanted after more than two years of deafness overlap substantially. Only 3 of 33 (9%) of the congenitally deaf children scored above 40% correct after 12 months of implant use.

Figure 5–14 compares the pre- and 12-month postimplant data. About 31 of the 53 (58%) children did not perform significantly above chance after 12 months of implant use. Twenty (38%) showed a statistically significant increase between preimplant and 12-month postimplant testing.

Osberger et al. (1991b) noted that 28 (prelingual and postlingual) children with the Nucleus implant averaged 50% (*sd* = 31) on the MTS word score. They also noted (Osberger et al. 1991a) that 11 children with the

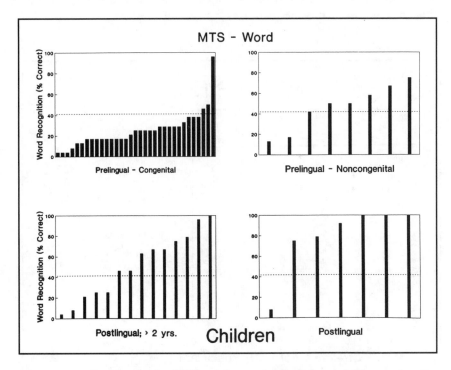

Figure 5–13. Results on the MTS-word test obtained from children using the Nucleus cochlear implant after 12-months of use (data from Staller et al., 1991b). Data above the dashed line represent a significance difference from chance (one-tailed test) at the 95% confidence level using the binomial model and 0 variance associated with chance .

Nucleus implant outperformed (mean = 44% correct, *sd* = 24) 11 children with the House implant (mean = 19% correct, *sd* = 17).

Boothroyd, Geers, and Moog (1991) provide a novel way of examining scores of cochlear-implanted children. The solid curvilinear line in Figure 5–15 (top) shows the average MTS word score of children using **hearing aids** as a function of their three-frequency-average hearing threshold. The data points in the lower right-hand corner are the performance of a different set of 53 children, again using **hearing aids**. Nearly all of these children failed to demonstrate word recognition. Figure 5–15 (bottom) shows the performance of the same 53 children after 12 months of use with the Nucleus **cochlear implant**. About one-third to one-half of these children perceived spectral information, as measured by this test. Boothroyd and colleagues also noted that performance of the implanted children was unrelated to their preoperative hearing thresholds. In addition, about 20% of the children performed like children using hearing aids with pure-tone thresholds of less than about 90 dB HL.

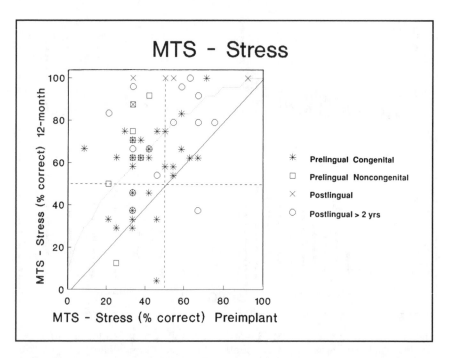

Figure 5–14. The results on the MTS-word test from children with the Nucleus cochlear implant comparing preimplant and postimplant (12 months) performance. (Data from Staller et al., 1991b.)

Staller et al. (1991a) reported that 16 children averaged 23% correct (*sd* = 10.1) on the Word Intelligibility by Picture Identification test (chance performance is 25%). Pre- and postlingual children were not distinguished. Similar results were reported by Tyler (1990) and Fryauf-Bertschy, Tyler, Kelsay, and Gantz (1992).

Staller et al. (1991b) reported that 54 children averaged 42% correct (*sd* = 19) (chance performance is 25%) on the Northwestern University Children's Perception of Speech test. Osberger et al. (1991b) reported that 22 children with the Nucleus implant averaged 44% correct (*sd* = 17).

In summary, there are large differences in the children's ability to identify words in a closed-set response format. Some of these differences may be related to the use of live voice testing, particularly because familiar talkers were used in some test situations. Perhaps as many as one-half of the children with the Nucleus cochlear implant demonstrate performance above chance. Some obtain high levels of performance (70–100% correct), whereas many others obtain no measurable benefit. Congenitally deaf children who have used their implant for only 12 months typically perform very poorly on this closed-set task.

OPEN-SET WORD RECOGNITION

Word perception without any knowledge of the possible set of response alternatives is much more difficult than closed-set recognition. Open-set testing also more closely represents the communication situations in real life. In natural speech perception we seldom are given four alternatives from which to select our response. Open-set word recognition, therefore, represents a better test of the actual speech-perception benefit.

Fifty children using the House implant were evaluated by Berliner, Tonokawa, Dye, & House, (1989). They used the 12 words in the GASP as stimuli and presented them without providing the children with the response alternatives. If any of these children had been administered the MTS or GASP previously, it could compromise the interpretation of this as a true open-set test. One child scored 9/12 items correct, three scored 8/12 items correct, and 4 scored 6/12 items correct. Staller et al. (1991b), also administering the GASP "open set," noted that 47 children averaged 24% correct (*sd* = 29). On the PB-K test, Staller et al. (1991b) reported that 25 children with the Nucleus cochlear implant averaged 12% correct (*sd* = 23). However, this may overestimate the typical ability because some of the test centers may have chosen not to test children whom they expected to score at chance on this difficult test. For example, only 25 children took the PB-K word test, 87 took the MTS word test, and 111 children took the Discrimination After Training test. Consistent with this contention is the lower scores reported by Osberger et al. (1991b), who noted that all 24 children studied by their group with the Nucleus implant averaged only 6% correct ($sd = 7$).

Staller et al. (1991a) reported that the 26 children who were administered the NU-6 test (designed for adults, Tillman & Carhart, 1966) averaged 4% correct ($sd = 9$).

Dowell et al. (1991) reported the speech-perception abilities of five (four were prelingual) of the better performers from 21 children implanted in Melbourne, Australia. Their scores on the AB word list (designed for adults; Boothroyd, 1968) were 30, 38, 39, 42, and 72% correct.

Thus, it would appear that a very small proportion of the children with cochlear implants obtained open-set word recognition after 12 months of use. However, in a few children high levels of word recognition have been observed. Most of the children are postlingually deafened, but a few were prelingually deaf.

SENTENCE PERCEPTION

Important differences exist between the perception of an isolated word and a continuous string of words (e.g., Summerfield, 1983). When an isolated word is presented the listener can devote seconds of processing time to evaluate, compare, and analyze the utterance. Continuous speech, however, must be processed quickly. This effect makes continuous speech more difficult to perceive than isolated words (Bilger, 1983). In addition, coarticulation can alter the acoustic characteristics of speech in sentences, sometimes changing the cues used to identify speech features.

However, there is another effect rendering sentences easier to perceive. The grammatical and vocabulary constraints imposed by language facilitates sentence perception, an advantage not present when individual words are used alone (see Boothroyd & Nittrouer, 1988; Miller, Heise & Lichten, 1951; for additional details).

Staller et al. (1991b) reported the results on the CID sentence test (designed for adults; Silverman & Hirsh, 1955) obtained from 43 subjects with 12-months experience with the Nucleus cochlear implant. The average score was 13% correct ($sd = 24$). Twenty-two (51%) recognized one or more correct words, with one child achieving 100% correct. Individual data for this group are shown in Figure 5–16. Congenitally and prelingual-noncongenital deafened children are not able to recognize many words in sentences without visual clues after 12 months of implant use. Three of the 17 postlingual more than 2 years children and 6 of the 8 postlingual children scored over 20% correct.

Staller et al. (1991a) noted that four children averaged 63% correct ($sd = 28$) on the BKB sentences, particularly high scores. Dowell et al. (1991)

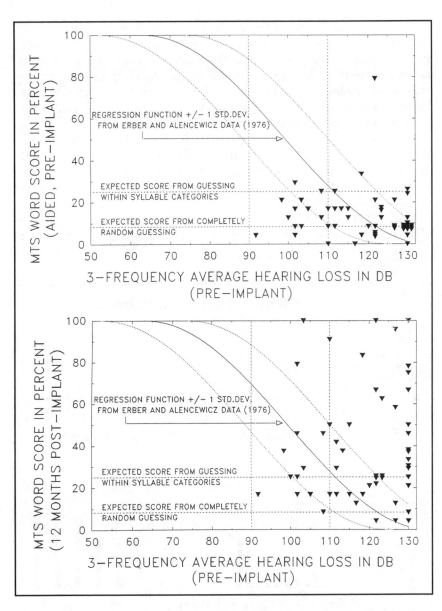

Figure 5–15. (Top) Preoperative data from children using hearing aids on the MTS-word test, as a function of their hearing threshold three-frequency average. (Bottom) Postoperative data from children using the Nucleus cochlear implant on the MTS-word test, as a function of their preimplant hearing threshold three-frequency average. See text for details. (Reprinted from Boothroyd, A., Geers, A. E., & Moog, J. S. (1991). Practical implications of cochlear implants in children. *Ear and Hearing, 12* (Suppl. 4), 81S–89S, with permission.)

reported that the 3 best of the 21 children in Melbourne scored 25, 35, and 75% correct on the same test, suggesting substantially lower scores in the Australian sample. The other 18 children failed to show any open-set recognition. It is possible that some of the children reported by Staller and colleagues from the multicenter trial were tested because there was some expectation that they would perform well, and others were not tested because of pessimistic expectations.

Berliner et al. (1989) reported on 41 children who used the House implant. They were required to answer the 10 questions on the GASP. One child scored 10/10, two scored 8/10, one scored 7/10, and two scored 6/10. Staller et al (1991a) noted that 21 children scored 29.5% correct ($sd = 39$) on the GASP questions.

Tyler (1990) used the closed-set Matrix sentence test in contrasting the results of 5 children with the Nucleus implant (Figure 5–17 top) to 10 of

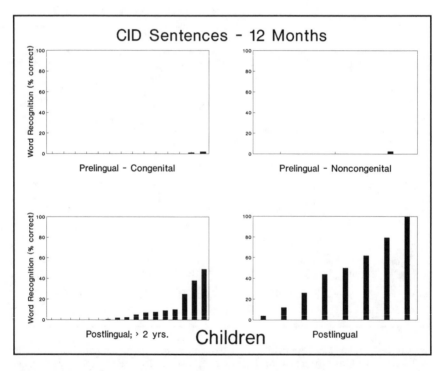

Figure 5–16. The performance of children with the Nucleus cochlear implant on the Central Institute for the Deaf Sentence test (data from Staller et al., 1991b). Each tic mark along the horizontal axis represents the results from one child. The absence of a bar indicates 0 percent correct. The test is open set.

the better children with the House cochlear implant (selected among over a hundred children) (Figure 5–17 bottom). On the easier Level A test, the one congenitally deaf child with the Nucleus implant scored higher than 9 of the 10 better children with the House implant.

In summary, sentence perception is beyond the abilities of many children who have used cochlear implants for 12 months. As with word perception, however, there are also several examples of prelingual and postlingual children who score above 50% correct.

VOWEL AND CONSONANT FEATURE PERCEPTION

Because vowels and consonants represent the building blocks to word recognition, it is important to carefully study their perception. This approach is particularly useful when the test is designed to elucidate the particular phonemes or speech features (see Dorman, Chapter 4) that are perceived and misperceived.

Geers and Moog (1991) reported that three children with the Nucleus implant averaged 32% above chance on the vowel subtest of the Phonetic Task Evaluation. On the consonant subset, the average performance for a 6-, 7-, and 10-year-old child was 8, 10, and 2% above chance on the features of manner, place, and voice.

Using the Change/No Change test, Osberger et al. (1991a) reported that 11 children with the House implant averaged 59% (*sd* = 18) and 61% (*sd* = 17) correct on the vowel-height and place subtests, and 11 children with the Nucleus implant averaged 88% (*sd* = 20) and 82% (*sd* = 17) correct, respectively. On the consonant subtests of voicing, manner and place, the children with the House implant scored 52% (*sd* = 6), 59% (*sd* = 14) and 65% (*sd* = 20) correct, respectively. The children with the Nucleus implant averaged 60% (*sd* = 14), 86% (*sd* = 14), and 77% (*sd* = 18) correct, respectively. All group differences were significant except the "place" difference. Similar scores for 28 children with the Nucleus implant were reported by Osberger et al. (1991b).

Boothroyd (1991) showed data from one 3-year-old implanted child with the Nucleus implant on the Imitative Test of Speech Pattern Contrast Perception. Perception of vowel height and place was greater than 70% correct, but consonant perception was poor.

Tyler (1990) assessed five children using the Nucleus implant on a closed set of 10 vowels in a /b/-vowel-/d/ context. An information transmission analysis indicated 39, 31, and 30% information transmitted for the features of second-formant frequency, first-formant frequency and duration, respectively. Four of the children were administered a 13-set consonant recognition task, in the /i/-consonant-/i/ context. An

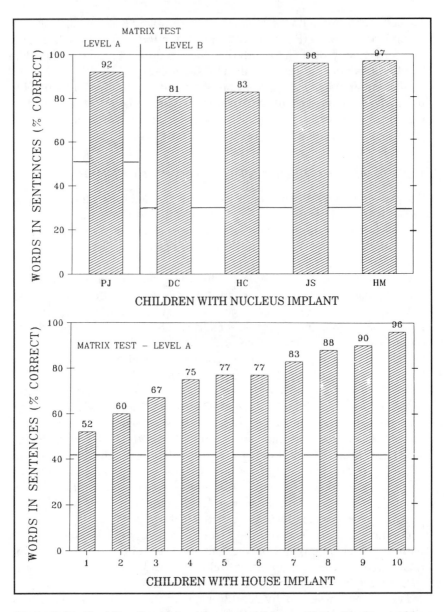

Figure 5–17. (Top) Results obtained from six children with the Nucleus cochlear implant on the Matrix test. (Bottom) The results from 10 of the better children with the House single channel implant. (Reprinted from Tyler, R. S., & Holstad, B. (1987). *A closed-set speech perception test for hearing-impaired children.* Iowa City: University of Iowa, with permission.)

information transmission analysis suggested that the nasal, voicing, and envelope features were best transmitted. The place feature was the most difficult to transmit. These observations are consistent with those made by Dowell et al. (1991), who reported data from four representative children who had used their implants for more than two years.

Tyler (1991) reported preliminary results from five children using the Nucleus implant on the Audiovisual Feature Test. An information transmission analysis indicated that voicing and nasality features were transmitted more effectively than frication, duration, and place features.

Osberger et al. (1991b) reported on 28 children using the Nucleus cochlear implant on the Indiana Minimal Pairs test. The average scores for vowel height and place were 79% (*sd* = 21) and 74% (*sd* = 22) correct, respectively, and for consonant manner, place and voicing were 65% (*sd* = 21), 64% (*sd* = 13) and 61% (*sd* = 19) correct, respectively (chance performance is 50%).

There are only limited data on the kinds of speech features perceived by children using cochlear implants. Some children appear to be able to make use of information about voicing, timing, and envelope cues. As with the adult patients, the transmission of information about formant frequencies and their trajectories, and frication, is more difficult to hear.

AUDIOVISUAL ENHANCEMENT

Perhaps the most practical advantage afforded by cochlear implants is the enhancement of lipreading. The perception of envelope time-intensity cues is sufficient to improve performance when combined with lipreading.

Staller et al. (1991b) reported data from 44 children using the Nucleus cochlear implant with the CID sentences in vision and audition-plus-vision. Twenty-five of 44 (57%) showed a statistically significant increase. On the WIPI test, however, they reported that only five children (13%) showed a significant enhancement.

Individual data from these children obtained on the WIPI test are shown in Figure 5–18 (top), which compares the vision-only to the vision-plus-audition scores. A wide range of vision-only scores are apparent for all groups. Data points above the diagonal represent an increase in lipreading ability provided by the implant. Although most children show an increase in the vision-plus-audition condition, only 8 out of 31 (26%) reach statistical significance. Figure 5–18 (bottom) shows the individual lipreading enhancement scores, calculated as the percentage of possible improvement (Tyler, 1991; Tyler, Opie, Fryauf-Bertschy, & Gantz, 1992; Walden, Erdman, Montgomery, Schwartz, & Prosek, 1981).

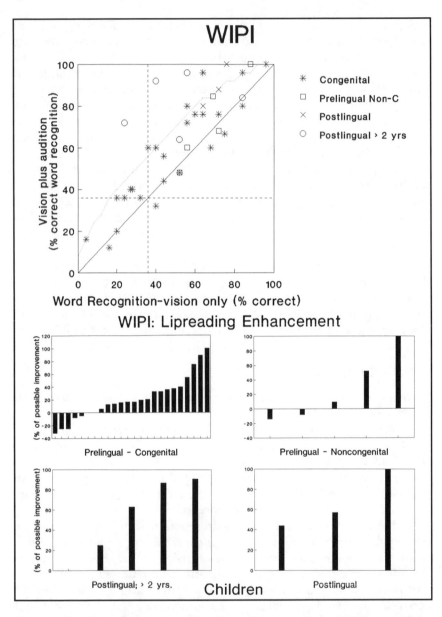

Figure 5–18. Vision alone and vision-plus-audition results on the Word Intelligibility by Picture Identification Test for children using the Nucleus cochlear implant (top). Data above the curved dotted line represent a significance increase in vision-plus-audition scores compared to vision-alone scores (one-tailed test) at the 95% confidence level using the binomial model (Thornton & Raffin, 1978). (Data from Staller et al., 1991b.) Audiovisual enhancement measured as the percentage of possible improvement on the WIPI test (bottom).

A very wide range of lipreading improvement was observed for the prelingual-congenital and prelingual-noncongenital groups. The better performance of the postlingual groups is evident.

Tyler et al. (1992) reported data from 12 children using the Nucleus device on the Audiovisual Feature Test. The results, shown in Figure 5–19, are divided into children who did not score above chance on the audition alone test (top) and those who did (bottom). The two groups show similar ranges in their lipreading scores. Across all features, there is an audiovisual enhancement over the lipreading score. This is true even in the group who failed to score above chance on the overall percent correct score. The audiovisual enhancement in the group who scored above chance in the audition condition was substantial for the voicing, nasality, and place features. The limited enhancement in lipreading in some children is difficult to understand. Many of the children were prelingually deaf, and lipreading enhancement may not be as great in this group because they lack templates for the acoustic and visual speech images, and the practice of integrating them. Another possibility may relate to the educational method used. Those children in "Combined" or "Total Communication" programs must watch both the face and the hands. This competition may hinder their ability to combine lipreading and auditory information.

PERFORMANCE AS A FUNCTION OF TIME

A large body of the results reported above are from children who have used their implants for only 12 months. It is of great interest to determine how speech perception of children with cochlear implants changes over time. Preliminary data from postlingually deafened adults shows that the greatest learning effects are for the first 6 to 18 months of use (Tye-Murray, Tyler, Woodworth, & Gantz, 1992; Tyler & Kelsay, 1990; Waltzman, Cohen, & Shapiro, 1986; see Dorman, Chapter 4), although some adults show improvement over much longer periods. Children, however, receive their implants with less experience listening to and coding speech. They are also typically fast learners. It is critical to determine if their performance stabilizes or even decreases after many years of electrical stimulation.

Staller et al. (1991b) reported the performance of a group of children implanted with the Nucleus device over a 36-month postoperative period. Figure 5–20 shows their results on a relatively simple task, the recognition of the talker gender, and of a more difficult one, the recognition of words on the Monosyllable-Trochee-Spondee test. On both tests, the performance increases at a very different rate for different children.

Fryauf-Bertschy et al. (1992) showed individual performance of 10 congenitally and three postlingually deafened children using the

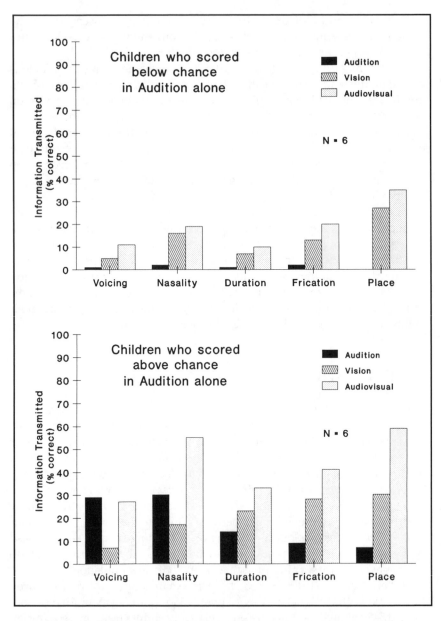

Figure 5–19. Audiovisual performance on the Audiovisual Feature Test on 6 children who scored at or below chance on the audition-alone condition (top) and on 6 children who scored above chance on the audition-alone condition. Averaged results are shown for the audition, vision, and audiovisual conditions. (Adapted from Tyler, Opie, Fryauf-Bertschy, & Gantz 1992.)

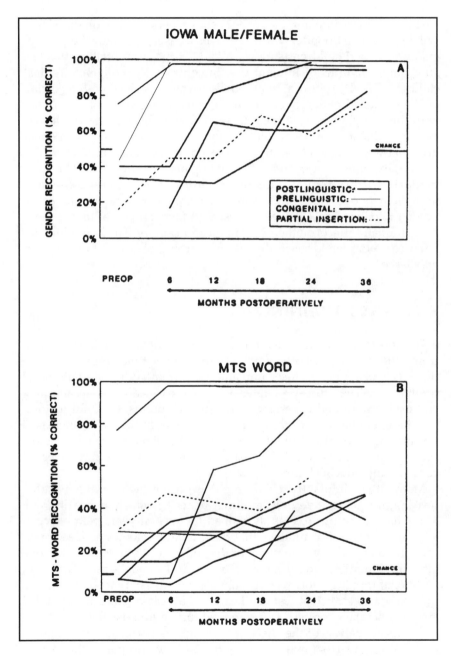

Figure 5–20. Performance over time for gender recognition (top) and the MTS-word test (bottom). (Adapted from Staller et al., 1991b.) Note that Staller et al., use 1/12 as the chance level on this test, whereas our approach is to use 1/4.

Nucleus cochlear implant. Figure 5–21 shows performance on the Mono-syllable-Trochee-Spondee word test over a 2-year period. The postlin-gually deafened children (subjects N11–N13) perform well on this test after only 6 months of implant use. In contrast, the congenitally deaf children (N1–N10) show a much slower learning curve than the postlin-gually deafened children. Some children require 2 years of experience with their implant before their scores fall significantly above chance. These results are consistent with the individual performance of 12 chil-dren followed over a 36-month period reported by Staller et al. (1991b).

Thus, experience over time with the implant is a critical variable, par-ticularly for prelingually deafened children. Most children show improvement over time, but long-term data and correlational studies are needed to determine if the levels of speech perception that they achieve have dramatic effects on their communication ability. The individual dif-ferences among children in the rate of learning to use the implant are very large.

EFFECTS OF TRAINING

It is important to distinguish the direct effect of the cochlear implant from other variables. For example, changes over time could be due to the effects of (1) the cochlear implant and formal auditory/audiovisual training (see Tye-Murray Chapter 3), (2) the cochlear implant and gen-eral exposure to and experience with speech sounds, (3) child matura-tion independent of receiving an implant or training, or (4) increased training and attention which might have occurred even without the cochlear implant. This is a vital issue in establishing the effectiveness of cochlear implants in children.

Many of the implanted children either do not hear anything with a hearing aid, or receive only minimal benefit from their hearing aid. Many have been unsuccessfully trained for several years before receiv-ing their implant. It is unlikely that the dramatic changes in speech-per-ception ability observed in many of the children (discussed above) soon after implantation would have occurred in these children because of additional training. However, it is appropriate to say that some children may have had sufficient residual hearing that was not adequately aided and may not have received sufficient auditory/audiovisual training.

A critical analysis of the effect of training was performed by Staller et al. (1991a), and is shown in Figure 5–22. They compared the perfor-mance of a group of 15 to 16 children before and after an 8-week preop-erative training period with that of the same children after 12 months of cochlear implant use. Performance for the Monosyllable-Trochee-

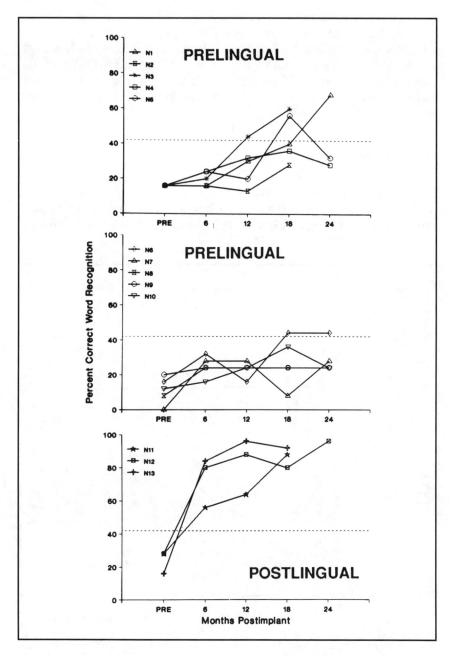

Figure 5–21. Performance over time of congenitally deaf (top two panels) and postlingually deaf (bottom panel) children. Each line represents data from a different child (Adapted from Fryauf-Bertschy et al., 1992.)

Spondee test shows the limited benefit of additional training in this group and the enhanced performance after using the implant.

Whether a child will benefit from additional auditory/audiovisual training depends on each individual child. It is the responsibility of the audiologist to ensure that the child is using the correct hearing aids, that they have been properly fit, that they remain in working order, and that they receive appropriate training.

EDUCATIONAL PLACEMENT

The educational placement of profoundly deaf children has been a controversial issue for many years (Lane, 1984). It is difficult to control all the possible factors in attempting to delineate which educational system is the best for

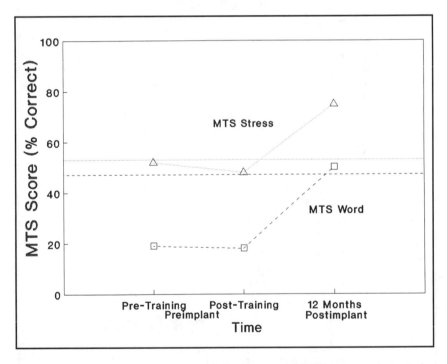

Figure 5–22. Performance of 15 and 16 children on the MTS stress and word test (respectively). Measurements were made before and after 8 weeks of training, prior to implantation. These measurements were repeated after 12 months of implant use (adapted from Staller et al., 1991a). Scores above the dotted and dashed line are significantly above chance at the 95% confidence level for the stress and word MTS test (respectively).

an individual child. Some initial attempts at comparing educational placements have been made in children with cochlear implants. Since they have more hearing than totally deaf children, the focus has been on comparing oral/aural schools with combined oral and an English-based sign system.

Berliner et al. (1989) studied children with the single-channel House device. They found that children in the oral/aural or cued speech systems generally performed higher than children in total communication programs, although there was substantial overlap.

Somers (1991) compared children trained in aural- or combined-educational environment. An attempt was made to match subgroups on important variables. All children became deaf before the age of three years, had similar language skills, and were between 4 and 9 years old. Recorded test materials included word, sentence, spondee, and pattern recognition. Figure 5–23 compares the results for children with hearing aids, cochlear implants (House and Nucleus), and a group of children who wore hearing aids although they had no usable hearing (a group considered to be the best control for the cochlear-implant group, since the other hearing-aid group would have had more hearing preoperatively than the cochlear-implant group). The totally deaf children with hearing aids performed the poorest and the combined-communication group also scored inferior to the other groups on a few tests. An additional comparison in that study between the two cochlear implant groups (six to seven children per group) suggested that the children with the Nucleus implant who received oral communication obtain the highest speech perception scores.

Osberger et al. (1991b) compared 12 children with the Nucleus implant using oral or cued-speech communication with 16 who were in total communication environments. Although scores were higher for children in the oral/cued group (see Osberger, et al., 1991b, Table 10), no significant differences were observed.

Staller et al. (1991b) compared the performance of 142 children using the Nucleus implant. The prelingually and postlingually deaf children were grouped according to those who obtained open-set word recognition to those who did not. They reported that more children in oral educational and mainstream programs were in the open-set speech-recognition category.

All of the above results should be treated with extreme caution, because it is difficult to match groups precisely for intellectual abilities, amount and quality of teaching, and auditory exposure in the home and at school. Furthermore, it may be that children who enter aural programs have more hearing and different skills than children who enter total-communication schools.

Some have argued that special schools should be established for children with cochlear implants. However, hearing-impaired children using cochlear implants, hearing aids, tactile aids or no assistive devices all deserve the same high-quality audiological and educational management. Furthermore, the introduction of cochlear implants has not created a new set of children requiring special attention. These profoundly hearing-impaired children were already present, and one would hope that the cochlear implant has facilitated their management.

Cochlear implants have not created a new issue regarding educational placement. The issue of whether an aural language or deaf language (such as American Sign Language in the United States) has not been altered by cochlear implants. What cochlear implants have done is provided additional hearing abilities to children who previously had very little or none. More children will now be considered appropriate for aural or aural/sign supported programs.

PREDICTING PERFORMANCE

It is important to determine if postoperative performance can be predicted based on some preimplant measurements. This might influence

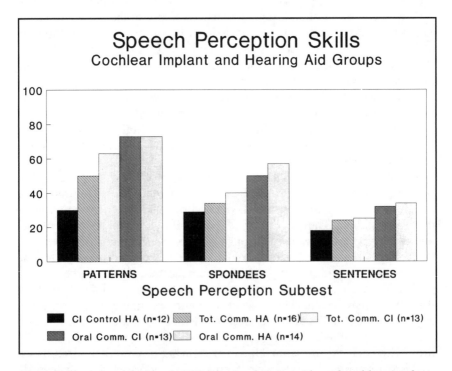

Figure 5–23. A comparison of children using hearing aids and cochlear implants in total communication and oral educational programs (see text). (Adapted from Somers, 1991.)

decisions about whether a child should receive an implant. For example, if it were certain that a child would derive dramatic benefit from a cochlear implant, then this might result in the child receiving the implant at a younger age. If the likelihood was poor that the child would derive much benefit, then tactile aids could be considered.

In this section, we consider the ability of biographical data to predict speech-perception results in children with cochlear implants. Other predictive measures are considered by Abbas (see Chapter 7), Dorman (see Chapter 4) and Shannon (see Chapter 8).

Staller et al. (1991a, 1991b) performed correlations on the results obtained from children with the Nucleus cochlear implant (the number of children was not specified). The most significant variable predicting speech perception was age at onset of deafness. That should not be too surprising considering that Staller and colleagues grouped prelingually and postlingually deafened children, and that performance between the two groups is dramatically different. The length of deafness was also significantly correlated with performance, but less so than age at onset. When the effects of age at onset were considered first (in a stepwise multiple regression analysis), the contribution of length of deafness was usually not significant (depending on the particular tests). The highest Pearson correlation was between age at onset of deafness and 'open-set' spondee recognition ($r = .697$; $r^2 = .486$).

In contrast to those observations, Osberger et al. (1991b) found a very small effect of years of deafness on performance and an even smaller effect of years of implant use. The 28 children tested were comprised of both prelingually and postlingually deaf children.

It is clear from our discussion above that congenitally deaf children do not perform as well as postlingually deaf children. It is of interest to examine the performance of noncongenitally deaf children as a function of their age at onset of profound deafness. Figure 5–24 shows that no relationship is apparent in either the WIPI lipreading enhancement measures or the MTS word scores with age at onset of profound deafness (data from Staller et al., 1991b).

Another important question is whether performance depends on the duration of profound hearing loss. The data presently available from congenitally deaf children is primarily with only 12 months of experience. Performance from this group is typically poor, and may underestimate and misrepresent any possible relation that may emerge after the children gain more experience. We can, however, examine this relation in the noncongenitally deafened population. Figure 5–25 (top) indicates that there is no relation with the MTS word recognition. There are few children who have been deaf more than 6 years who obtain high levels of word recognition on the CID sentences (Figure 5–25, bottom).

It is noteworthy that attempts at predicting speech-perception performance of postlingually deafened adults using cochlear implants have

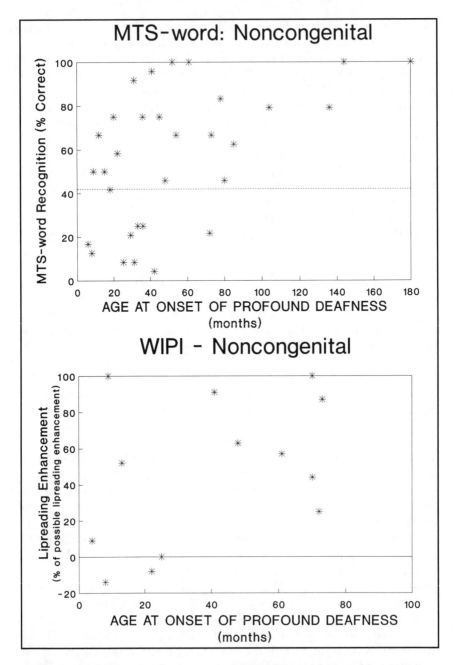

Figure 5–24. Performance of noncongentially deafened children with the Nucleus cochlear implant as a function of their age at onset of profound deafness for the MTS-word score (top) and lipreading enhancement on the WIPI test (bottom).

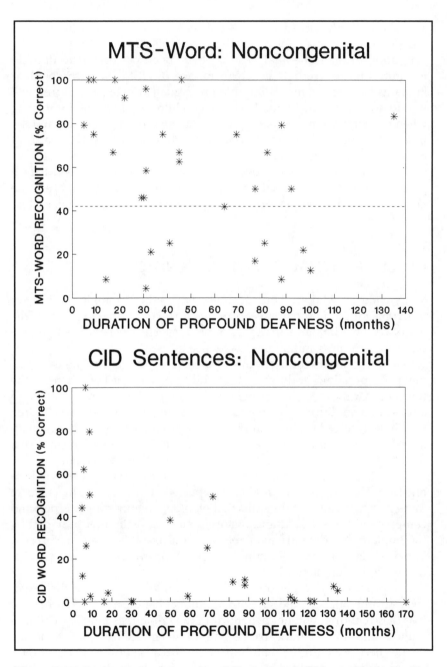

Figure 5–25. Performance of noncongentially deafened children with the Nucleus cochlear implant as a function of their duration of profound deafness for the MTS-word score (top) and word recognition in sentences with the CID sentence test.

also shown high correlations with speech perception and length and onset of deafness (e.g., Spivak & Waltzman, 1990; Tyler, 1991).

It is unfortunate the analyses that have been performed to date do not allow us to predict the performance of children with cochlear implants beyond the indication that prelingually deafened children will not do as well as postlingually deafened children. It will be interesting when the correlations are performed on the two populations separately. In addition, most of the data are from children with only 12 months of experience, possibly before many have reached their full potential. The preliminary data, however, suggest that the correlation between speech perception and other variables will not be high. This means that the ability to predict the performance for a particular individual will be very difficult.

CHILDREN WITH MULTIPLE HANDICAPS

Many children who are born deaf also have other disabilities, either at birth or acquired in the first years of life. It is worthwhile to consider the use of cochlear implants in these populations. Here we discuss two possibilities, blindness and intellectual deficiencies.

One of the major contributions of a cochlear implant is the enhancement of lipreading abilities. Blind children will not benefit from the implant in this way. Nevertheless, there have been some deaf-blind adults (Martin, Burnett, Himelick, Phillips, & Over, 1988) and children who have received cochlear implants. They demonstrate environmental-sound and audition-alone speech recognition. Some may have a visual field that is very narrow and show an audiovisual enhancement.

Another issue is whether children with cognitive deficiencies will benefit from the implant. It might be expected that they might perform more poorly because of the skills that would be required to interpret and comprehend the reduced and distorted electrical stimulus provided by the implant. No data are available that address this question directly. However, even a limited amount of speech or everyday sound perception could be very helpful.

It appears that two general statements can be made about the use of cochlear implants in children with additional handicaps. First, it may be that these children will not benefit from the implant as much as children without additional handicaps. Second, these children frequently have a greater need for additional auditory input because of the effects of their other handicaps. It is likely that any benefit received may be particularly important to their quality of life.

IMPLICATIONS FOR SELECTION CRITERION

Several factors are relevant to the selection of children for cochlear implantation. Many factors can influence performance. For example Hellman et al. (1991) are developing a profile that includes chronological age, duration of deafness, medical-radiological findings, multiple handicapping conditions, functional hearing level, speech-language abilities, family structure and support, parent-child expectations, educational environment, availability of support services, and cognitive learning style. These factors can have a critical impact on performance, but insufficient data are available at this time to use them to reject a child for implantation because of the duration of deafness or educational placement, for example. If the child is old enough to show some positive interest in obtaining a cochlear implant, or if the parents do when the child is too young to demonstrate a positive or negative interest, then the selection criteria should be based on speech-perception tests.

Children should be fit with appropriate hearing aids and provided with aural rehabilitation during a suitable time period to determine what levels of speech-perception ability they can achieve with their hearing aid. What is a "suitable time" will depend on each child. Their speech-perception abilities should be compared to the measured abilities of similar children using cochlear implants. For example, the child's performance on the MTS stress test could be compared with the data shown in Figure 5–11. If the child was congenitally deaf and scored 75% correct on the MTS stress test, then there is about a 20% chance that performance would be improved after one year of experience with the cochlear implant.

Unfortunately, there is only limited data of this type available. In addition it is usually not presented separately for congenital, prelingual noncongenital, and postlingual populations. Furthermore, it would be desirable to have data from tests that are not susceptible to learning effects, such as closed-set tests that include a large set of items (like the WIPI). Producing such a data set, and therefore the utilization of appropriate selection criteria, is more complicated for many children under 4 years of age and is not presently possible for children under 2 years of age (see also Tye-Murray, Chapter 3 and Abbas, Chapter 7).

CONCLUSION

In this chapter we have provided some suggestions regarding the administration and interpretation of speech perception tests for young children. These guidelines are critical for the determination of success of children using cochlear implants. We also reviewed many of the speech perception tests available for children, to provide a broad appreciation of which tests are available and which test areas need further development. A review of results on children with cochlear implants suggests that, on average, children using the Nucleus implant outperform those using the House implant. It is also true that, on average, postlingually deafened children perform better than prelingually deaf children. Most of the gathered data are from children with only 12 months of experience with the implant. The next few years will be critical to determine what levels of performance these children reach after 3 or 4 years of experience and whether these levels of speech perception dramatically influence their lifestyles.

ACKNOWLEDGMENTS

The author was supported, in part, by the National Institutes of Health grant DC00242; grant RR59 from the General Clinical Research Centers Program, Division of Research Resources, NIH; and a grant from Lions Clubs of Iowa, International Exchange Rehabilitation

I wish to thank Holly Fryauf-Bertschy, Danielle Kelsay, Jane Opie, Karen Kirk, and Nancy Tye-Murray for helpful discussions on this topic, as well as useful comments on earlier drafts of this manuscript. I also wish to thank Steve Staller for sharing individual data and Aaron Thornton, Marilyn Demorest, and George Woodworth who made valuable comments about statistical issues.

REFERENCES

Bench, J., & Bamford, J. (1979). *Speech-hearing tests and the spoken language of hearing-impaired children*. London: Academic Press.

Berliner, K. I., & Eisenberg, L. S. (1985). Methods and issues in the cochlear implantation of children: An overview. *Ear and Hearing, 6* (Suppl. 3), 6S–13S.

Berliner, K. I., Tonokawa, L. L., Dye, L. M., & House, W. F. (1989). Open-set speech recognition in children with a single-channel cochlear implant. *Ear and Hearing, 10*(4), 237–242.

Bilger, R. C. (1983). Perceptions from electrical stimulation. In C. W. Parkins & S. W. Anderson, (Eds.), *Cochlear prostheses: An international symposium* (pp. 206). New York: New York Academy of Sciences.

Bilger, R., Black, F., Hopkinson, N., Myers, E., Payne, J., Stenson, N., Vega, A., & Wolf, R. (1977). Evaluation of subjects presently fitted with implanted auditory prostheses. *Annals of Otology, Rhinology, and Laryngology, 86* (Suppl. 38), 92–140.

Bilger, R. C., & Hopkinson, N. T. (1977). Hearing performance with the auditory prosthesis. *Annals of Otology, Rhinology, and Laryngology, 86* (Suppl. 38) 76–91.

Boothroyd, A. (1968). Developments in speech audiometry. *Sound, 2*, 3–10.

Boothroyd, A. (1984). Auditory perception of speech contrasts by subjects with sensorineural hearing loss. *Journal of Speech and Hearing Research, 27*, 134–144.

Boothroyd, A. (1986). *A three-interval, forced-choice test of speech pattern contrast perception.* New York: City Uniersity of New York and Lexington Center.

Boothroyd, A. (1991). Assessment of speech perception capacity in profoundly deaf children. *The American Journal of Otology, 12* (Suppl.), 67–72.

Boothroyd, A., Geers, A. E., & Moog, J. S. (1991). Practical implications of cochlear implants in children. *Ear and Hearing, 12* (Suppl.4), 81S–89S.

Boothroyd, A., & Nittrouer, S. (1988). Mathematical treatment of context effects in phoneme and word recognition. *Journal of the Asoustical Society of America, 84,* 101–114.

Clark, G. M., Tong, Y. C., & Patrick, J. F. (1990). Cochlear prostheses. New York: Churchill Livingstone.

Craig, W. N. (1964). Effects of preschool training on the development of reading and lipreading skills of deaf children. *American Annals of the Deaf, 109,* 280–296.

Danley, M. J., & Fretz, R. J. (1982). Design and functioning of the single-electrode cochlear implant. *Annals of Otology Rhinology, and Laryngology, 91* (Suppl. 91), 21–26.

De Filippo, C. L. (1988). Tracking for speechreading training. *The Volta Review, 90*(5), 215–237.

De Filippo, C. L., & Scott, B. L. (1978). A method for training and evaluating the reception of ongoing speech. *Journal of the Acoustical Society of America, 63,* 1186–192.

Dorman, M. F., Dankowski, K., McCandless, G., & Smith, L. (1989). Identification of synthetic vowels by patients using the Symbion multichannel cochlear implant. *Ear and Hearing, 10,* 40–43.

Dorman, M. F., Hannley, M. T., Dankowski, K., Smith, L., & McCandless, G. (1989). Word recognition by 50 patients fitted with the Symbion multichannel cochlear implant. *Ear and Hearing, 10,* 44–49.

Dowell, R. C., Dawson, P. W., Dettmen, S. J., Shepherd, R. K., Whitford, L. A., Seligman, P. M., & Clark, G. M. (1991). Multichannel cochlear implantation in children: A summary of current work at the University of Melbourne. *The American Journal of Otology, 12* (Suppl.), 137–143.

Dreschler, W. A., & Plomp, R. (1985). Relations between psychophysical data and speech perception for hearing-impaired subjects. *Journal of the Acoustical Society of America, 78,* 1261–1270.

Dunn, L. M. (1965). *Peabody Picture Vocabulary Test.* Minneapolis, MN: American Guidance Service Inc.

Elliott, L., & Katz, D. (1980). *Development of a new children's test of speech discrimination.* St. Louis, MO: Auditec.

Erber, N. P. (1980). Use of the Auditory Numbers Test to evaluate speech perception abilities of hearing-impaired children. *Journal of Speech and Hearing Disorders, 45,* 527–532.

Erber, N. P. (1982). *Auditory training.* Washington, DC: Alexander Graham Bell Association for the Deaf.

Erber, N., & Alencewicz, C. (1976). Audiologic evaluation of deaf children. *Journal of Speech and Hearing Disorders, 41,* 256–267.

Finitzo-Hieber, T., Matkin, N. D., Cherow-Skalka, E., & Gerling, I. J. (1977). *Sound Effects Recognition Test.* St. Louis, MO: Auditec.

Fryauf-Bertschy, H., Tyler, R. S., Kelsay, D., & Gantz, B. J. (1992). Performance over time of congenitally deaf and postlingually deafened children using a multichannel cochlear implant. *Journal of Speech and Hearing Research, 35,* 913–920.

Geers, A. E., & Moog, J. S. (1987). Predicting spoken language acquisition in profoundly deaf children. *Journal of Speech and Hearing Disorders, 52*(1), 84–94.

Geers, A. E., & Moog, J. S. (1989). Evaluating speech perception skills: Tools for measuring benefits of cochlear implants, tactile aids, and hearing aids. In E. Owens & D. K. Kessler, (Eds.), *Cochlear implants in young deaf children* (pp. 227–256). Boston: College-Hill Press.

Geers, A. E., & Moog, J. S. (1991). Evaluating the benefits of cochlear implants in an education setting. *The American Journal of Otology, 12,* (Suppl.), 116–125.

Haskins, H. A. (1949). *A phonetically balanced test of speech discrimination for children.* Unpublished masters thesis, Northwestern University, Evanston, IL.

Hellman, S. A., Chute, P. M., Kretschmer, R.E., Nevins, M.E., Parisier, S. C., & Thurston, L. C. (1991). The development of a children's implant profile. *American Annals of the Deaf, 136*(2), 77–81.

Henderson, W. G., Fisher, S. G., Cohen, N., Waltzman, S., Weber, L., & the VA Cooperative Study Group on Cochlear Implantation (1990). Use of principal components analysis to develop a composite score as a primary outcome variable in a clinical trial. *Controlled Clinical Trials, 11,* 199–214.

Jerger, S., Jerger, J., & Lewis, S. (1981). Pediatric speech intelligibility test. II. Effect of receptive language age and chronological age. *International Journal of Pediatric Otorhinolaryngology, 3,* 101–118.

Jerger, S., Lewis, S., Hawkins, J., & Jerger, J. (1980). Pediatric speech intelligibility test. I. Generation of test materials. *International Journal of Pediatric Otorhinolaryngology, 2,* 217–230.

Kirk, K. I. (1990). *Gap-duration discrimination identification of stop consonants in normal-hearing impaired listeners.* Unpublished manuscript, University of Iowa, Iowa City,

Knutson, J. F., Hinrichs, J. V., Tyler, R. S., Gantz, B. J., Schartz, H. A., & Woodworth, G. (1991a). Psychological predictors of audiological outcomes of multichannel cochlear implants: Preliminary findings. *Annals of Otology, Rhinology, and Laryngology, 100*(10), 817–822.

Knutson, J. F., Schartz, H. A., Gantz, B. J., Tyler, R. S., Hinrichs, J. V., & Woodworth, G. (1991b). Psychological change following 18-months of cochlear implant use. *Annals of Otology, Rhinology, and Laryngology, 100*(10), 877–882.

Lane, H. (1984). *When the mind hears: A history of the deaf.* New York: Vintage.

Lane, H. (1990). Cultural and infirmity models of deaf Americans. *Journal of the Academy of Rehabilitative Audiology, 23,* 11–26.

Lutman, M. E., & Clark, J. (1986). Speech identification under simulated hearing-aid frequency response characteristics in relation to sensitivity, frequency resolution and temporal resolution. *Journal of the Acoustical Society of America, 80,* 1030–1040.

Martin, E. L., Burnett, P. A., Himelick, T. E., Phillips, M. A., & Over, S . K. (1988). Speech recognition by a deaf-blind multi-channel cochlear implant patient. *Ear and Hearing, 9* (2), 70–74.

McCormick, B. (1977). *The toy discrimination test: An aid for the screening of hearing of children above the mental age of 2 years.* London: Public Health.

Mecklenburg, D., Shallop, J., & Ling, D. (1987). *Phonetic task evaluation* unpublished manuscript, Cochlear Corporation, Englewood, CO.

Miller, G. A., Heise, C. A.,.& Lichten, D. (1951). The intelligibility of speech as a function of the context of the test material. *Journal of Experimental Psychology, 41,* 329–335.

Miller, G. A., & Nicely, P. E. (1955). An analysis of perceptual confusions among some English consonants. *Journal of the Acoustical Society of America, 27,* 338–352.

Moog, J. S., & Geers, A. E. (1990). *Early Speech Perception Test.* St. Louis, MO: Central Institute for the Deaf.

Moog, J. S., & Geers, A. E. (1991). Educational management of children with cochlear implants. *AAD/Reference, 136*(2), 69–76.

Osberger, M. J., Miyamoto, R. T., Zimmerman-Phillips, S., Kemink, J. L., Stroer , B. S., Firszt, J. B., & Novak, M. A. (1991a). Independent evaluation of the speech perception abilities of children with the Nucleus 22-Channel cochlear implant system. *Ear and Hearing, 12* (Suppl. 4), 66S–80S.

Osberger, M. J., Robbins, A. M., Miyamoto, R. T., Berry, S. W., Myres, W. A., Kessler, K. S., & Pope, M. L. (1991b). Speech perception abilities of children with cochlear implants, tactile aids, or hearing aids. *American Journal of Otology, 12* (Suppl.), 105–115.

Owens, E., & Raggio, M. (1987). The UCSF tracking procedure for evaluation and training of speech reception by hearing-impaired adults. *Journal of Speech and Hearing Disorders, 52*, 120–128.

Plant, G. L. (1983). *The PLOTT Test.* Sydney, Australia: National Acoustic Laboratories.

Ross, M., & Lerman, J. (1971). *Word Intelligibility by Picture Identification.* Pittsburgh: Stanwix House, Inc.

Ross, M., & Randolph, K. (1990). A test of the auditory perception of alphabet letters for hearing-impaired children: The APAL Test. *Volta Review, 92*(5), 237–244.

Silverman, S. R., & Hirsh, I. (1955). Problems related to the use of speech in clinical audiometry. *Annals of Otology, Rhinology and Laryngology, 64*, 1234–1244.

Somers, M. N. (1991). Speech perception abilities in children with cochlear implants or hearing aids. *American Journal of Otology, 12* (Suppl.), 174–178.

Spivak, L. G., & Waltzman, S. B. (1990). Performance of cochlear implant patients as a function of time. *Journal of Speech and Hearing Research, 33*, 511–519.

Staller, S. J., Beiter, A. L., Brimacombe, J. A., Mecklenburg, D. J., & Arndt, P. (1991a). Pediatric performance with the Nucleus 22-channel cochlear implant system. *American Journal of Otology, 12* (Suppl.), 126–136.

Staller, S. J., Dowell, R. C., Beiter, A. L., & Brimacombe, J. A. (1991b). Perceptual abilities of children with the Nucleus 22-channel cochlear implant. *Ear and Hearing, 12*(4), 34S–47S.

Stelmachowicz, P. G., Jesteadt, W., Gorga, M. P., & Mott, J. (1985). Speech perception ability and psychophysical tuning curves in hearing-impaired listeners. *Journal of the Acoustical Society of America, 77*(2), 620–627.

Summerfield, Q. (1983). Audiovisual speech perception, lipreading and artificial stimulation. In M. E. Lutman & M. P. Haggard (Eds.), *Hearing science and hearing disorders* (pp. 132–182). London: Academic Press.

Thielemeir, M. A. (1984). *The Discrimination After Training Test.* Los Angeles: House Ear Institute.

Thornton, A. R., & Raffin, M. J. M. (1978). Speech-discrimination scores modeled as a binomial variable. *Journal of Speech and Hearing Research, 21*, 507–518.

Tillman, T. W., & Carhart, R. (1966). *An expanded test for speech discrimination utilizing CNC monosyllabic words.* Northwestern University Auditory Test No. 6 Technical Report No. SAM-TR-66-55. USAF School of Aerospace Medicine, Brooks Air Force Base, Texas.

Trammell, J., Farrar, C., Francis, J., Owens, S., Schepard, D., Thies, T., Witlen, R., & Faist, L. (1981). *Test of auditory comprehension.* North Hollywood, CA: Foreworks.

Tye-Murray, N., & Tyler, R. S. (1988). A critique of continuous discourse tracking as a test procedure. *Journal of Speech and Hearing Disorders, 53*, 226–231.

Tye-Murray, N.,Tyler, R. S., Woodworth, G., & Gantz, B. J. (1992). Performance over time with a Nucleus or Ineraid cochlear implant. *Ear and Hearing*, in press.

Tyler, R. S. (1990). Speech perception with the Nucleus cochlear implant in children trained with the auditory/verbal approach. *American Journal of Otology, 11*(2), 99–107.

Tyler, R. S. (1991). What can we learn about hearing aids from cochlear implants. *Ear and Hearing, 12*(Suppl. 6), 177S–186S.

Tyler, R. S. (1992). Cochlear implants and the Deaf culture. (in press). *American Journal of Audiology.*

Tyler, R. S., Berliner, K., Demorest, M., Hirshorn, M., Luxford, W., & Mangham, C. (1986). Clinical objectives and research-design issues for cochlear implants in children. *Seminars in Hearing, 7*(4), 433–440.

Tyler, R. S., Fryauf-Bertschy, H., & Kelsay, D. (1991). *Audiovisual Feature Test for Young Children.* Iowa City: The University of Iowa.

Tyler, R. S., & Holstad, B. (1987). *A closed-set speech perception test for hearing-impaired children.* Iowa City: University of Iowa.

Tyler, R. S., & Kelsay, D. (1990). Advantages and disadvantages perceived by some of the better cochlear implant patients. *American Journal of Otology, 11*(4), 282–288.

Tyler, R. S., Moore, B. C. J., & Kuk, F. K. (1989). Performance of some of the better cochlear-implant patients. *Journal of Speech and Hearing Research, 32,* 887–911.

Tyler, R. S., Opie, J. M., Fryauf-Bertschy, H., & Gantz, B. J. (1992). Future directions for cochlear implants. *Journal of Speech Language Pathology and Audiology, 16*(2), 151–164.

Tyler, R. S., Preece, J. P., & Lowder, M. W. (1983). *The Iowa Cochlear Implant Test Battery.* Iowa City: University of Iowa.

Tyler, R. S., Preece, J. P., & Tye-Murray, N. (1986). *The Iowa Phoneme and Sentence Tests.* Iowa City, Iowa: The University of Iowa.

Tyler, R. S., Summerfield, Q., Wood, E. J., & Fernandes, M. A. (1982). Psychoacoustic and phonetic temporal processing in normal and hearing-impaired listeners. *Journal of the Acoustical Society of America, 72,* 740–752.

Walden, B., Erdman, S., Montgomery, A., Schwartz, D., & Prosek, R. (1981). Some effects of training on speech recognition by hearing-impaired adults. *Journal of Speech and Hearing Research, 24,* 207–216.

Waltzman, S. B., Cohen, N. L., & Shapiro W. H. (1986). Long-term effects of multichannel cochlear implant usage. *Laryngoscope, 6,* 1083–1087.

Wang, M. D., & Bilger, R. C. (1973). Consonant confusions in noise: A study of perceptual features. *Journal of the Acoustical Society of America, 54,* 1248–1266.

CHAPTER 6

Speech Production
EMILY A. TOBEY

Speech perception and speech production are intrinsically linked to one another in the communication chain. As Figure 6–1 illustrates, the conveyance of an idea from a speaker to a listener involves linguistic, physiologic, and acoustic processes. A speaker selects an abstract auditory perceptual representation and activates complex interactions between the cerebrum, basal ganglia, and cerebellum in order to prepare the activation of motor nerves and muscle groups. Activation of muscles leads to articulator movements that serve to modulate the air stream and alter the cavity configurations of the vocal tract. Complex proprioceptive, tactile, and auditory feedback systems assist in regulating these complex interactions. Auditory feedback to the speaker may be provided by air-conducted or bone-conducted signals. The combined effects of these activities are rapidly varying acoustic outputs which are internally monitored by the speaker and received by a listener who, in turn, processes the signals via peripheral and central auditory mechanisms to arrive at the auditory perceptual representation intended by the speaker. Investigations of speech production probe these various levels through measurements of the muscles, movement of the articulators, the acoustic output or listener's perceptions.

Evidence for within speaker linkages between speech production and perception derives from a variety of sources including experiments that seek to disrupt auditory feedback in normal-hearing listeners and examine the consequences to speech production. Experimental disruptions include delaying the airborne acoustic signal presented to the auditory periphery in order to introduce a temporal mismatch between airborne and bone-conducted signals (Fairbanks, 1955), increasing the intensity of background noise (see Lane & Tranel, 1971 for a review), or frequency-shifting vocal output (Elman, 1981). Speech changes in response to these experimental disruptions are explained in several ways. One of the initial explanations assigns a primary role for auditory feedback and proposes it modifies or controls speech motor gestures in a closed feedback system (Fairbanks, 1955). More recently, investigators argue that auditory feedback contributes a secondary role to the regulation of speech motor gestures since auditory information often arrives after the end of the movements it is to correct under normal speaking conditions (Borden, 1979).

Since primary or secondary intrinsic linkages between speech perception and production are evident in normal-hearing individuals, one also would anticipate linkages in speech perception and production in profoundly hearing-impaired individuals. Poorer receptive vocabulary skills are seen

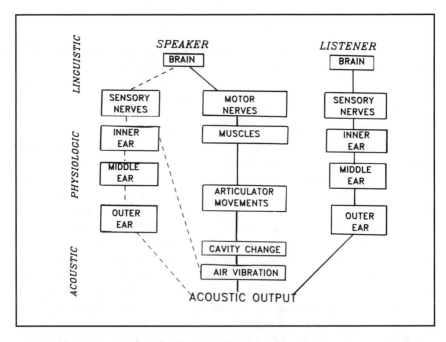

Figure 6–1. A schematic representation of the various levels of linguistic, physiologic, and acoustic processes involved in communication is shown. A speaker will receive sensory feedback from tactile and proprioceptive receptors, as well as auditory feedback delivered via air and bone conduction. A listener, in turn, receives the acoustic output of the speaker and processes the signal in order to receive the linguistic content of the speaker's message.

in individuals with pure-tone thresholds of 105 dB HL or greater: These individuals score slightly below half the normal rate of receptive-vocabulary acquisition of normal-hearing individuals (Boothroyd, Geers, & Moog, 1991). Boothroyd (1985) reports differences in speech intelligibility as a function of hearing loss, even among children classified as profoundly hearing impaired. Although numerous studies demonstrate positive relationships between degree of hearing impairment and the severity of abnormal oral-communication skills, the relationships are not entirely straightforward. Stark and Levitt (1974) report profoundly hearing-impaired children who score well on perceptual tests measuring suprasegmental aspects did not necessarily score well on the production of similar features; however, children who score high on production of suprasegmental features always score average to above average on the perception tests. As Osberger et al. (1991) conclude, good perceivers are not always good producers but good producers are generally good perceivers.

The lack of a clear one-to-one correspondence between perceptual and production skills occurs in profoundly hearing-impaired speakers, in part, because of the interactive effects of two auditory paths (air and bone) providing feedback on an abnormally produced speech output. The lack of one-to-one correspondence makes it difficult to predict how cochlear implants designed to translate acoustic properties of speech into electrical parameters as a means of mimicking aspects of normal audition and perception will influence speech production. Additional chapters in this volume (see Dorman, Chapter 4 and Tyler, Chapter 5) discuss the speech-perception capabilities of individuals using cochlear implants. This chapter will turn its attention to speech production and explore how studies examining the influence of cochlear implants on speech production provide important theoretical and clinical information regarding the linkages of perception and production.

Cochlear implants are designed to provide auditory information to individuals experiencing profound hearing impairments and who receive limited perceptual benefit from more traditional prosthetic devices, such as hearing aids. Yet, a variety of external factors may influence the effectiveness of these devices. A wide variety of abnormal speech and language behaviors appear as the consequence of profound hearing impairment. Several factors appear to influence the severity of abnormal behaviors including the amount of residual hearing, the age of hearing loss onset, and the length of profound hearing impairment. Although an intensive literature base exists regarding the abnormal speech-production characteristics of profound hearing-impaired speakers (see Osberger & McGarr, 1982 for a review), far less is known about the speech characteristics of individuals with severe, moderate, or minimal hearing impairments. Thus, very little information is available to guide one in anticipating what to expect of speech production as a speaker moves from a profound hearing impairment to a severe impairment or a moderate impairment when using a cochlear implant. Further complications arise when considering the interactions of age of onset on speech production. Disruption in the normal reception of auditory information during the early periods of speech and language acquisition results in devastating consequences to spoken communication skills. Isolating the precise effects of profound hearing impairment on a child's speech-production is difficult given the concurrent development of anatomical, physiological, and cognitive processes. Deprivation of the auditory code in young children reduces their opportunity to develop important perceptual contrasts which contribute to the linguistic knowledge base of their language. As clinicians, should we expect the same magnitude or type of speech changes in individuals using cochlear implants who have limited experience with the auditory code versus individuals who may have extensive linguistic and auditory experience prior to receiving profound hearing impairments? Portions of this chapter will review the speech characteristics of postlingually deafened adults and young children in order to explore the similarities and differences in these populations as a means of setting the stage for examining the effects of cochlear implants on their speech.

Two of the major difficulties encountered in reviewing the speech-production characteristics of these populations is the dearth of standardized instruments measuring speech production and the lack of speech-production norms for individuals with varying degrees of hearing impairment. One need only contrast the wide number of instruments used to estimate perceptual performance to the few instruments available for assessing speech production in individuals with hearing impairments to recognize the enormity of the problem. To further complicate the situation, clinicians are interested in tracking speech-production performance longitudinally. Repeated administration of the same instrument multiple times reduces the internal validity of the measures and always leads one to question if performance has truly changed or has the client learned the task. Poor inter- and intrajudge reliabilities also appear in speech-production measures as judges are required to make decisions on speech that is, in many cases, virtually unintelligible. This chapter also will explore how these factors limit our ability to make clinical expectations regarding the influence of cochlear implants on the development or maintenance of speech production.

INFLUENCE OF AUDITORY FEEDBACK ON VOCAL OUTPUT

Auditory feedback appears critical for acquiring the sounds of speech. Young children explore a variety of phonetic features prior to modeling their vocal output to speakers around them through the use of auditory feedback and, thus, acquire the sound contrasts incorporated in their language. Profound hearing impairments occurring during these exploratory periods result in reduced phonetic repertoires fraught with errors and lead to inappropriately produced phonemes. Developmentally, auditory feedback allows children to make comparisons between their speech and adult models in order to develop the phonemic categories of their language.

The role of auditory feedback within the control strategies used after speech and language are developed, however, remains controversial. Some investigators (Fairbanks, 1955; Lee, 1950) propose that speech gestures are actively modified or controlled by auditory feedback since experimental conditions such as delayed auditory feedback (a disruption of speech production when the airborne acoustic signal is delayed in time) (Fairbanks, 1955) and the Lombard effect (an increase in vocal effort in the presence of loud background noise) (see Lane & Tranel, 1971 for a review) create changes in speech output. Borden (1979) argues that auditory information fails to play an active, primary role in the normal moment-to-moment control of speech, principally because the time constants involved in audition are long and the information tends to arrive after the end of the movements it is to correct. Instead, investigators propose auditory feedback serves as a calibrator for other sensory systems, such as proprioception, more likely to be responsible for the moment-to-moment adjustments of speech gestures (for examples see, Cowie & Douglas-Cowie, 1983; Zimmermann & Rettaliata, 1981). Additional evidence suggesting auditory information is weighted less heavily in adult speakers is found in the literature exploring the speech-production characteristics of postlingually deafened adults. In these studies reviewed later in this chapter, one finds speech deteriorates but is not completely eliminated. It is the systematic deterioration, rather than elimination, that provides support indicating auditory feedback serves as a calibrator (or tuning device) for other feedback mechanisms contributing to the moment-to-moment control of speech.

EFFECTS OF DEAFNESS ON VOCAL OUTPUT IN ANIMALS

We also can investigate how auditory feedback influences vocal output in animals. Animal studies provide us the opportunity to separate the effects of deafness on vocal output alone from the interaction of deafness on linguistic factors conveyed via vocal output in humans. Experimental studies in animals confirm the complexity of reduced auditory feedback on the development of vocal output. Several studies examining the vocal output of artifically deafened felines and birds report similar consequences to those observed in profoundly hearing-impaired children.

Reductions in suprasegmental and segmental aspects of vocal output occur following deafness in many animal species. For example, hearing sensitivity in normal kittens increases rapidly between days 6 and 10 after birth (Ehret & Romand, 1981). Kittens deafened early in life produce louder cries than normal-hearing kittens between days 9 and 23 postdeafening and from day 82 onward (Romand & Ehret, 1984). Totally deaf cats produce cries twice as loud as normal-hearing cats at 30 and 50 days postdeafening and cries of the deaf cats are nearly 6 times louder than normal-hearing cats at 1 year postdeafening (Shipley, Buchwald, & Carterette, 1988). Thus, totally deaf cats do not cease vocalizing; instead, their vocal output contains several deviant features.

Early deafening also appears to affect fundamental frequencies and harmonic structure of cat cries. Shipley et al. (1988) report the fundamental frequencies of deaf kittens at 30 days post-deafening were about 250 Hz higher than for normal-hearing animals. Kittens deafened shortly after birth produce greater amplitudes than normal-hearing kittens in low-frequency harmonics up to day 42 and greater amplitudes in higher harmonics from day 82 onward (Romand & Ehret, 1984). Normal-hearing kittens produce a variety of cries with rapid frequency or amplitude modulations; however, deafened kittens fail to acquire these features within the same time frame as normal-hearing kittens. Thus, early deafening in kittens adversely affects the development of some suprasegmental properties (intensity, fundamental frequency and harmonic structure) and some aspects related to segmental properties (such as the rapid frequency and amplitude modulations shaping the cries into syllabic-type structures).

A far more complex picture of the interactions of auditory feedback on suprasegmental and segmental vocal development is observed in birds. Removal of the cochlea, rendering a bird deaf, does not appear to adversely influence the development of turkey gobbling (Schleidt, 1964), chicken calls (Konishi, 1963), or ring dove calls (Nottebohm & Nottebohm, 1971). Konishi (1964; 1965) found several songbirds developed abnormal song patterns after deafening, including the American robin, Mexican junco, and white-crowned sparrow. In a series of elegant studies conducted by Marler and his colleagues (Marler, 1981; Marler & Sherman, 1983; Marler & Tamura, 1964; Searcy & Marler, 1987), the songs of swamp and song sparrows were examined in birds reared in acoustic isolation, deafened early in life, and receiving normal auditory feedback. Early deafening appears to influence the gross syntactical organization (a combination of different notes) and the frequency characteristics of the notes as shown in Figure 6–2. Examinations of the fine structures of the notes and syllable-like structures reveal further degradation in early deafened sparrows.

Species specificity in song structure (i.e., characteristics that appear in one species but not the other) was maintained in some instances of the deaf birds. For example, deaf swamp sparrows averaged songs of 2.7 s and deaf song sparrows averaged songs of 1.7 s. This pattern closely resembled the innate calls produced by birds raised in acoustic isolation and not allowed to hear songs from other birds (i.e., innate song duration for song sparrows was 2.9 s and 2.0 s for swamp sparrows) (Marler & Sherman, 1983). Species specificity was not maintained in other instances such as the notes produced per song. Deaf song sparrows produce a greater number of notes (an average of 16.6) than deaf swamp sparrows (an average of 12.1); however, the opposite was true in the innate calls of song and swamp birds raised in acoustic isolation. Swamp sparrows averaged 19.8 notes per song and song sparrows averaged 10.4 notes per song. Studies examining adult song sparrows responses to

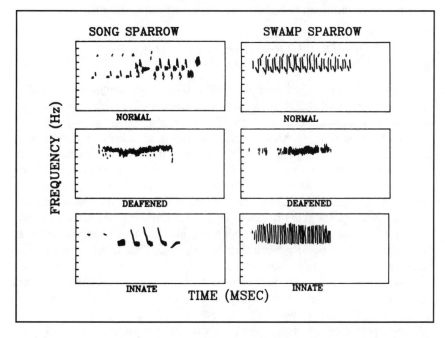

Figure 6–2. A spectrographic representation of three types of swamp sparrow and song sparrow calls are shown. The middle panel depicts the calls of birds deafened by removal of their cochleae early in life. The bottom panel shows an example of innate calls which occur when the birds are raised in isolation and have no contact with other birds of their species. The top panel demonstrates the complex patterns produced by birds with normal hearing and who have contact with other birds of their species. (Adapted from Marler, 1991.)

songs of male song sparrows reared in acoustic isolation or deafened early in life revealed the territorial males responded more aggressively to the isolated males than to the songs of deaf males. Deaf songs evoked almost no response from adult female song sparrows (only 1 out of 29 birds preformed a solicitation display).

Collectively, studies of some animals reveal deterioration in the suprasegmental and segmental properties of vocal output following deafness. These studies suggest that early deafness has a number of vocal output consequences that are not necessarily linguistically bound. Alterations in speech production may be expected in overall intensity levels, the range and mean fundamental frequency, the overall duration of segments, and the complexity of the syllabic-like structures. If auditory feedback is critical for developing or controlling these variables in species other than humans, one might also anticipate that similar parameters will be adversely effected in humans. The following sections review the vocal output characteristics of postlingually deafened adults and in children with profound hearing impairments.

SPEECH-PRODUCTION CHARACTERISTICS IN POSTLINGUALLY DEAFENED ADULTS

Alterations to suprasegmental properties of speech are evident in postlingually deafened adults. Postlingually deafened men, ranging in age from 42 to 69 years, produce significantly higher fundamental frequencies than normal-hearing male speakers of similar ages (Leder, Spitzer, & Kirchner, 1987). Horii (1982) finds significantly higher fundamental frequencies in hard-of-hearing female speakers than normal-hearing control subjects; however, Kirk and Edgerton (1983) report lower fundamental frequencies in two deaf female speakers when compared to matched control subjects. Normal-hearing speakers produce higher fundamental frequencies while reading a passage than when speaking, but hard-of-hearing speakers failed to show a similar relationship (Horii, 1982). The magnitude of these fundamental frequency changes can be quite dramatic. For example, fundamental frequencies are higher for one of Waldstein's (1990) speakers than the norms for 6-year-old children (the age the speaker became deaf) or adolescent girls (the age of the speaker at the time of study).

Measures of period-to-period fundamental frequency variability (jitter) are lower in adventitiously deaf adults than in normal-hearing speakers, further suggesting adventitiously deaf adults experience difficulty with fine phonatory control (Lane & Webster, 1991). Poor phonatory control is evident on stress and prominence features. Postlingually deafened adults are 43% more variable in pitch than in normal-hearing adults, regardless if the pitch measurements are acquired on stressed or unstressed vowels (Lane & Webster, 1991). Postlingually deafened adults produce stressed vowels with higher fundamental frequencies than normal-hearing speakers, and the differences are particularly exaggerated by stress placement. Increases in variability appear when deaf speakers are requested to place pitch variations in sentences: greater fundamental frequency variability occurs on prominent syllables in deaf speakers than normal-hearing speakers.

Fewer studies are available examining intensity measures in postlingually deafened adults. Leder et al. (1987c) report significantly greater intensities are produced by postlingually deafened than normal-hearing males. Standard deviations were two-to-three times greater in the postlingually deafened adults, suggesting they produced greater intensity fluctuations during speech. These data are in contrast to those of Kirk and Edgerton (1983) who compared the ranges of relative intensity (subtracting the minimum from maximum decibel produced) and standard deviations in two male and female deaf speakers. Male and female deaf speakers produced similar intensity ranges and variability measures to normal-hearing controls.

Difficulties with temporal parameters also are apparent in the speech of postlingually deafened adults. Significantly longer sentence durations have been observed by a number of investigators (Kirk & Edgerton, 1983; Lane & Webster, 1991); however, a similar pattern of decreasing overall durations as a function of the type of sentence (declarative or interrogative) was observed in normal and postlingually deafened adults (Waldstein, 1990). Significantly longer syllables (Lane & Webster, 1991; Leder et al., 1987b) and pause durations (Lane & Webster, 1991) contribute to the overall lengthening of sentence durations in postlingually-deafened adults. Postlingual deafness also appears to influence consonant and vowel production. In extensive studies conducted with postlingually deafened adults, Cowie and colleagues (Cowie & Douglas-Cowie, 1983; Cowie, Douglas-Cowie, & Kerr, 1982) found the most common substitutions involved voiced for voiceless plosives and labiodental fricatives. Additional errors included hypernasality, omissions of consonants with mid and posterior places of articulation, affricate reduction, and the inappropriate use of palatal fricatives. Vowels tended to be more centralized: [i] tended to sound like [I] and [ɛ] tended to sound like [æ]. Although they found many of the same error patterns in postlingually deafened adults that occur in prelingually deafened children (Smith, 1975), the errors were roughly 75% more common in the prelingually deafened children.

Difficulties with plosive and fricative production also are verified in acoustic studies investigating the speech of postlingually deafened adults. Lane and Webster (1991) report postlingually deafened adults fail to differentiate /ʃ/ for /s/. In addition, they found a lack of differentiation in burst spectra for plosive consonants. Restrictions in the range of voice-onset times associated with voiceless stop consonants appears in postlingually deafened speakers (Waldstein, 1990). Observations such as these lead Lane and Webster (1991) to suggest that postlingual deafness results in systematic errors of phonetic implementation rather than errors in phonological planning.

Additional evidence suggesting postlingually deafened adults experience difficulty with phonetic implementation is found in the acoustic characteristics of vowels. Formant-frequency measures indicate a restricted vowel space, although not as restricted as that associated with prelingually deaf speakers (Shukla, 1989; Svirsky & Tobey, 1991; Waldstein, 1990). Adventitiously deaf speakers are less consistent in their productions and demonstrate greater variability from token to token (Svirsky & Tobey, 1991; Waldstein, 1990). Overall vowel durations are typically longer in postlingually deafened adults than in normal-hearing adults; however, temporal relationships associated with tense and lax vowels are maintained (Waldstein, 1990). There also is some evidence to suggest that length of deafness influences vowel characteristics: Waldstein (1990) found greater deviations in vowel targeting and durations in two individuals who acquired deafness at early ages.

Taken overall, the similarity between the vocal output consequences of deafness in animals and postlingually deafened adults is striking. Both experience alterations in suprasegmental and segmental aspects. Changes in suprasegmental properties are evident in alterations of intensity, fundamental frequencies, and temporal characteristics. Changes in segmental properties are present in consonants and vowels in humans and in the frequency/amplitude shapings of syllabic-like calls in other species. Now let us turn our attention to the speech characteristics of children with profound hearing impairments.

SPEECH-PRODUCTION CHARACTERISTICS OF PROFOUNDLY HEARING-IMPAIRED CHILDREN

An extensive review of the literature on the speech-production characteristics of profoundly hearing-impaired speakers may be found in Osberger and McGarr (1982). In this section, we will highlight a few of the features associated with the speech production of profoundly hearing-impaired children. Many investigators report hearing-impaired children use excessively high pitches (Angelocci, Kopp, & Holbrook, 1964; Martony, 1968) and inappropriate variations in fundamental frequency (Monsen, 1979; Smith, 1975). Abnormal temporal patterns associated with stress are found in profoundly hearing-impaired speakers. Durations of unstressed syllables are shorter than those associated with stressed syllables in hearing-impaired speakers; however, the proportional shortening is generally smaller than in normal-hearing speakers (Osberger & Levitt, 1979; Stevens, Nickerson, & Rollins, 1978). McGarr and Harris (1980) observed that hearing-impaired speakers intentionally lengthened stressed vowels relative to unstressed vowels, but the intended stress patterns were not always correctly perceived by listeners.

Reduced sound repertoires containing multiple errors are characteristic of profoundly hearing-impaired children. Substitutions of one sound for another, omissions, and distortions frequently occur (Osberger & McGarr, 1982). Visible consonants produced in the front of the mouth are used more frequently than less visible consonants produced in the back of the mouth (Carr, 1953; Gold, 1980; Lach, Ling, Ling, & Ship, 1970; Nober, 1967; Smith, 1975). Profoundly hearing-impaired speakers correctly produce 37% of front and 14% of back consonants (Champagne, 1975). Voicing errors occur, although studies differ as to the direction of the error (i.e., voiced for voiceless or vice versa) (Hudgins & Numbers, 1942; Mangan, 1961; Nober, 1967; Smith, 1975). Manner errors, including nasal-oral substitutions, often appear in the speech of profoundly hearing-impaired children (Markides, 1970; Smith, 1975). Vowels also are produced with errors. Front vowels appear to be produced with more errors than back vowels, suggesting profoundly hearing-impaired children may have difficulty with tongue position (Nober, 1967; Smith, 1975). Difficulties in regulating tongue height are also observed. Profoundly hearing-impaired children produce a greater number of errors on high or mid vowels than vowels with low tongue height positions (Geffner, 1980; Smith, 1975).

There also are indications that the speech-production skills of congenitally deafened children differ from those of children who have exposure to the auditory code and language prior to deafness. To characterize those differences, two studies are presented in depth. The first explores the speech deterioration noted in a 5-year-old child, and the second compares the speech development of identical twins, one who has normal hearing and the other who experiences a profound hearing impairment.

Case 1: Speech Characteristics of A Postlingually Deafened Child

One of the most comprehensive studies detailing the phonetic disintegration following hearing impairment tracked the speech of a 5-year-old boy who suffered a profound hearing loss following haemophilis influenza meningitis (Binnie, Daniloff, & Buckingham, 1982). Pure-tone audiometry revealed no responses in the child's left ear and responses in the right ear were obtained at the upper limits of the audiometer. No responses were obtained to bone-conducted stimuli. The child received amplification; however, only 50–60 dB HL aided speech detection thresholds were ever obtained. Speech recordings were initiated 6 weeks after detection and continued to be sampled at 2-week intervals for 9 months. Abnormal phonetic quality and reduced intelligibility were observed by the final test session; however, most intended sounds remained present and continued to contain features representative of their phonemic class. Generalized slowing of speech was noted over the 9-month test period. Overall word durations increased from a mean of 646 to 986 ms and variability, as measured by standard deviations, increased from 185 to 344 ms. The deafened child's words were approximately 10% longer during the first recorded session and 97% longer by the seventh recording session than values reported for normal-hearing children (Smith, 1978). Further examination revealed that 97% of the word utterances contained more syllables than intended and all but four instances of the new syllables were created by insertion of the schwa vowel, /ʌ/.

Following 9 months of profound hearing impairment, utterances were produced with a monotonous, high-pitched, and less inflected voice. Comparisons of fundamental frequency across the test sessions indicated an initial mean fundamental frequency of 424 Hz during the first session, a peak of 477 Hz in session five, and a mean of 399 Hz in session seven. Standard deviations ranged from 76–138 Hz, with the largest standard deviation occurring in the seventh session. The deaf child produced nearly an octave above the mean fundamental frequencies of normal-hearing 5-year-olds (Weinberg & Zlatin, 1970). The range of fundamental frequencies used also declined.

Segmental sound production was significantly altered. Consonant production was exaggerated, vowels were diphthonized, consonant clusters were reduced, and assimilation nasality (perceived as hypernasality) was noted during the last three recording sessions. Syllabification, cluster reduction, and over aspiration rarely were seen in the first recording session but encompassed nearly 90% of the utterances in the final test session. Overall intelligibility was rated at approximately 50% during the first three recording sessions and deteriorated to 30–35% during the last four sessions. The child's speech was approximately 30% less intelligible than the speech of a normal-hearing adult during the first session and deteriorated an additional 20% by session seven.

Case 2: Phonetic Development in Twins with Differing Auditory Function

Kent and colleagues (Kent, Osberger, Netsell, & Hustedde, 1987) explored the phonetic development in two identical male twins, one with normal hearing and the other with a severe-to-profound hearing loss bilaterally. The hearing-impaired child failed an audiometric screening at birth, and the loss was confirmed by auditory brainstem response audiometry and behavioral evaluation at 3 months. The child was fitted with binaural, behind-the-ear hearing aids and provided habilitation services. Speech samples of the twins were acquired at 8, 12, and 15 months. Comparisons indicated significant differences in formant frequencies, consonant repertoires, and syllable structures between the two infants.

Measures of the peak fundamental frequency acquired within syllables indicated the hearing-impaired child had a higher modal value and slightly larger range of frequencies than his normal-hearing twin during the first session. These differences continue to be present in the two later recordings. In addition, phonatory contributions within a single utterance often changed markedly. Formant frequencies of vowel-like productions produced by the normal-hearing twin indicated a steady reconfiguration of the vowel quadrilateral in a manner paralleling the previously reported developmental stages (Kent & Murray, 1982). Quite a different pattern, however, was associated with the hearing-impaired twin as shown in Figure 6–3. A greater restricted vowel formant-frequency region was observed at 15 months than at 8 months.

Qualitative and quantitative differences also were apparent in syllabic structures. At 8 months, the hearing-impaired twin produced primarily vowel or diphthonal syllables with a predominance of /ae/ vowels while no vowel or diphthonal syllables were produced by the normal-hearing twin. Instead, the normal-hearing twin produced primarily consonant-vowel structures formed with five different vowels. Additional comparisons acquired at 15, 20, and 24 months indicated a preponderance of vowel and vowel-vowel structures in the hearing-impaired child's repertoire from age 8 to 20 months. Consonant-vowel syllables increased in number by 20 months and expanded to consonant-vowel-consonant-vowel structures by 24 months. Contrastively, the hearing twin produced a much wider variety of syllable structures even at 8 months than were produced by the hearing-impaired twin. A reduction in the type of syllable structures produced occurred for the normal-hearing twin over time and reflected the phonological requirements of his increasing vocabulary. However, the hearing-impaired twin produced syllabic structures at 24 months that barely overlapped the syllabic structures produced by the normal-hearing infant at 8 months.

Consonant features also were significantly different across the two infants. At 8 months, the hearing-impaired infant produced predominately stops with occasional bilabial trills. Further diversification of features was evident at 24 months; however, the majority of productions were alveolar (77%) with few occurrences of dental (1%), velar (0%), or glottal (1%)

places. The normal-hearing twin produced a variety of consonants including fricatives and stops at several places of articulation. A wide range of
places of articulation was evident at 24 months and included bilabials
(43%), alveolars (22%), dentals (13%), velars (7%), and glottals (9%).

Speech repertoires are severely reduced in postlingually deafened and
congenitally deafened children, as exemplified by the studies reviewed
above. Errors appear on both segmental and suprasegmental levels. As
in other animal species, profound hearing impairments result in higher
than normal fundamental frequencies and longer durations. Syllabic
structures are adversely influenced and failed to show the variety of features associated with normal-hearing speakers. Consonant and vowel
productions also are replete with errors and contribute to reductions in
overall speech intelligibility.

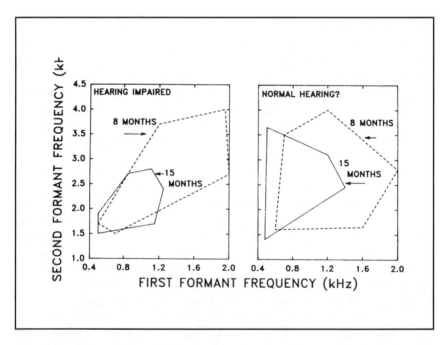

Figure 6–3. First and second formant frequency vowel spaces are shown for normal hearing and hearing-impaired twins. The left panel depicts the vowel space
produced by the hearing-impaired twin at 8 months and 15 months of age. The
right panel illustrates the vowel space of the normal hearing twin at similar ages.
Although the vowel spaces are different for the twins even at 8 months, differences in vowel spaces are accentuated by 15 months. The hearing-impaired twin
shows a greatly reduced vowel space relative to his normal hearing sibling.
(Adapted from Kent et al. 1987.)

EFFECTS OF COCHLEAR IMPLANTS ON SPEECH PRODUCTION

Taken collectively, elimination of auditory feedback during the formative years of development results in poorer regulation of fundamental frequency, intensity, and duration. These features, however, often are coded in the processing strategies used in many cochlear implants. One might hypothesize that cochlear implants will provide information useful for regulating these features and assist in the development of more nearly normal intonation, stress, and rhythm patterns. Segmental performance also is adversely effected with reduced or eliminated auditory feedback. As discussed in greater detail in Chapters 4 (Dorman) and 5 (Tyler) in this volume, cochlear implants may provide important feedback regarding the critical timing relationships distinguishing voiced-voiceless decisions, spectral cues associated with manner and place of articulation, and spectral/timing cues distinguishing many vowels. Thus, one might anticipate changes occurring to these parameters in speakers using cochlear implants.

SPEECH-PRODUCTION CHARACTERISTICS OF ADULT COCHLEAR-IMPLANT USERS

Initial observations of speech production following cochlear implantation were usually a secondary observation with the major emphasis of studies being placed on reception abilities. Significant improvement in speech intelligibility was reported in 4 out of 12 users of a House single-channel cochlear implant (Bilger et al., 1977) and in users of the Vienna device (Hochmair-Desoyer, 1981). Following these initial observations, Kirk and Edgerton (1983) examined the suprasegmental properties of four postlingually deafened adults who received a House cochlear implant. They observed more nearly normal fundamental frequencies in two male and two female single-channel users after using the implants for time periods ranging from 2 to 8 years. Inconsistent temporal alterations were noted in the users postimplantation: one user continued to prolong utterances, two users produced shorter utterances, and one user produced longer utterances. Fundamental-frequency declination and rate of articulation improved in the utterances of a Swedish female after 2 years use with an extra-cochlear implant (Plant & Oster, 1986). Ball and Faulkner (1989) also report fundamental-frequency ranges approached normal values with less irregular glottal periodicity in eight adults using a single-channel extra-cochlear implant that provided information regarding speakers fundamental frequency.

Alterations in fundamental frequency, duration, and intensity parameters are evident in the reacquisition of contrastive stress demonstrated in a single patient using a House single-channel implant (Leder et al., 1986). Contrastive stress represents a task where a noun is changed to a verb (e.g., CONvert versus conVERT). Prior to implantation, the patient was unable to produce contrastive stress. Significantly higher fundamental frequencies for initial and final stressed syllables were observed relative to unstressed syllables 1 day after implantation. Four months later, higher fundamental frequencies for stressed syllables was accompanied by greater intensities and longer durations signalling a more nearly normal relationship. Listeners failed to assign the stress appropriately prior to implantation; however, stress was correctly identified postimplantation. Similar observations of more appropriate strategies for producing stress postimplantation were observed in an adolescent user of the Nucleus multichannel implant (Tartter, Chute, & Hellman, 1989). Tartter and her colleagues noted an inappropriate reduction in unstressed-syllable durations prior to implantation that became more normal after implantation.

Lane, Perkell, Svirsky, and Webster (1991) recently explored how feedback from a Ineraid multichannel cochlear implant influenced speech breathing in three deaf adults. Significant changes in mean airflow were observed in all three speakers postimplantation, as shown in Figure 6–4. Postimplantation, significant alterations to the average volume of air expended per syllable were evident in two of the three speakers. Comparisons of these values to those of normal-hearing speakers and congenitally deafened speakers suggested the changes in average airflow and mean volume of air per syllable moved in more normal directions postimplantation.

Longitudinal measurements have been made of fundamental frequencies, intensities, duration, and formant frequencies in the same speakers examined by Lane and Webster (1991). Changes were apparent in all the values measured after implantation; however, the changes varied greatly from individual to individual (Perkell, Lane, Svirsky, & Webster, submitted). In three out of four speakers, significant changes in first-formant frequencies were found postimplantation. Second-formant frequencies decreased for two speakers, remained constant for one speaker, and increased for one speaker postoperatively. Low vowels appear to account for more of the first-formant decreases indicating the speakers used higher tongue positions postoperatively. Second-formant frequency changes primarily involved front vowels and were in directions more nearly normal for three of the four speakers who received perceptual benefit from the implant. Three of the speakers demonstrated large tense-lax duration contrasts prior to implantation and preserved a similar (but less exaggerated) pattern postimplantation. Significant lowering of fundamental frequencies were observed postimplantation in two speakers with abnormally high pitches preimplant. A decrease in intensity was apparent in all speakers.

Although on the surface it would appear that these are rather a potpourri of findings, Perkell and his colleagues have proposed a model to account for the findings. They suggest that vowel production is influenced not only by age at deafening and perceptual performance with an implant but also by mechanical relationships between duration, fundamental frequency, and first-formant frequencies; acoustic and aerodynamic relationships between airflow and intensity; postural interactions with changes in speaking rate, fundamental frequency, and intensity; and compensatory strategies used to exaggerate tense/lax vowel contrasts. In their model, they suggest three interacting components. In the first component, speakers discriminate gross aspects of the waveform such as speaking rate, fundamental frequency, and intensity and in turn, make postural adjustments that alter these parameters. For example, it appears that increasing speaking rate results in a decrease in vowel

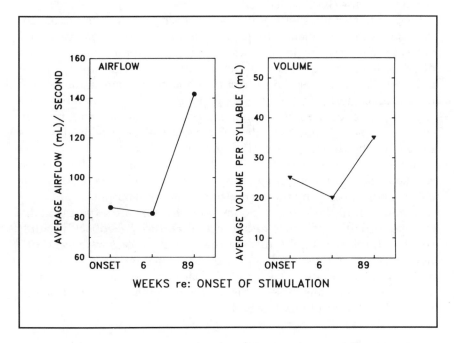

Figure 6–4. Average airflow is shown on the left panel and average volume of air expended per syllable is shown on the right panel for three postlingually deafened adults while reading passages prior to receiving stimulation from a Ineraid cochlear implant and various times after stimulation. (Adapted from Lane & Webster, 1991.)

duration. A reduction in vowel duration could influence tongue height since the tongue might not have sufficient time to lower and, hence, result in a decrease in first-formant frequencies. In the second component, it is hypothesized that the adjustments observed in the first component are complexly linked to additional parameters which result in further speech changes such as alterations to formant values and breathiness. Thus, the increases in tongue height associated with the reduced speaking rate may lead to increase tension of the vocal folds because more anterior tongue positions, in turn, move the hyoid bone forward which, in turn, pulls the strap muscles and consequently increase the tension on the vocal folds (Honda, 1983). The exaggerated pattern of intrinsic pitch (i.e., higher pitches for high vowels and lower pitches for low vowels) may be due to tongue pull when auditory feedback is absent. The tongue-pull effect is less dramatic when auditory feedback is provided via a cochlear implant. In the third component, speakers adjust their articulation to convey (or maintain) dimensions associated with phonemic contrasts, such as the durational patterns associated with tense/lax distinctions.

Longitudinal studies with adult users of cochlear implants reveal subtle changes in fundamental frequency, duration, airflow, intensity, and vowel formant frequencies. Studies examining the speech characteristics of adult users of cochlear implants suggest information from the implants serves to assist the speakers in phonetic implementation rather than phonological targeting, per se. Experience with the auditory code and linguistic features, in conjunction with information provided by cochlear implants, appears to allow some speakers to develop strategies for enhancing dimensions underlying linguistic contrasts associated with contrastive stress and tense/lax distinctions. These studies suggest speakers use information from cochlear implants to initiate a "domino" chain of adjustments in order to fine tune their vocal outputs.

In addition to these studies, some investigators are experimentally manipulating the presence or absence of auditory feedback in adult cochlear-implant users by turning the speech processors on and off. Information from these studies provide additional insight on the role of auditory feedback after speech and language are developed. In the next section, we will review these studies and highlight how they expand our knowledge about auditory feedback.

EXPERIMENTAL STUDIES IN ADULT COCHLEAR-IMPLANT USERS

Experimental manipulations of the type of auditory stimulation provided by cochlear implants have been used to explore the interactions of auditory feedback on speech production. Svirsky and Tobey (1991) compared formant frequencies of vowels produced by a single female user of a Nucleus multichannel cochlear implant without auditory stimulation (speech processor turned off) to those produced with auditory stimulation (the processor turned on). Higher first-formant frequencies were observed when the processor was on versus off in five of the eight vowels. Significant shifts in second-formant frequencies also were observed for /I/, /ɛ/, /o/, and /ɚ/. In a reversal of the conditions (processor on followed by processor off), significant shifts in first-formant frequencies were found for four out of the eight vowels and in second-formant frequencies for three of the vowels. As shown in Figure 6–5, formant frequencies for /u/ and /ae/ failed to become significantly more neutralized during the off condition but the "intermediate" vowels of /I/ and /ɛ/ became more neutralized and demonstrated considerable overlap. Observations from this study suggest some vowel formant-frequencies shift in the absence of auditory feedback and the shifts may be more dramatic in intermediate, rather than point vowels, per se. But more important, this study experimentally demonstrates that the absence of auditory feedback influences some speech parameters more than other parameters.

In a second study investigating the apparent lability of intermediate vowels in conditions with and without auditory feedback, the vowel /ɛ/ was produced under three feedback conditions (Svirsky & Tobey, 1991). Two of the conditions paralleled the first study and the third condition presented auditory feedback via a single channel. The third condition allowed the investigators to explore if the speech changes observed for this vowel in the processor on-versus-off conditions were related to the content of the auditory signal or merely a response to stimulation of the auditory nerve, per se, regardless of the information content of the signal. In one speaker, significantly lower first-formant frequencies were observed when a complete array of information was presented via the implant (see Figure 6–6). Significantly higher first formants were observed when the implant was turned off or provided only a single channel of auditory information. Significantly lower second-formant frequencies were observed in the absence or restricted auditory feedback conditions relative to the condition providing the map used daily by the speaker. In the second speaker, a similar decrease in second-formant frequencies was observed when the processor was turned off or providing only a single channel of feedback. First-formant frequencies were significantly higher when a single channel or no feedback was presented. These data suggest the type of stimulation is important: nonspectral stimulation provided by the single-channel map failed to elicit the formant frequencies seen when speaker's daily map (F0-F1-F2) was used. Thus, it appears that, at least in some talkers, the context of auditory feedback may be important for some aspects of production. The rapid changes in vowel parameters also suggests the calibration role of auditory feedback may occur within relatively short temporal windows of a few seconds or less.

To examine the size of the temporal windows associated with auditory feedback, vowel production was investigated with three adult users of a Richards implant who were asked to turn off their speech processors for 24 hours (Svirsky, Lane, Perkell, & Webster, submitted). This study explored whether a day long period of auditory deprivation resulted in speech changes and if so, what type of changes occurred. Vowel production was examined in five conditions: (1) after the speech processor was turned off for 24 hours, (2) turned immediately on, (3) after 15 minutes of use, (4) turned immediately off, and (5) after the pro-

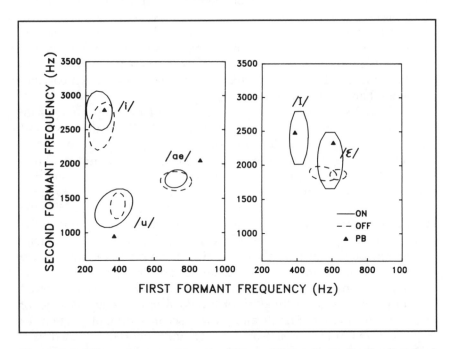

Figure 6–5. Ellipses incorporating the 99% confidence limits for the first- and second-formant frequencies are shown for five vowels. Ellipses in the left panel represent the values obtained three vowels, /i/, /æ/, and /u/, made in extreme positions in the vocal tract. The ellipses in the right panel represent the values obtained for two vowels, /ɪ/ and /ɛ/, produced in less extreme positions in the vocal tract. Solid lines represent values obtained with the speech processor turned on and dashed lines represent the values obtained with the speech processor turned off. Values for a normal hearing speaker are depicted by the triangles. Considerable overlap of values is evident for the intermediate vowels. (Adapted from Svirsky & Tobey, 1991.)

cessor was turned off for 15 minutes. Intensity measures obtained after the 24-hour deprivation period were 5–7 dB more intense than measures acquired during the last postimplant session of a longitudinal study investigating the speech characteristics of the users (Perkell et al., submitted). For two of the three users, the intensity values were similar to their preimplant values. Turning the speech processor on resulted in intensity levels which fell within one standard error of the mean of the last postimplant session. Thus, intensity changed in similar directions and magnitudes for the rapid on-off conditions, as was observed in the longitudinal study contrasting pre- and postimplantation.

Vowel-nuclei durations also changed as a function of processor status, although the pattern of change was not uniform across the three speakers. Two users demonstrated shorter durations when the speech processor was turned on relative to when the processor was turned off. However, in at least one speaker, the reductions in duration were not uniform

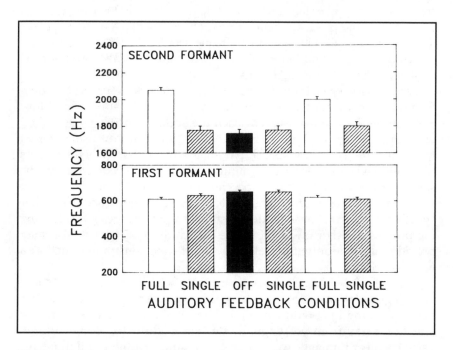

Figure 6–6. Means and standard errors for first and second formant frequencies for the vowel /ɛ/ are shown. First-formant frequencies are displayed in the lower panel and second-formant frequencies are displayed in the upper panel. Clear bars represent the values obtained with a full map (F0-F1-F2) used daily by the speaker. Striped bars represent the values obtained when the auditory stimulation was restricted to a single channel of stimulation. Solid bars represent the values obtained when the processor was turned off. (Adapted from Svirsky & Tobey, 1991.)

across all vowels. Instead, this person reduced three lax vowels (/ɪ/, /ɛ/, and /ʊ/) by approximately 25% more than three tense vowels (/i/, /a/, and /u/) when the processor was turned on after 24 hours deprivation. Duration measures also indicated different durational strategies were used by the speakers. One speaker demonstrated values that separated tense-lax pairs even after 24 hours of auditory deprivation; however, values increased further after the processor was turned back on and decreased substantially when the processor was turned off again. A second user had small variations in duration when the processor was turned on and off suggesting the subject failed to use duration to contrast tense-lax vowels. The third speaker's responses fell between the other two subjects.

Fundamental and formant frequencies also responded to the processor on-versus-off conditions. Fundamental frequencies were higher after 24 hours of auditory deprivation and dropped when the processor was turned on. Formant frequencies also showed a different pattern of responses across speakers. One speaker failed to show systematic changes in vowel space as a function of the processor being turned on versus off. A second speaker demonstrated small shifts in formant frequencies for /ɪ/, /ʊ/, /a/, and /ɛ/ reflecting higher and posterior articulation. A third speaker showed primarily shifts in the first-formant dimension for some vowels.

Overall, greater changes in speech parameters were observed when the processor was turned on immediately following 24 hours of auditory deprivation than were observed when the speech processor was turned off after 24 hours of non-use followed by 30 minutes of use. After 24 hours of non-use, many speech parameters were reset when speakers were allowed to experience 30 minutes of auditory feedback from the speech processor. Many of the speech parameters maintained their reset values immediately after the speech processor was turned off. Other speech parameters, however, demonstrated rapid changes when turning the processor either on or off suggesting auditory feedback also may provide information within relatively short time constraints, such as a few seconds or less.

Auditory feedback appears to interact with the control of some suprasegmental and segmental properties of speech production within both short- and long-term temporal windows. However, as we turn our attention away from postlingually deafened adults to young children using cochlear implants, we must keep in mind that these children have less linguistic and auditory experience. As discussed earlier, auditory feedback allows young children to compare their productions with adult models in order to develop the skilled speech gestures necessary to produce the sounds of their language. Thus, the series of tasks facing a young child are quite different than those experienced by an adult famil-

iar with the rules of a language and the skilled gestures needed to produce that language. Theoretically, auditory feedback from cochlear
implants should be used by young children to develop phonemic elements, as well as to fine tune the phonetic implementation involved in
their production.

SPEECH CHARACTERISTICS OF COCHLEAR-IMPLANTED CHILDREN

One of the first difficulties a clinician encounters when evaluating the
speech-production skills of children using cochlear implants is the lack
of normative speech-production data as a function of degree of hearing
impairment. The absence of normative data makes it difficult to predict
what speech features should be acquired and when they should be
acquired. Professionals are interested in tracking speech performance
longitudinally; however, the dearth of materials results in multiple
administrations of the same instrument. Multiple administrations
reduce the internal validity of testing instruments since it is difficult to
separate out learning of the test from a true change in performance.
Additional problems associated with inter- and intrajudge reliabilities
occur as clinicians attempt to grapple with transcribing or judging
speech samples that are basically unintelligible. Nonetheless, several
attempts to document speech-production changes over time in children
with cochlear implants are underway and constitute a initial step
towards providing information useful for comparisons with other hearing-impaired populations.

Measures Of Speech Production

Several approaches have been initiated to examine and track the speech
and language skills in deaf children receiving cochlear implants. One
approach has been to use a test battery composed of instruments typically used with hearing-impaired or normal-hearing children to measure
progress (Geers & Moog, 1991; Kirk & Hill-Brown, 1985; Tobey,
Angelette et al., 1991; Tobey, Carotta, Kienle, & Musgrave, 1986; Tobey &
Hasenstab, 1991; Waltzman et al., 1990). Examples of the type of instruments used with hearing-impaired children include the *Phonetic Task
Evaluation* (Mecklenburg, Shallop, & Ling, 1987), *Fundamental Speech Skills
Test* (Levitt, 1987), the *Central Institute of the Deaf (CID) Inventory* (Moog,
1989), the *CID Picture-Speech Intelligibility Evaluation* (Monsen, Moog, &
Geers, 1988), the *Phonetic Level Speech Evaluation* (Ling, 1976), and the
Phonologic Level Speech Evaluation (Ling, 1976). A second approach has
focused on eliciting speech samples and developing various phonetic

transcription systems to categorize the utterances (Carney, Firszt, & Johnson, 1990; Pancamo & Tobey, 1989; Osberger et al., 1991; Tobey, Pancamo, Staller, Brimacombe, & Beiter, 1991). These approaches have explored the use of metaphonological transcriptions used to code the pre-speech vocalizations of infants, traditional phonetic transcriptions, reduced phonetic feature transcriptions, and indications of speech versus nonspeech utterances. A third approach examined the acoustic characteristics of speech produced prior to implantation and at various times postimplantation (Murchison & Tobey, 1989; Tartter et al., 1989). In these studies, the acoustic features of vowels and consonants have been examined in order to determine how experience with a cochlear implant influences vowel formant frequencies and spectral/temporal properties of consonants. A fourth approach has probed the development of spoken communication rule systems, such as pragmatics, semantics, syntax and morphology (Hasenstab & Tobey, 1991).

Many of the instruments selected for use with children with cochlear implants probe a child's ability to imitate suprasegmental properties of speech including variations in duration, intensity, and fundamental frequency. Other instruments are selected because they inquire about a child's ability to imitate segmental properties such as vowel and diphthong production, simple consonants, and consonant blends. Elicited, rather than imitative, responses are also included as a means of assessing a child's ability to use suprasegmental and segmental aspects without a clinician's model. Thus, imitative tasks mimic the more traditional clinical model of providing a stimulus and examining how closely a child models it and elicited tasks examine how well a child may generalize a skill to produce it in the absence of a model.

Performance of Cochlear-Implanted Children on Imitative Speech Tasks

One of the most widely used imitative tasks has been the *Phonetic Level Speech Evaluation* which was developed to provide a framework for training and tracking speech performance in hearing-impaired children (Ling, 1976). The *Phonetic Level Speech Evaluation* consists of two major subdivisions: a division assessing suprasegmental performance and a division assessing segmental performance. The nonsegmental division assesses a child's ability to imitate sounds of varying loudness, duration, and pitch. Performance is scored as a consistently correct production, an inconsistently correct production, or an error. The segmental division seeks to inquire if the child may differentiate different sounds in isolation (such as bi, bo), reliably repeat multiple utterances (e.g., bibibibi), alternate two or more syllables at a reasonable rate (e.g., bebo), and vary the syllables in duration, loudness, or pitch. The types of segments assessed include vowels and diphthongs, simple consonants in all positions with different vowels, and consonant blends in all positions with all vowels. As in the nonsegmental division, performance is scored to indicate error, inconsistently correct, and consistently correct productions. To adapt the *Phonetic Level Speech Evaluation* as a tool for tracking speech-production performance quantitatively over time, Kirk and Hill-Brown (1985) devised a numeric system shown in Table 6–1. Error productions across all categories tested were scored a "0." Inconsistently correct productions of suprasegmental tokens were awarded a "1," and consistently correct productions were awarded a "2." Imitation of segmental skills was scaled to reflect the increasing difficulty of each of the tasks. For example, numeric scores of sounds repeated in isolation were similar to those used for nonsegmental scoring but repeated syllables received a "3" for inconsistently correct and a "4" for consistently correct productions. The highest score on a given trial was used: If a child was awarded a "2" for producing /bi/ consistently in isolation and a "3" for inconsistently repeating it (i.e., /bibibi/), the highest score was taken.

Table 6–1. *Numeric scoring system used to quantify responses on the Phonetic Level Evaluation.* Scores for each subsection are tallied and an overall composite score is acquired by adding each of the subsections*

Test Measures Score	Score
Nonsegmental Subtest	
Consistent error productions	0
Inconsistently correct productions	1
Consistently correct productions	2
Segmental Subtest	
Consistent error productions	0
Isolated Syllables	
Inconsistently correct productions	1
Consistently correct productions	2
Repeated Multiple Syllables	
Inconsistently correct productions	3
Consistently correct productions	4
Alternating Syllables	
Inconsistently correct productions	5
Consistently correct productions	6
Pitch Varying Syllables	
Inconsistently correct productions	7
Consistently correct productions	8

Adapted from Kirk & Hill-Brown (1985).
* Ling (1976)

Figure 6–7 illustrates the mean nonsegmental performance prior to implantation and at two periods postimplantation of children who received the House single-channel cochlear implant (Kirk & Hill-Brown, 1985). The House implant provides information regarding the timing and intensity of speech, as well as limited pitch information. Since suprasegmental properties of speech are carried by variations in intensity, duration, and fundamental frequencies, the physical parameters coded by the implant provide important suprasegmental cues. As shown in Figure 6–7, there was a general tendency for nonsegmental scores to improve after implantation. Small, but consistent, increases in the ability to imitate sounds of varying durations, intensities, and pitches were observed.

Increases in segmental imitation also were observed in children using the House implant as shown in Figure 6–8 (Kirk & Hill-Brown, 1985). Increases in the ability to imitate vowels and diphthongs were observed 6

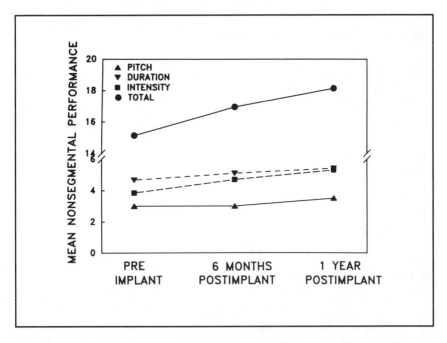

Figure 6–7. Mean nonsegmental performance on the *Phonetic Level Speech Evaluation* is illustrated for children using a House cochlear implant prior to implantation and at two times postimplantation. Total nonsegmental performance steadily increases over the postimplantation test periods. Scores are higher for duration and intensity manipulations than pitch manipulations at all test periods. (Adapted from Kirk & Hill-Brown, 1985.)

months and 1 year after use with the implant. Similarly, increases in the ability to imitate simple consonants and consonant blends were evident postimplantation. Examination of performance as a function of age at the time of implant revealed the majority of significant increases in performance occurred for children who were between the ages of 2 and 5 years when implanted. Significant increases were observed 6 months postimplant in the abilities to imitate vocal duration, pitch, intensity, vowels and diphthongs, and simple consonants. Continued increases in performance were noted for all parameters, except pitch, one year postimplantation. Children implanted between the ages of 6 and 12 years demonstrated significant increases in overall segmental imitation, which were due primarily to increases in the ability to imitate simple consonants.

Nonsegmental and segmental performance in children implanted with the Nucleus multichannel cochlear implant (Wearable Speech Processor coding F0-F1-F2) also show gains in performance after implantation (Tobey, Angelette et al., 1991). Tobey and Hasenstab (1991) found a

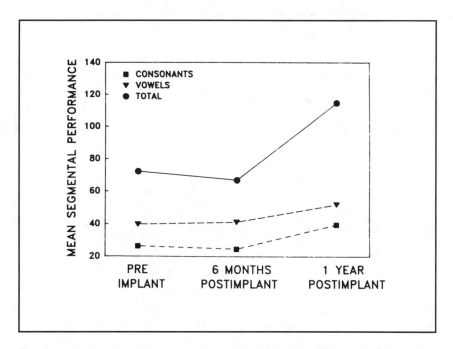

Figure 6–8. Overall segmental performance on the *Phonetic Level Speech Evaluation* significantly increases after one year's use with a House cochlear implant. Higher segmental scores are found for the imitation of vowels than simple consonants, although performance for both sections significantly increases with implant use. (Adapted from Kirk & Hill-Brown, 1985.)

trend for increased ability to imitate nonsegmental features over a two year period of time, as shown in Figure 6–9. Paired comparisons of children tested prior to implantation, and after 1 and 2 years experience indicated a significant increase in performance postimplantation; however, no significant differences were found between the two postoperative testing sessions. A steady increase in segmental performance was observed for the population of children after implantation (Figure 6–9). Paired comparisons of scores acquired from children tested preimplant and across three or four, 6-month postimplant sessions showed significant increases in performance at each postimplant session.

Clinical categories outlined in Table 6–2 were developed to provide a means of determining the clinical significance of the speech-production performance observed in children using a multichannel cochlear implant on the *Phonetic Level Speech Evaluation* (Staller, 1990; Staller, Beiter, & Brimacombe, 1991; Staller, Gibson et al., 1991; Tobey, Angelette et al., 1991). Clinical categories were formed by tabulating scores in the fashion suggested by

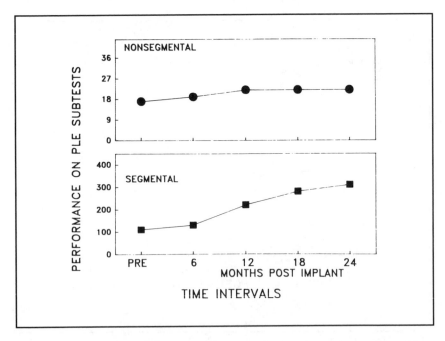

Figure 6–9. Mean performance of children using a Nucleus multichannel cochlear implant on the nonsegmental portion of the *Phonetic Level Speech Evaluation* is depicted in the upper panel. Performance on the segmental subtest is depicted in the lower panel. Segmental scores appear to steadily increase with increased usage of the cochlear implant. (Adapted from Tobey & Hasenstab, 1991.)

Kirk and Hill-Brown (1985) and examining what elements of the test were incorporated in such scores. "Clinical improvement" was arbitrarily judged to have occurred if a child's postimplantation score fell in a higher clinical category than their preoperative score. No clinical improvement was judged to occur if a child's postimplantation score fell in the same category or a lower category as their preimplantation score. Clinical improvement was observed in nonsegmental performance postimplantation in 31.1% of the 61 children tested (Tobey, Angelette et al., 1991). Average scores prior to implantation were 14.9 and 20.9 after implantation. A breakdown of the population into noncongenitally (chronological age and length of deafness differed) and congenitally (chronological age and length of deafness were the same) deafened children revealed 44% of the noncongenitally and 11.1% of the congenitally deafened children increased their nonsegmental performance by one or more "clinical categories." A similar comparison of segmental performance found 66.7% of the children improved by one or more "clinical categories" after a year's use with the multichannel cochlear implant. Mean performance before implantation was 102.9 and 179.1 after implantation. Improvements were found for 70.4% of the noncongenitally and 60.1% of the congenitally deafened children. Additional comparisons of nonsegmental and segmental performance were also made across two age groups. Significant clinical improvements in the ability to imitate nonsegmental features were found for 33.4% of the younger children and 17% of the older children. Postimplantation, 73% of the younger children and 50% of the older children showed clinical improvement for segmental imitation.

Table 6–2. *Clinical categories of the Phonetic Level Speech Evaluation* used to demonstrate and monitor changes in performance over time*

Category	Scores
Nonsegmental Performance	
Inconsistent productions	0–14
Consistent productions	15–28
Segmental Performance	
Inconsistent vowel productions	0–18
Consistent vowel productions	19–36
Consistent vowel and inconsistent consonant	37–52
Consistent vowel and visible consonants	53–104
Consistent vowel and inconsistent nonvisible consonants	105–208
Consistent simple consonants	209–416
Consistent simple and inconsistent consonant blends	417–832

Adapted from Tobey, Angelette et al. (1991).
* Ling (1976)

Another instrument which has been used to track the progress of speech-performance skills in children receiving cochlear implants is the *Phonetic Task Evaluation* (Mecklenberg et al., 1987). This measure evaluates a child's ability to imitate speech contrasts including pitch, manner, place, voicing, and vowels. Geers and Moog (1991) found higher *Phonetic Task Evaluation* scores for three children ages 6, 7, and 10 years after using a multichannel cochlear implant for a year. Scores for the 7-year old child were greater than one standard deviation improvement after 1 year's use. Geers and Moog (1991) also investigated the children's performance on the *Fundamental Speech Skills Test* (Levitt, 1987) and observed the greatest increase in performance for the 6-year-old cochlear-implant child.

Postimplant performance on imitative tasks assessing segmental aspects of speech production suggest that auditory feedback provided by cochlear implants may assist children in beginning to develop phonemic elements and refining the articulatory gestures necessary to produce the elements. The relatively poor performance of suprasegmental imitation, however, is puzzling. Given cochlear implants provide fairly robust cues related to suprasegmental features, one would have expected greater strides in performance than were evident in these studies. It may be possible that less strides were made in the imitation of suprasegmental features because the clinical emphasis in most (re)habilitation programs is on sound structure rather than on suprasegmentals (see Tye-Murray, Chapter 3). However, closer examination of these observations is warranted.

Performance of Cochlear-Implanted Children on Elicited Measures

Speech samples are routinely elicited by clinicians using a variety of materials, such as pictures, toys, or games. Samples are consequently phonetically transcribed and analyzed using a variety of techniques. One technique which has been used to describe the elicited speech of cochlear-implant children is the *Phonologic Level Speech Evaluation* (Ling, 1976). In this evaluation, responses are judged as in error, inconsistently correct or consistently correct. Kirk and Hill-Brown (1985) quantified these as "0," "1," and "2," respectively. Evaluation of children receiving a single-channel cochlear implant revealed higher nonsegmental scores at 6 months and 1 year postimplantation than prior to implantation, as shown in Figure 6–10. At 6 months postimplant, children demonstrated significant increases in breath control, intensity control, vowel duration and consonant duration. After 1 year using the implant, improvements were also noted in phrasing and stress. Segmental performance also showed steady improvement with increased cochlear implant use. The main increases in performance were found for vowels and diphthongs and simple consonants. As in the case of the imitative performance of these children, the greatest gains in performance were found for the children implanted between the ages of 2 to 5 years. Children implanted between the ages of 6 and 12 had higher nonsegmental and segmental skills relative to the younger children. Although this group of children demonstrated increased performance postimplant, the amount of change was less than the youngest group.

Tobey and colleagues (Tobey, Angelette et al., 1991; Tobey & Hasenstab, 1991) expanded the numeric system developed by Kirk and Hill-Brown for the *Phonologic Level Speech Evaluation* to include four "clinical categories" for judging progress. Scores were taken from the Kirk and

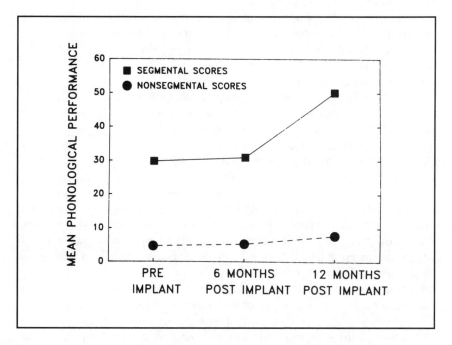

Figure 6–10. Mean performance on the nonsegmental and segmental portions of the Phonologic Speech Level Evaluation are shown for children using a House single channel cochlear implant. Segmental scores significantly increase between 6 months and a year's use with the implant. Small increases in nonsegmental performance also are evident between 6 months and 1 year's use with the House device. (Adapted from Kirk & Hill-Brown, 1985.)

Hill-Brown (1985) scoring system and "clinical categories" were devised to reflect the type of speech acts incorporated by the scores. **Category 1: Consistent Vowels and Limited Consonants** consisted of scores ranging from 0 to 20 and typically represented the production of a few visible consonants and vowels. **Category 2: Consistent Vowels and Large-set of Consonants** consisted of scores 21 to 50 and represents a greater variety of consonants in combinations with vowels. **Category 3: Simple Consonants and Inconsistent Word Initial Blends** included scores between 51 and 88 and represented the occasional use of initial consonant blends. **Category 4: Simple Consonants and Inconsistent Word Final Blends** consisted of scores between 89 and 110 and represented production incorporating a wide set of vowels and consonants. Performance was arbitrarily judged clinically improved if a child's score fell in a higher clinical category postimplant than preimplant. No improvement was judged to have occurred if the child's performance remained in the same clinical category or fell to a lower clinical category.

Evaluation of the phonologic skills revealed a little over half the children (55.6%) improved their scores more than one clinical category postimplantation. Mean performance of the children preoperatively was 34.3 and after 1 year's use, scores averaged 51.2. Increased segmental performance was observed for 61.4% of the congenitally deafened and 55.6% of the noncongenitally deafened children. Comparisons between children implanted between the ages of 2 and 9 versus 10 through 17 years revealed 66.9% of the younger children improved their segmental performance and only 47% of the older children improved their performance. Although these studies provide evidence that segmental skills are increasing in children using cochlear implants, they fail to specify precisely what is increasing.

To partially address this limitation, the consonant repertoires of children using a Nucleus multichannel cochlear implant (Wearable Speech Processor using a F0-F1-F2 coding strategy) were investigated in 29 children, ranging in age from 3.8 to 17.5 years (Pancamo & Tobey, 1989; Tobey, Pancamo et al., 1991). Speech samples were phonetically transcribed and matrices were constructed which assigned a 1 when a phoneme occurred (regardless of the number of times it occurred) and a 0 if it never occurred. Comparisons of productions collected prior to and 1 year following implantation revealed more children produced stop, fricative, glide, and nasal consonants 1 year postimplant (Tobey, Pancamo et al., 1991). As one might anticipate, prior to implantation, a significantly greater number of older profoundly hearing-impaired children produced consonants than younger children. Significantly greater numbers of children in the three youngest age groups (less than 5 years, 6–9 years, 9–11 years) produced stop consonants one year postimplant (Figure 6–11). No significant increases in the number of older children (12 years and older) were observed postimplantation for the production of stop consonants, in part, because nearly all the children were producing stop consonants prior to implantation.

One way of evaluating the influence of the implant versus possible maturational effects is to compare the postimplant performance of the youngest groups to the preimplant performance of the next older group. For example, over 70% of the children 5 years and younger produced stop consonants postimplantation but only 56% of the children in the 6–9-year-old group produced stops prior to implantation. Similarly, 72% of the 6–9-year-olds produced stop consonants postimplantation compared to 55% of the children in the 9–11-year-old group preimplant. Figure 6–12 illustrates the percentage of children producing the stop consonants as a function of place of articulation before and after implantation. A greater proportion of children produced the more visible, front consonants than the less visible, velar consonants: a finding similar to other studies investigating profoundly hearing-impaired speech. Although the proportion of children producing the

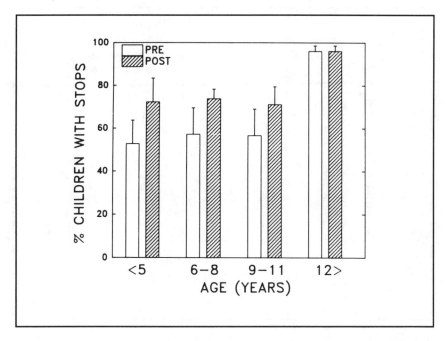

Figure 6–11. Mean percentage of children across four age groups producing stop consonants before and after implantation are shown. Percentage of children producing stop consonants prior to implantation are represented by the clear columns and percentage of children producing stop consonants postimplant are shown in striped columns. (Adapted from Pancamo & Tobey, 1989.)

voiced stop consonants did not change postimplant, the proportion of children producing the voiceless cognates was significantly greater postimplant.

A similar overall age pattern is observed for nasal consonants, as well (Figure 6–13). A greater proportion of children 12 years and older produce nasal consonants than children 5 years and younger. The more visible bilabial and alveolar nasals, /m/ and /n/ occurred more frequently than the velar /ŋ/ prior to implantation; however, a significantly greater proportion of children produced the bilabial and velar consonant postimplant (Figure 6–14). The proportion of children using the nasal-velar consonant remains small postimplant reflecting its usage in English. That is, this consonant typically appears in a medial or final position and profoundly hearing-impaired children often omit consonants in these positions.

A fewer proportion of younger children produced fricative or glide consonants as illustrated in Figures 6–15 and 6–16. In part, these lower proportions may reflect developmental factors since fricatives and glides

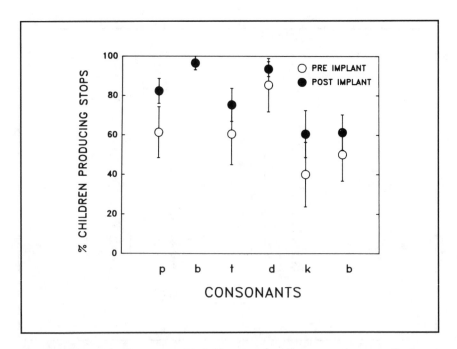

Figure 6–12. Mean percentage of children producing stop consonants displayed as a function of place of articulation and voicing. Significantly more children produced stop consonants postimplant, with the greatest increases occurring for the voiceless stop consonants. (Adapted from Pancamo & Tobey, 1989.)

are acquired later than stop and nasal consonants. Significant increases, however, are observed in the proportion of children producing these consonants postimplant. Figure 6–17 depicts the proportion of children producing the various fricatives as a function of place of articulation and voicing. A significant increase in the proportion of children producing fricatives increases postimplant for all sounds, but the voiced /ð/ and /z/. Sounds which occur less frequently in English (i. e., /θ/ and /ʒ/) are produced by fewer children regardless of implant condition. Four out of five glides also are produced by a greater proportion of children postimplant, as shown in Figure 6–18. Significantly more children produce /j/, /l/, /r/, and /w/, although the number of children producing /r/ postimplant is significantly fewer than for the other tokens.

Performance on elicited, rather than imitative, measures suggest many of the children are increasing the range of sounds in their repertoires. Moreover, the greatest strides in performance are observed for young children who fall within the critical period of speech and language

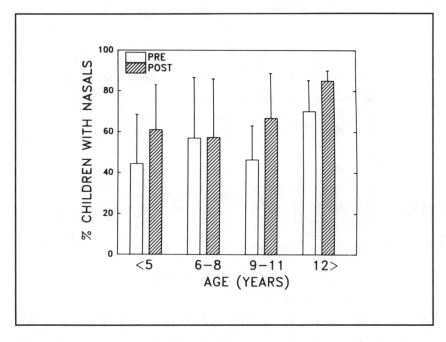

Figure 6–13. Mean percentage of children across four age groups producing nasal consonants before and after implantation are shown. Percentage of children producing nasal consonants prior to implantation are represented by the clear columns and percentage of children producing stop consonants postimplant are shown in striped columns. (Adapted from Pancamo & Tobey, 1989.)

development suggesting auditory augmentation via cochlear implants enhances the use of many sounds. Postimplant, greater numbers of children are producing the information bearing elements of speech, consonants. Information from the cochlear implant appears to assist more children in producing voiceless consonants, perhaps by providing temporal cues related to vowel length (i.e., vowels are longer following voiced stop consonants than voiceless stops). But are these changes sufficient to increase the overall intelligibility of their speech?

Increased intelligibility scores were found postoperatively in children using the Nucleus cochlear implant (Staller, 1990; Staller, Gibson et al., 1991; Tobey, Angelette et al., 1991). Speech intelligibility of 17 children improved from 18.1% preoperatively to 33.5% 1 year postoperatively, on a task modeled after McGarr (1983). In this task, children are asked to read 36 sentences varying in length and contextual cues. Overall performance is determined by the number of key words correctly identified by judges. The measure is conservative, in that only

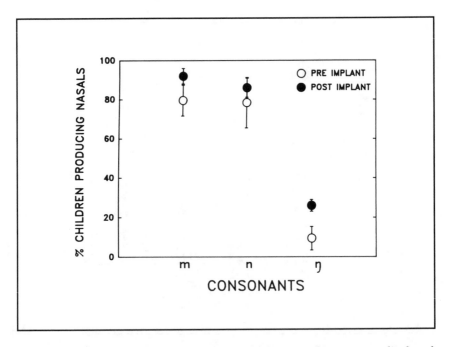

Figure 6–14. Mean percentage of children producing nasal consonants displayed as a function of place of articulation. Significantly more children produced nasal consonants postimplant; however, fewer children produced the velar consonant, /ŋ/, than the bilabial (/m/) or alveolar (/n/) nasal consonants. (Adapted from Pancamo & Tobey, 1989.)

key words are scored rather than the total number of words. It is limited in its use because children need to be able to read. Prior to implantation, speech intelligibility was remarkably similar to other reports of 18.7% (Smith, 1975), 20.7% (Brannon, 1964), 19% (John & Howarth, 1965), and 19.1% (Markides, 1970). The nearly doubling of performance postoperatively suggests feedback from the cochlear implant, in conjunction with the aural-(re)habilitation programs, may aid in increasing speech intelligibility. However, one must also recognize that increases in intelligibility are small and most children remained less than 50% intelligible.

Phonetic Analyses of Speech Performance in Cochlear-implanted Children

Osberger et al. (1991) have examined speech samples from three experimental groups of children who used either the House single-channel cochlear

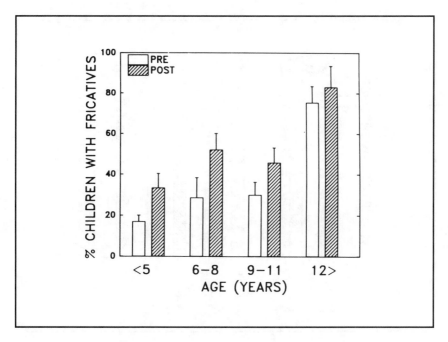

Figure 6–15. Mean percentage of children across four age groups producing glide consonants before and after implantation are shown. Percentage of children producing glide consonants prior to implantation are represented by the clear columns and percentage of children producing glide consonants postimplant are shown in striped columns. (Adapted from Pancamo & Tobey, 1989.)

implant, the Nucleus 22-electrode cochlear-implant system, or the Tactaid II, a two-channel vibrotactile aid. Each of the children received intensive speech-production training during the first 6 to 9 months of device use. Performance from these groups was contrasted to a control group of children using Tactaid II devices who received only the minimal training provided in their school program.

Three methods of analyses were devised to measure the samples. The first measure was designed to capture the pre-device characteristics of the children who produced primarily isolated sounds or single-syllable utterances with unidentifiable phonemes or sounds. Sounds were classified as speech, nonspeech, or speech-like. Nonspeech sounds included lip smacking, inhalation, lip popping, growls, "raspberries," ingressive air streams, trilled sounds and sigh/exhalation. Speech-like utterances primarily represented vocalic segments, segments with nasal quality, or glottal fry utterances. Calculations were consequently made of the percentage of vocalizations produced, the percentage of phonetic approxi-

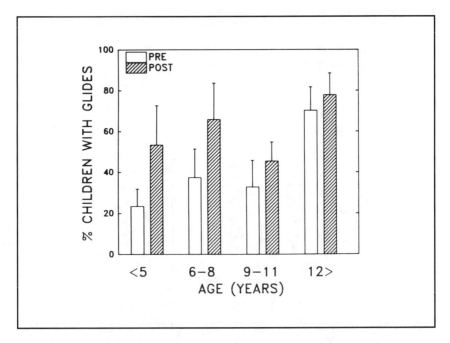

Figure 6–16 Mean percentage of children across four age groups producing fricative consonants before and after implantation are shown. Percentage of children producing fricative consonants prior to implantation are represented by the clear columns and percentage of children producing fricative consonants postimplant are shown in striped columns. (Adapted from Pancamo & Tobey, 1989.)

mations (determined from the speech and speech-like tokens) and the percentage of phonetic productions (determined from the speech tokens).

As Figure 6–19 depicts, the frequency of occurrence of vocalizations, phonetic approximations, and phonetic productions was essentially the same for the Tactaid and House device users in the pre-device condition. The number of phonetic productions was slightly less for the control group and for the Nucleus users in the pre-device condition; however, these two groups showed the greatest increase in phonetic productions after 1 year's use with the devices. The greatest changes in the Nucleus group occurred during the initial 6 months. Although this group showed the greatest improvement, only 67% of their utterances were judged to be phonetic productions. Children with House cochlear implants showed less substantial changes in performance in the latter 6 months of use. An additional type of analysis was conducted on the phonetic inventories of the children. In this case, frequency of occurrences were calculated on the consonant features by place, manner, and voicing. As shown in Figure 6–20, all four groups produced a higher percentage of stop, followed by nasal, consonants than other manner consonants prior to device use and

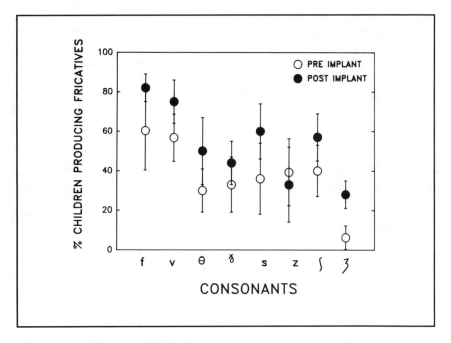

Figure 6–17. Mean percentage of children producing fricative consonants displayed as a function of place of articulation. Significantly more children produced fricative consonants postimplant. (Adapted from Pancamo & Tobey, 1989.)

after 1 year's use. The pattern of performance was used to establish a clinical goal designed to reduce the number of stop and nasal consonants and increase the number of fricatives and glides. Users of the House cochlear implant reduced the use of nasals and demonstrated minimal changes in fricatives and glides after a year's use; however, they also demonstrated increased use of stop consonants. Nucleus users produced a greater number of stop consonants in the 12-month testing period than in the pre-device period. These children produced fewer nasal consonants and a greater number of fricatives and glides in the postimplant condition relative to the preimplant condition.

Examinations of the types of place-of-articulation used by children showed a predominance of labial/labiodental productions, shown in Figure 6–21. Since alveolar/dental sounds occur more frequently in the speech of normal-hearing children, a clinical goal was established to increase the use of alveolar/dental sounds and a decrease in bilabial/labial sounds. Following training, this pattern was evident in the Nucleus implant users 12 months postimplantation. A similar pattern of performance, however, was not apparent in the House implant users.

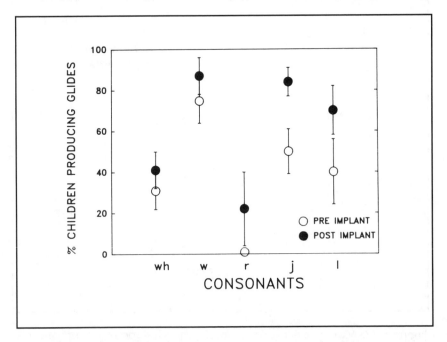

Figure 6–18. Mean percentage of children producing glide consonants displayed as a function of place of articulation. (Adapted from Pancamo & Tobey, 1989.)

Instead, these children increased the number of labial/labial dental consonants and decreased the number of dental/alveolar consonants.

Acoustic Studies of Speech Production in Cochlear-Implanted Children

Tartter et al. (1989) extensively examined the acoustic characteristics of a profoundly postlingually deafened teenager before implantation and various times after implantation of a Nucleus multichannel cochlear implant. These investigators found significantly higher fundamental frequencies occurred 1 day, 3 months, and 1 year postimplant than preimplant. Average durations decreased significantly across the postimplant testing sessions. Voice-onset times (a temporal measure reflecting the coordination of the upper and laryngeal articulators) demonstrated two categories prior to implantation: voice-onset times were longer for voiceless consonants than voiced consonants. This pattern did not reliably change over the year. Vowels were not

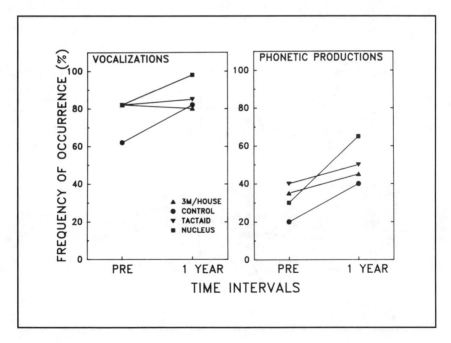

Figure 6–19. The frequency of occurrence of vocalizations and phonetic productions are shown for four groups of subjects before and after prosthetic device use. The frequency of occurrence for vocalizations is shown in the left panel and the frequency of occurrence of phonetic productions is shown in the right panel. (Adapted from Osberger et al., 1991.)

significantly longer before voiced than unvoiced consonants at any of the test sessions. The only evidence of place of articulation production changes was found in measures where the burst and frication spectra filled only a small portion of the spectrum (i.e., > 4k Hz). Vowel formant-frequency measures revealed a constriction of the vowel space.

Other investigators (Fourakis, Geers, & Tobey, 1990) have examined the acoustic properties of vowels and investigated the possibility of developing metrics for measuring progress of children using cochlear implants, tactile aids and hearing aids. These authors applied a three-dimensional auditory-perceptual space (Miller, 1988) defined by the first three significant prominences in the short-term spectrum of the vowel, as well as the fundamental frequency. These values are used to determine the x, y, and z coordinates of vowels. The values produced by the children were compared to an ideal three-dimensional representation determined for the Peterson and Barney (1952) values of children. When the prosthetic devices were compared for significant differences

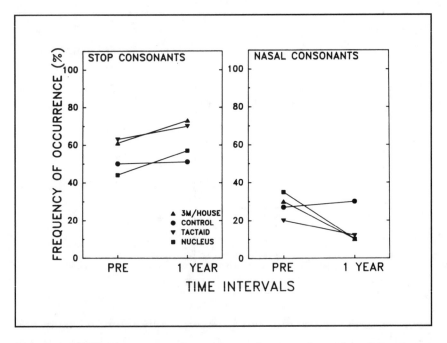

Figure 6–20. The frequency of occurrence of stop and nasal consonants are shown for four groups of subjects before and after prosthetic device use. The frequency of occurrence for stop consonants is shown in the left panel and the frequency of occurrence for nasal consonants is shown in the right panel. (Adapted from Osberger et al., 1991.)

between pre- and posttest scores, cochlear-implant users showed significant improvement on three out of five vowels, hearing-aid users showed improvement for two out of five vowels, and tactile-aid users showed no improvement for any vowel. Productions were also compared for two test sessions contrasting performance with the devices turned on versus off. The cochlear-implanted and tactile aided children produced three out of five vowels further from the target values during the device off condition. No differences were found for the child using the hearing aids.

In an experimental study contrasting the production of vowels produced with an implant turned on versus off, Tobey and her colleagues (Murchison & Tobey, 1989; Tobey, Angelette et al., 1991) examined the production of the word "head" in 10 children using the Nucleus device. Recordings were obtained during the first annual postoperative evaluation. Samples were acquired with the implant turned on, immediately after the implant was turned off, 20 minutes after the implant was

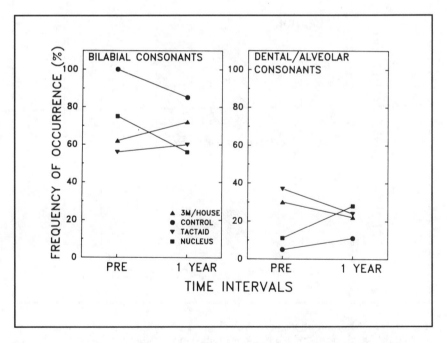

Figure 6–21. The frequency of occurrence of bilabial and dental/alveolar consonants are shown for four groups of subjects before and after prosthetic device use. The frequency of occurrence for bilabial consonants is shown in the left panel, and the frequency of occurrence for dental/alveolar consonants is shown in the right panel. (Adapted from Osberger et al., 1991.)

turned off, and immediately after the implant was turned back on. As shown in Figure 6–22, the overall duration of the tokens was significantly longer in the absence of feedback from the implant and returned to shorter values when the implant was turned back on. Changes in fundamental frequencies were evident between the two off conditions. First-formant frequencies showed an "early-late" effect (see Figure 6–23). That is, first-formant frequencies were comparable in the first two on-off conditions; however, after 20 minutes of deafness, the first formants were lower and did not increase when the implant was turned back on. Second-formant frequencies significantly decreased during the two processor off conditions relative to the processor on conditions.

Investigations of relatively "long-term" and "short-term" effects of cochlear implants suggest some aspects of vowel production may be influenced by feedback delivered by a cochlear implant. We emphasize

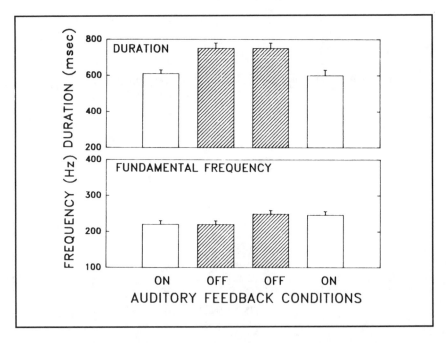

Figure 6–22. Mean durations of the vowel token, /ɛ/ are shown for 10 children producing the word "head" with a Nucleus multichannel cochlear implant turned on vs. off (upper panel). Samples were collected with the speech processor turned on, turned immediately off, after 20 minutes with the processor off, and immediately after the processor was turned back on. Overall durations were significantly longer when the implant was turned off. Mean fundamental frequencies are shown in the lower panel. Significantly higher fundamental frequencies were observed after the processor was turned off for 20 minutes. (Adapted from Murchison & Tobey, 1989.)

the phrase, "some aspects" since it does not appear that all vowels are equally influenced or influenced in similar fashions. Longitudinal studies indicated significant changes on only three out of five vowels (Fourakis et al., 1990). Examinations of vowels produced when auditory feedback is removed relatively rapidly by turning the speech processor off also indicated three out of five vowels were farther from target values when auditory feedback was absent (Fourakis et al., 1990). An additional study concentrating on a single vowel token revealed several parameters were labile to the presence or absence of auditory feedback. These parameters included changes in fundamental frequency, overall token duration, and formant frequencies (Murchison & Tobey, 1989; Tobey, Angelette et al., 1991). Although these two studies support the lability of some vowel parameters to the presence or absence of auditory feedback, the differences in design (single-subject vs. group) make it difficult to specify the various types of strategies used by children. It remains unclear if some

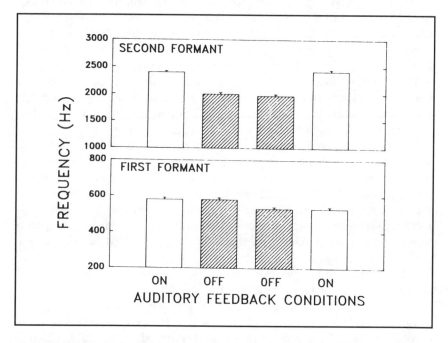

Figure 6–23. Mean formant frequencies of the vowel token, /ɛ/ are shown for ten children producing the word "head" with a Nucleus multichannel cochlear implant turned on vs. off. Samples were collected with the speech processor turned on, turned immediately off, after 20 minutes with the processor off, and immediately after the processor was turned back on. First formant frequencies are shown in the lower panel and second formant frequencies are shown in the upper panel. (Adapted from Murchison & Tobey, 1989.)

vowels will improve more than others and what type of time frame is needed to observe the improvements. Future investigations incorporating processor on-off conditions within longitudinal designs may assist in answering some of these concerns.

Spoken Language Performance in Children with Cochlear Implants

Concerns with the segmental performance of vowels and consonants represent the tip of the iceberg. Clinicians are equally concerned regarding influence of cochlear implants on the development of the five-rule systems of pragmatics, semantics, morphology, syntax, and phonology. Only two investigations (Hasenstab, 1989; Hasenstab & Tobey, 1991) have examined these rule systems in cochlear-implanted children, in part, because it is difficult to assess these systems in children who are, for most practical purposes, unintelligible. Hasenstab and Tobey (1991) describe the spoken communication skills of four children, two who lost their hearing around 3 years of age and two who had profound hearing losses present at birth. One child, 6.5 years old, lost her hearing at age 4 years and was implanted with a Nucleus multichannel cochlear implant 14 months later. Deficits were observed across all five-rule systems prior to implantation. Reacquisition and further development of the rule systems were evident 18 months postimplant. Age appropriate pragmatics, syntax, and semantics were observed, although the child continued to experience difficulty with the subtle meanings of words.

A second child, deafened at age 19 months, had 3-year's experience with the multichannel cochlear implant. Prior to implantation, sign language was used to provide receptive input but expressive output deteriorated and the child was considered noncommunicative. Spoken communication was used exclusively after 3-year's use with the implant. Pragmatic skills were determined to be age-appropriate; however, her semantic rule system was limited in vocabulary. Misarticulations characterized her phonology rule system and also affected her morphology system.

A third child with a profound congenital hearing loss was implanted at age 5 years after using amplification for 10 months. After 2.5-year's experience with the implant, the child demonstrated age-appropriate pragmatic and syntactic rule systems. Semantics were restricted in terms of vocabulary but phonology was well developed. In contrast, a fourth child who also had a profound congenital hearing loss and was implanted at age 5 years, used a mixture of sign language and spoken communication. Restrictions were found in all rule systems, although an increase in intelligible function words and phrases were emerging.

These examples serve to illustrate the difficulty of assessing linguistic rule systems in children who experience reductions in speech intelligibility. The examples highlight the enormity of the restrictions occurring in spoken language in children with profound hearing impairment and suggest the rate of acquisition of the rule systems is slow even following implantation. Acquisition of speech in children with cochlear implants appears to require the integration of phonetic and prosodic characteristics of speech with social and cognitive factors in order to continue developing effective use of linguistic rule systems for oral communication. Intervention plans for children with cochlear implants should include strategies for assisting in the development of these rule systems.

CLINICAL IMPLICATIONS FOR CHILDREN AND ADULTS WITH COCHLEAR IMPLANTS

WHAT DO WE KNOW NOW?

Before moving our attention to the future, it is practical to stop for a moment and summarize where we currently stand. Experiments in other animal species suggest the absence of auditory feedback results in a reduced repertoire of vocal output. The internal structures of the reduced repertoire are composed of higher fundamental frequencies, greater intensities, and signals of longer duration. In addition, the envelope shaping of cries in deaf animals lacks the rapid frequency and amplitude modulations seen in normal-hearing animals. If one examines the communicative effectiveness of such signals (as in those studies examining the response of territorial male or female birds to the songs of deaf birds), one must conclude the reduced repertoires are also communicatively "unintelligible." That is, the deaf songs fail to elicit the same type of responses that songs produced by normal-hearing birds elicit.

The similarity between the aberrant physical parameters of the vocal output of deaf animals and man is striking. Animal studies allow one to eliminate linguistic factors in order to isolate the direct effects of deafness on vocal output. Postlingually deafened adults typically experience higher fundamental frequencies, greater intensities, and longer durations. Difficulties with subtle phonetic implementation also is observed in consonant and vowel productions. The combined effect of these alterations on overall speech intelligibility remains controversial. For example, Goehl and Kaufman (1984) report the speech of five adults with acquired hearing losses ranging from 60–110 dB HL showed "no clinically significant deterioration of speech sound production," although they tempered their conclusions by stating changes occurred in "nonlinguistic parameters such as voice quality, pitch, loudness, and timing." Following the publication of this study, several responses appeared arguing that there are specific, identifiable articulatory effects correlated with adventitious deafness (see for example, Cowie, Douglas-Cowie, & Stewart, 1986; Zimmermann & Collins, 1984). Significant deterioration in overall speech intelligibility, however, has been observed in a young postlingually deafened child (Binnie et al., 1982) suggesting a relationship between the age of onset of deafness and length of deafness to the severity of aberrant speech parameters.

The complexity of this relationship is observable in young children with profound hearing impairments. One of the consequences of profound hearing impairment early in life is a significant reduction in the amount and content of vocal output. Children often appear to fail to grasp the concepts of articulatory targets and their associated phonological rule systems. Observations of nonspeech and speech-like elements suggest the vocalizations of children with profound hearing impairments may not be guided by linguistic units such as phonemes or the phonetic categories of vowels and consonants. Higher fundamental frequencies, greater intensities, and longer durations accompanied the poor segmental performance which, in turn, influence overall speech intelligibility. Thus, the development of oral communication skills in humans experiencing deafness during the critical periods of speech and language are hampered by a lack of articulatory/phonemic targets, as well as, poor phonetic implementation of those targets.

In postlingually deafened adults, auditory feedback from cochlear implants appears to influence some suprasegmental and segmental parameters. Auditory feedback from cochlear implants fails to influence all speech-production parameters equally. Studies contrasting speech before and after implantation demonstrate changes in intensity, fundamental frequency, and duration. Auditory feedback via a cochlear implant also influences different parameters in vowel production before and after implantation. Depriving individuals of auditory feedback by turning the speech processor on versus off demonstrates the lability of some speech parameters. Changes in formant frequencies, intensity, fundamental frequency, and durations are evident after relatively long periods of auditory deprivation (24 hours) or relatively short periods (within a few seconds).

Studies contrasting longitudinal and rapid changes in speech parameters in the same adult subjects suggest the parameters which change longitudinally also are the same parameters which change quickly when auditory feedback is eliminated by turning the speech processor off. Although it appears some speech parameters are influenced more than others by auditory feedback delivered via a cochlear implant, there is a great deal of variability across subjects as to which of these parameters change. The lack of a consistent pattern across all adult subjects suggests performance may be influenced by several factors including the number of remaining auditory nerve fibers, the number of electrodes inserted, perceptual performance with the implant, and the length of profound hearing loss. Central auditory systems appear relatively intact in postlingually deafened adults, although cochleas are nonfunctioning (Born & Rubel, 1985; Hinojosa & Marion, 1983). Differences in auditory perception across adult subjects are often attributed to differences in peripheral neural patterns (see Abbas, Chapter 7). It is not clear how individual differences in peripheral auditory neural patterns contribute to the differences in phonetic implementation strategies postimplant, however.

Interactions between peripheral and central auditory neural patterns and speech production in young children are even less clear. If central auditory mechanisms are needed, one must questioned if they are impaired in congenitally deaf children or if they will develop when presented with atypical patterns of electrical stimulation. Variability in speech-production performance across individual children is probably linked to the amount of intact peripheral and central auditory neural patterns, in conjunction with, individual differences associated with linguistic, social, and cognitive factors.

Individual differences are found in children with cochlear implants, although the greatest changes in speech performance appear at segmental levels, rather than in changes to fundamental frequencies, intensities, or durations. Longitudinal studies suggest sound acquisition may advance but it is not entirely clear what sounds will be developed first and whether some sounds will be more labile or responsive to auditory feedback from a cochlear implant than other sounds. Comparisons of sounds produced with the speech processor turned on versus off result in changes to many speech parameters; however, the lack of a systematic pattern either across sounds or across different children suggest complex interactions across linguistic, motoric, sensory, and cognitive domains. Data from the studies examining the temporal course of deterioration in adult users of cochlear implants suggest further deterioration the longer the period of auditory deprivation. Thus, one might anticipate even greater deterioration in speech skills in young children using cochlear implants if auditory feedback is removed since these children experience difficulty with phonological, as well as, phonetic implementation.

CLINICAL IMPLICATIONS

Qualitative and quantitative changes in speech-production skills are evident in a large number of children using cochlear implants. Recent data on speech production with patients using cochlear implants suggest that suprasegmental and segmental properties of speech are influenced by the auditory feedback provided by the implant. Clinical assessment of speech production should include a thorough evaluation of both properties, in conjunction with, assessments of receptive and expressive language rule systems.

Although suprasegmental performance tends to be higher following implantation, it appears to plateau after implantation and no further improvement is observed (Tobey, Angelette et al., 1991). This finding is surprising given that auditory cues for prosodic, nonsegmental properties may be coded by implants in several ways. Plateaus in performance may occur as children shift their attention to more advanced communication skills, such as accurate sound production, however, suprasegmental aspects should not be ignored within the overall clinical plan. One procedure which may serve as a reasonable model for designing a clinical intervention program highlighting suprasegmental production is described by Osberger (1988). She adapted Ling's (1976) approach in order to develop a three-stage model to improving suprasegmental control. The three stages included production on an imitative basis following an auditory model, production on demand following a visual cue, and discrimination where a teacher produced a prompt, the child imitated the prompt, and then pointed to the symbol corresponding to the teacher's prompt. One of the parameters included in the program included durational control where long and short durations were trained in order to model the relationship between stressed and unstressed syllables. Durational patterns were first taught with nonsense syllables in phrase structure and gradually expanded to include real words. Investigations of this type of procedure revealed the discrimination task is difficult and may not be appropriate for all children (particularly young preschool children). Similarly, the use of nonsense syllables did not always facilitate production of target speech patterns with words but did serve as a useful strategy for some children. Regardless of these limitations, the approach described by Osberger could form the skeleton of a clinical intervention plan for improving suprasegmental performance in cochlear-implanted children.

Significant improvements in sound production are evident in many of the children receiving cochlear implants and may be further accentuated by training specifically designed to enhance spoken communication skills (Osberger et al., 1991). Clinical goals might include: (a) the elimination of inappropriate speech or speech-like sounds, (b) the increased production of phonetic structures and syllables, (c) the increased usage of less visible places of articulation, (d) developing a more diverse set of manner-of-production consonants, and (e) an increased usage of high-front vowels. Clinical goals should stress the acquisition of articulatory targets, as well as, developing speech contrasts. As these skills develop, clinical intervention should incorporate procedures to develop the rule systems of phonology, morphology, semantics, syntax, and pragmatics.

As mentioned earlier, clinical intervention for postlingually-deafened adults is controversial (see for example, Goehl & Kaufman, 1984; Zimmermann & Collins, 1984; Cowie et al., 1986). Postlingually deafened adults rarely demonstrate difficulties with phonological parameters but, instead, experience difficulty in the implementation of the articulatory gestures underlying the phonemes. Studies contrasting speech before and after implantation reveal systematic changes in physical parameters contributing to suprasegmental and some segmental properties. Auditory feedback from cochlear implants appears to be useful in monitoring some parameters that are thought to have less alternative feedback from taction or proprioception. The type of auditory information provided by an implant also appears important. Limiting the information to a single channel delivered by a multichannel cochlear implant fails to elicit the same type of production responses that a full complement of information (F0-F1-F2) does (Svirsky & Tobey, 1991). Thus, auditory stimulation, per se, is not sufficient. Instead, it appears that the content of the feedback also is critical.

Whereas one of the long-term goals for children with cochlear implants is increasing speech intelligibility, the goals for postlingually deafened adults using cochlear implants are quite different since overall speech intelligibility may be preserved or minimally diminished. Studies examining speech-production performance in postlingually deafened adults suggest the age of onset is critical and may outweigh length of deafness (Waldstein, 1990). Phonetic and phonemic accuracy may diminish greatly if deafness occurs in childhood (Binnie et al., 1982) or adolescence (Plant, 1984). In individuals deafened early in life, clinical intervention may be a useful accessory following implantation and serve to increase the rate of change in segmental and suprasegmental parameters observed to change with implant experience. In individuals deafened later in life, clinical intervention following implantation might provide a structure environment for reacquiring subtle phonetic skills. However, these suggestions must be taken cautiously since the issue of speech-production training in adults with cochlear implants has yet to be experimentally investigated.

FUTURE DIRECTIONS FOR RESEARCH IN SPEECH PRODUCTION IN PERSONS WITH COCHLEAR IMPLANTS

The complexity of these issues serve as a challenge to clinicians and researchers. As Boothroyd queried in a discussion following a presentation of possible assessment tools for examining the speech-production skills of children with cochlear implants, "How do you approach speech management in an essentially novel population that has gone through many developmental milestones without auditory sensory input and now is suddenly provided with information that was not available previously? The intervention with this novel population may be quite different from what is generally thought of as being appropriate" (Boothroyd discussion in Tobey et al., 1986, p. 416).

To improve our assessment and management of this novel population, studies are needed in several critical areas. Studies are needed to develop standardized assessment tools for monitoring speech-production performance since there are no instruments currently available that have been standardized on hearing-impaired individuals. Clinical researchers are limited by the lack of normative data examining the interactions of chronological age and hearing level upon speech-production skills. Thus, it is difficult to predict how speech might be expected to change as a child moves from a profound hearing impairment to a severe or moderate impairment when fitted with prosthetic devices, including cochlear implants. Normative data for hearing-impaired populations of various severities would provide a meaningful baseline against which one could assess the influence of cochlear implant upon speech development.

Hierarchies of instruments are needed to track a hearing-impaired child's performance longitudinally. Ideally, the hierarchy would incorporate measures of phonetic, phonological, semantic, pragmatic, morphological, and syntactic rule systems. The hierarchy of measures should be predictive of eventual performance on higher-level measures. Information of this type would allow clinicians to address two critical questions. First, what are the speech-production skills of profoundly hearing-impaired children and second, how much better are the speech-production skills after implantation?

Additional experimental studies contrasting speech produced with and without the speech processor turned on also are needed. These experimental studies afford an investigator the luxury of manipulating an independent variable (presence or absence of auditory feedback) and determining its direct effects on dependent variables. Longitudinal studies incorporating this type of paradigm might tell us what speech parameters are likely to change, which parameters need extensive remediation in order to evoke change, and which parameters may never change. Information from these types of studies may provide the framework necessary for designing appropriate intervention programs.

Linkages between speech perception and production are evident in normal-hearing and in hearing-impaired speakers. However, the paucity of studies clearly detailing perceptual and productive performance on the same subjects makes it difficult to predict the impact auditory feedback from a cochlear implant might have upon speech production. The lack of a clear one-to-one correspondence between perceptual and production skills emphasizes the need to incorporate measures of both in the evaluation and intervention of profoundly hearing-impaired individuals. Similar considerations apply to the study of cochlear implants and their influence upon speech and language.

Studies also are needed to explore the appropriate methods to include in intervention programs. How effective are drills versus providing a child multiple opportunities to self-initiate gestures? How much time should be spent on developing speech contrasts as opposed to specific articulatory contrasts? What are the best methods for achieving generalization and retention of skills outside the clinical setting? Should speech intervention be provided adult users, and if so, what should the intervention include?

SUMMARY

The purpose of this chapter has been to review the recent literature addressing the speech-production characteristics of children and adults using cochlear implants. The major points covered in this chapter are summarized below.

1. The vocal output of deaf animals is remarkably similar to the vocal characteristics of profoundly hearing-impaired children and deaf adults. Changes in suprasegmental and segmental aspects of vocal output occur in humans and animals. The remarkable similarity supports the appropriateness of additional animal studies investigating the effects of deafness and cochlear implants upon the vocal output of animals. Such studies will allow investigators to model the linkages between the auditory and motor systems used in production. Methodical longitudinal studies may reveal important information regarding how age of onset and length of deafness influence vocal abilities.

2. The suprasegmental and segmental errors observed in postlingually deafened adults suggest difficulty with articulatory implementation, rather than phonological selection.

3. Profoundly hearing-impaired children experience a broad range of abnormal speech and language behaviors including reduced phonemic repertoires containing multiple errors.

4. Fundamental frequencies, intensities, and durations approach more normal values in postlingually deafened adults using

cochlear implants. Following implantation, postlingually deafened adults demonstrate changes in airflow and in some parameters associated with vowel production.

5. Experimental studies contrasting speech produced with a cochlear implant turned on versus off demonstrate some parameters of vowel production are more labile than other parameters. In addition, these studies suggest the content of the auditory feedback is important and the calibration role of auditory feedback may occur within relatively short temporal windows, as well as, longer temporal windows.

6. Higher suprasegmental and segmental performance is found in children using cochlear implants. Suprasegmental performance appears to plateau within the first year of use with an implant; however, improvements in segmental performance appear to occur with additional experience with the implants.

7. Comparisons of sounds produced with and without the speech processor turned on reveal children experience difficulties maintaining vowel production in the absence of auditory feedback; however, the lack of a systematic pattern across individual children suggest complex interactions between linguistic, motoric, sensory, and cognitive domains.

8. Speech intelligibility appears to nearly double after implantation relative to preimplant scores in children using cochlear implants; however, intelligibility remains below 50%. The rate of acquisition of linguistic rule systems remains slow following implantation.

9. Clinical intervention appears to assist some children using cochlear implants in decreasing the proportion of nonspeech tokens relative to speech tokens.

10. A critical need continues to exist for studies producing standardized testing instruments, establishing normative data for children of various ages with varying levels of hearing impairment, and examining the role of auditory feedback in postlingually deafened adults.

The advent of more widespread use of cochlear implants holds great promise for stimulating research investigating the role of auditory feedback and the viability of cochlear implants for providing such feedback. Continued investigations of speech production in cochlear-implant users will provide mechanisms for improving the clinical management of profoundly hearing-impaired children and adults. In addition, experimental studies contrasting speech produced with and without cochlear implants will continue to extend our current theoretical knowledge regarding the role of auditory feedback on speech production.

ACKNOWLEDGMENT

Preparation of this manuscript was supported, in part, by a National Institutes of Health Academic Research Enhancement Award (R15DC00037).

REFERENCES

Angelocci, A., Kopp, G., & Holbrook, H. (1964). The vowel formants of deaf and normal and hearing eleven to fourteen year old boys. *Journal of Speech and Hearing Disorders, 29,* 156–170.

Ball, V., & Faulkner, A. (1989). Speech production of postlingually deafened adults using electrical and acoustic speech pattern prostheses. *Speech, Hearing, and Language: Work in Progress (U.C.L.), 3,* 13–32.

Bilger, R., Black, F., Hopkins, N., Myers, E., Payne, J., Stenson, N., Vega, A., & Wolf, R. (1977). Evaluation of subjects presently fitted with implanted auditory prostheses. *Annals of Otology, Rhinology, and Laryngology, 86,* 1–76.

Binnie, C., Daniloff, R., & Buckingham, H. (1982). Phonetic disintegration in a five-year old following sudden hearing loss. *Journal of Speech and Hearing Disorders, 47,* 181–189.

Boothroyd, A. (1985). Auditory capacity and the generalization of speech skills. In J. Lauter (Ed.), Speech planning and production in normal and hearing-impaired children. *ASHA Reports, 15,* 8–14.

Boothroyd, A., Geers, A., & Moog, J. (1991). Clinical Implications of Cochlear implants in children. *Ear and Hearing,* (Suppl. 12), 81S–89S.

Borden, G. (1979). An interpretation of research on feedback interruption during speech. *Brain and Language, 7,* 302–319.

Born, D., & Rubel, E. (1985). Afferent influences on brainstem auditory nuclei of the chicken: Neuron number and size following cochlear removal. *Journal of Comparative Neurology, 231,* 435–445.

Brannon, J. (1964). Visual feedback of glossal motions and its influence on the speech of deaf children. Unpublished doctoral dissertation, Northwestern University, Chicago, IL.

Carney, A., Firszt, J., & Johnson, C. (1990). Longitudinal changes in speech intelligibility in children with cochlear implants. *ASHA, 32,* 120(A).

Carr, J. (1953). An investigation of the spontaneous speech sounds of five-year-old deaf-born children. *Journal of Speech and Hearing Disorders, 18,* 22–29.

Champagne, S. (1975). A study on the relationship between articulatory ability and spoken language of deaf and hard-of-hearing adolescent children. Unpublished master's thesis. The Ohio State University, Columbus, OH.

Cowie, R. & Douglas-Cowie, E. (1983). Speech production in profound postlingual deafness. In M. Lutman & M. Haggard (Eds.), *Hearing Science and Hearing Disorders* (pp. 183–231). New York: Academic Press.

Cowie, R., Douglas-Cowie, E., & Kerr, A. (1982). A study of speech deterioration in postlingually deafened adults. *Journal of Laryngology and Otology, 96,* 101–112.

Cowie, R., Douglas-Cowie, E., & Stewart, P. (1986). A response to Goehl and Kaufman. *Journal of Speech and Hearing Disorders, 51,* 183–187.

Ehret, G., & Romand, R. (1981). Postnatal development of absolute auditory thresholds in kittens. *Journal of Comparative Physiology and Psychology, 95,* 304–311.

Elman, J. (1981). Effects of frequency-shifted feedback on the pitch of vocal productions. *Journal of Acoustical Society of America, 70,* 45–50.

Fairbanks, G. (1955). Selected vocal effects of delayed auditory feedback. *Journal of Speech and Hearing Research, 20,* 333–345.

Fourakis, M., Geers, A., & Tobey, E. (1990). Acoustic evaluation of vowels produced by hearing impaired children. *Journal of Acoustical Society of America, 88,* S175(A).

Geers, A., & Moog, J. (1991). Evaluating the benefits of cochlear implants in an education setting. *American Journal of Otology,* (Suppl. 12), 116–125.

Geffner, D. (1980). Feature characteristics of spontaneous speech production in young deaf children. *Journal of Communication Disorders, 13,* 443–454.

Goehl, H., & Kaufman, D. (1984). Do the effects of adventitious deafness include disordered speech. *Journal of Speech and Hearing Disorders, 49,* 58–64.

Gold, T. (1980). Speech production in hearing-impaired children. *Journal of Communication Disorders, 13,* 397–418.

Hasenstab, S. (1989). The multichannel cochlear implant in children. *Topics in Language Disorders, 4,* 45–59.

Hasenstab, S., & Tobey, E. (1991). Language development in children receiving Nucleus multichannel cochlear implants. *Ear and Hearing,* (Suppl. 12), 55S–65S.

Hinojosa, R., & Marion, M. (1983). Histopathology of profound sensorineural deafness. In C. Parkins & S. Anderson (Eds.), Cochlear Prostheses: An international symposium. *Annals of the New York Academy of Sciences, 405,* 450–484.

Hochmair-Desoyer, I. (1981). Four years experience with a cochlear prosthesis *Medical Progress of Technology, 8,* 107–119.

Honda, K. (1983). Relationship between pitch control and vowel articulation. In D. Bless & J. Abbs (Eds.), *Vocal fold physiology: contemporary research and clinical issues.* San Diego: College-Hill Press.

Horii, Y. (1982). Some fundamental frequency characteristics of oral reading and spontaneous speech by hard-of-hearing young women. *Journal of Speech and Hearing Research, 25,* 608–610.

Hudgins, C., & Numbers, F. (1942). An investigation of the intelligibility of the speech of the deaf. *Genetic Psychology Monographs, 25,* 289–392.

John, J., & Howarth, H. (1965). The effect of time distortions on the intelligibility of deaf children's speech. *Language and Speech, 8,* 127–134.

Kent, R., & Murray, A. (1982). Acoustic features of infant vocalic utterances at 3, 6, and 9 months. *Journal of Acoustical Society of America, 72,* 353–365.

Kent, R., Osberger, M., Netsell, R., & Hustedde, C. (1987). Phonetic development in identical twins differing in auditory function. *Journal of Speech and Hearing Research, 52,* 64–75.

Kirk, K., & Edgerton, B. (1983). The effects of cochlear implant use on voice parameters. *Otolaryngological Clinics of North America, 16,* 281–292.

Kirk, K., & Hill-Brown, C. (1985). Speech and language results in children with a cochlear implant. *Ear and Hearing, 6,* 36S–47S.

Konishi, M. (1963). The role of auditory feedback in the vocal behavior of the domestic fowl. *Z. Tierpsychologia, 20,* 349–367.

Konishi, M. (1964). Effects of deafening on song development in two species of juncos. *Condor, 66,* 86–102.

Konishi, M. (1965). Effects of deafening on song development in American robins and black-headed grosbeaks. *Z. Tierpsychologia, 22,* 284–599.

Lach, R., Ling, D., Ling, A., & Ship, N. (1970). Early speech development in deaf infants. *American Annals of the Deaf, 118,* 43–45.

Lane, H., Perkell, J., Svirsky, M., & Webster, J. (1991). Changes in speech breathing following cochlear implants in postlingually deafened adults. *Journal of Speech and Hearing Research, 34,* 526–533.

Lane, H., & Tranel, B. (1971). The Lombard Sign and the role of hearing in speech. *Journal of Speech and Hearing Research, 14,* 677–709.

Lane, H., & Webster, J. (1991). Speech deterioration in postlingually deafened adults. *Journal of Acoustical Society of America, 89*(2), 859–866.

Leder, S., Spitzer, J., & Kirchner, J. (1987a). Speaking fundamental frequency of postlingually profoundly deaf adult men. *Annals of Otology, Rhinology, and Laryngology, 96,* 322–324.

Leder, S., Spitzer, J., Milner, P., Flevaris-Phillips, C., Richardson, F., & Kirchner, J.C. (1986). Reacquisition of contrastive stress in an adventitiously deaf speaker using a single-channel cochlear implant. *Journal of Acoustical Society of America, 79*(6),1967–1974.

Leder, S., Spitzer, J., Milner, P., Flevaris-Phillips, C., Kirchner, J., & Richardson, F. (1987c). Voice intensity of prospective cochlear implant candidates and normal-hearing adult males. *Laryngoscope, 97,* 224–227.

Leder, S., Spitzer, J., Kirchner, J., Flevaris-Phillips, C., Milner, P., & Richardson, F. (1987b). Speaking rate of adventitiously deaf male cochlear implant candidates. *Journal of Acoustical Society of America, 82*(3), 843–846.

Leder, S., & Spitzer, J. (1990). A perceptual evaluation of the speech of adventitiously deaf adult males. *Ear and Hearing, 11*(3), 169–175.

Lee, B. (1950). Some effects of side tone delay. *Journal of Acoustical Sociel of America, 22,* 639–640.

Levitt, H. (1987). Fundamental Speech Skills Test. New York: City University of New York.

Liberman, A., Cooper, F., Shankweiler, D., & Studdert-Kennedy, M. (1967). *Perception of the speech code. Psychological Review, 74,* 431–461.

Ling, D. (1976). *Speech and the hearing impaired child: Theory and practice.* Washington, DC: Alexander Graham Bell Association.

Mangan, K. (1961). Speech improvement through articulation testing. *American Annuals of the Deaf, 106,* 391–396.

Markides, A. (1970). The speech of deaf and partially hearing children with special reference to factors affecting intelligibility. *British Journal of Disorders of Communication, 5,* 126–140.

Marler, P. (1981). Birdsong: The acquisition of a learned motor skill. *Trends in Neurosciences, 4,* 88–94.

Marler, P., & Sherman, V. (1983). Song structure without auditory feedback: Emendations of the auditory template hypothesis. *The Journal of Neuroscience, 3*(3), 517–531.

Marler, P., & Tamura, M. (1964). Culturally transmitted patterns of vocal behavior in sparrows. *Science, 146,* 1483–1486.

Martony, J. (1968). On the correction of the voice pitch level for severely hard of hearing subjects. *American Annals of the Deaf, 113,* 195–202.

Mecklenberg, D., Shallop, J., & Ling, D. (1987). *Phonetic task evaluation.* Englewood, CO: Cochlear Corporation.

McGarr, N. (1983). The intelligibility of deaf speech to experienced and inexperienced listeners. *Journal of Speech and Hearing Research, 26,* 451–458.

McGarr, N., & Harris, K. (1980). Articulatory control in a deaf speaker. *Haskins Laboratories Status Report on Speech Research, SR-63/64,* 309-322.

Miller, J. (1988). Auditory-perceptual analysis of selected syllables. *Journal of Acoustical Society of America, 84,* S154(A).

Monsen, R. (1979). Acoustic qualities of phonation in young hearing-impaired children. *Journal of Speech and Hearing Research, 22*, 270–288.

Monsen, R., Moog, J., & Geers, A. (1988). The Picture Speech Intelligibility Evaluation. St. Louis: Central Institute of the Deaf.

Moog, J. (1989). The CID Phonetic Inventory. St. Louis: Central Institute of the Deaf.

Murchison, C., & Tobey, E. (1989). Rapid changes in speech production with and without auditory stimulation. *Proceedings of the Second Annual Southeastern Allied Health Research Symposium*, 260–268. Louisiana State University Medical Center: New Orleans, LA.

Nober, H. (1967). Articulation of the deaf. *Exceptional Children, 33*, 611–621.

Nottebohm, F., & Nottebohm, M. (1971). Vocalizations and breeding behavior of surgically deafened ring doves, <u>Streptopelia risoria</u>. *Animal Behavior, 19*, 313–327.

Osberger, M. (1988). Development and evaluation of some speech training procedures for hearing impaired children. *Speech of the Hearing Impaired: Research, Training and Personnel Preparation*, 333–348.

Osberger, M., & Levitt, H. (1979). The effect of timing errors on the intelligibility of deaf children's speech. *Journal of Acoustical Society of America, 66*, 1316–1324.

Osberger, M., & McGarr, N. (1982). Speech production characteristics of the hearing impaired. In N. Lass (Ed.), *Speech and language: Advances in basic research and practice*, New York: Academic Press.

Osberger, M., Robbins, A., Berry, S., Todd, S., Hesketh, L., & Sedey, A. (1991). Analysis of the spontaneous speech samples of children with a cochlear implant or tactile aid. *American Journal of Otology*, (Suppl. 12), 173–181.

Pancamo, S., & Tobey, E. (1989). Effects of multichannel cochlear implant upon sound production in children. *Proceedings of the Second Annual Southeastern Allied Health Research Symposium*, pp 319–330. Louisiana State University Medical Center: New Orleans, LA.

Perkell, J., Lane, H., Svirsky, M., & Webster, J. (Submitted). Speech of cochlear implant patients: A longitudinal study of vowel production. *Journal of Acoustical Society of America.*

Peterson, G., & Barney, F. (1952). Control methods used in a study of the vowels *Journal of Acoustical Society of America, 24*, 175–184.

Plant, G. (1984). The effects of an acquired profound hearing loss on speech production. *British Journal of Audiology, 18*, 39–54.

Plant, G., & Oster, A. (1986). The effects of cochlear implantation on speech production. A case study. STL-QPSR, 1, 65–83.

Romand, R., & Ehret, G. (1984). Development of sound production in normal, isolated, and deafened kittens during the first postnatal months. *Developmental Psychobiology, 17*(6), 629–649.

Searcy, W., & Marler, P. (1987). Response of sparrows to songs of deaf and isolation-reared males: Further evidence for innate auditory templates. *Developmental Psychobiology, 20*(5), 509–519.

Schleidt, W. (1964). Uber die Spontaneitat von Erbkoordinationen. *Z. Tierpsychologia, 21*, 235–356.

Shipley, C., Buchwald, J., & Carterette, E. (1988). The role of auditory feedback in the vocalizations of cats. *Experimental Brain Research, 69*, 431–438.

Shukla, R. (1989). Phonological space in the speech of the hearing impaired. *Journal of Communication Disorders, 22*, 317–325.

Smith, B. L. (1978). Temporal aspects of English speech production: A developmental perspective. *Journal of Phonetics, 6*, 37–68.

Smith, C. (1975). Residual hearing and speech production in deaf children. *Journal of Speech and Hearing Research, 18*, 795–811.

Staller, S. (1990). Perceptual and productive abilities in profoundly deaf children with multichannel cochlear implants. *Journal of American Academy for Audiology, 1*, 1–3.

Staller, S., Beiter, A., & Brimacombe, J. (1991). Children and multichannel cochlear implants. In *Cochlear Implants: A Practical Guide*, (pp. 283–321). Whurr Publishers Limited: London.

Staller, S., Gibson, A., Beiter, A., Chute, P., Goin, D., Portmann, M., & Schwartzman, G. (1991). Cochlear implants in children: results and complications. In I. Kaugman Arenberg (Ed.), *Proceedings of the Third International Symposium and Workshops on the Surgery of the Inner Ear* (pp. 1–4). Amsterdam: Kugler and Ghedini Publications.

Stark, R., & Levitt, H. (1974). Prosodic feature perception and production in deaf children. *Journal of Acoustical Society of America, 55*, S23(A).

Stevens, K., Nickerson, R., & Rollins, A. (1978). On describing the suprasegmental properties of the speech of deaf children. In D. McPherson & M. Davids (Eds.), *Advances in prosthetic devices for the deaf: A technical workshop* (pp. 134–155). Rochester, NY: National Technical Institute for the Deaf.

Svirsky, M., & Tobey, E. (1991). Effect of different types of auditory stimulation on vowel formant frequencies in multichannel cochlear implant users. *Journal of Acoustical Society of America, 89*, 2895–2904.

Svirsky, M., Lane, H., Perkell, J., & Webster, J. (Submitted). Effects of short-term auditory deprivation on speech production in adult cochlear implant users. *Journal of Acoustical Society of America.*

Tartter, V., Chute, P., & Hellman, S. (1989). The speech of a postlingually deafened teenager during the first year of use of a multichannel cochlear implant. *Journal of Acoustical Society of America, 86*, 2113–2121.

Tobey, E., Carotta, C., Kienle, M., & Musgrave, G. (1986). Speech production considerations in the management of children receiving cochlear implants. *Seminars in Hearing, 7*, 407–422.

Tobey, E., & Hasenstab, S. (1991). Effects of a Nucleus multichannel cochlear implant upon speech production in children. *Ear and Hearing*, (Suppl. 12), 48S–54S.

Tobey, E., Angelette, S., Murchison, C., Nicosia, J., Sprague, S., Staller, S., Brimacombe, J. & Beiter, A. (1991). Speech production in children receiving a multichannel cochlear implant. *American Journal of Otology*, (Suppl. 12), 164–172.

Tobey, E., Pancamo, S., Staller, S., Brimacombe, J., & Beiter, A. (1991). Consonant production in children receiving a multichannel cochlear implant. *Ear and Hearing, 12*, 23–31.

Waldstein, R. (1990). Effects of postlingual deafness on speech production: Implications for the role of auditory feedback. *Journal of Acoustical Society of America. 88*(5), 2099–2114.

Waltzman, S., Cohen, N., Spivak, L., Ying, E., Brackett, D., Shapiro, W., & Hoffman, R. (1990). Improvement in speech perception and production abilities in children using a multichannel cochlear implant. *Laryngoscope, 100*, 240–243.

Weinberg, B., & Zlatin, M. (1970). Speaking fundamental frequency characteristics of five- and six-year old children with mongolism. *Journal of Speech and Hearing Research, 13*, 418–425.

Zimmermann, G., & Collins, M. (1984). The speech of the adventitiously deaf and auditory information: A response to Goehl and Kaufman (1984). *Journal of Speech and Hearing Disorders, 6*, 220–221.

Zimmermann, G., & Rettaliata, P. (1981). Articulatory patterns of an adventitiously deaf speaker: Implications for the role of auditory information in speech production. *Journal of Speech and Hearing Research, 24,* 169–178.

CHAPTER 7

Electrophysiology
PAUL J. ABBAS

Acoustic stimulation of the normal ear produces a traveling wave of vibration in the cochlea, which selectively stimulates hair cells along the length of the basilar membrane according to the frequency of the stimulus. The activated hair cells in turn release chemical neurotransmitters to their associated terminals which generate action potentials on the auditory-nerve fibers. Action potentials then propagate along the length of the nerve fiber, transmitting information to brainstem nuclei. A cochlear implant bypasses this normal processing of sound by the cochlea and stimulates auditory-nerve fibers directly. Since the normal pattern of excitation of neurons is so complex, no artificial device is yet capable of reproducing the normal pattern of neural responses to sound in a deaf individual.

To understand the functioning and the limitations of a cochlear implant, it is important to be familiar with the electrophysiological responses of single neurons in the normal auditory system. As more individuals with significant amounts of residual hearing are receiving cochlear implants, decisions concerning implantation are going to be more dependent on the comparison between hearing-impaired individuals with amplification and those with cochlear implants. An understanding of the underlying physiological responses in the impaired auditory system provides a basis for comparisons between these two groups.

There are several noninvasive test procedures which rely on physiological measures of auditory function. These tests, such as the electrically evoked brainstem response, generally use far-field measures of neural response, that is, the summed activity of a population of neurons are measured rather than the action potentials from single neurons. Several of these far-field measures may have clinical utility in choosing candidates for cochlear implants, fitting the implant to an individual, and diagnosing hardware problems.

This chapter summarizes both single neuron and far-field responses. First, data from single neurons are discussed. Topics include the responses to sound stimuli, some ways in which these responses change with hearing impairment, and the differences in neural response to acoustic and electric stimulation. Single-unit data are limited to animal studies but far-field evoked response measures can be made in both animals and humans. The discussion of far-field measures provides a basis for comparison among species. Finally, several applications of far-field measures to human cochlear-implant users are discussed.

RESPONSE PROPERTIES OF AUDITORY-NERVE FIBERS

This section is organized into subsections dealing with specific response properties of the single neurons in auditory-nerve response. In each subsection, the discussion includes data from normal-hearing experimental animals, data from animals with induced hair cell pathology (when available), and data from animals stimulated by a cochlear implant.

The number of neurons in the auditory nerve varies across animal species but is generally on the order of 10,000 neurons. Each neuron synapses on hair cells in a particular region of the cochlea. For descriptive purposes, these neurons are separated into larger, more numerous Type I cells which innervate inner hair cells and smaller Type II cells which innervate outer hair cells (Spoendlin, 1973). The experiments summarized below usually entail placing a microelectrode into the auditory nerve of an anesthetized animal to isolate the electrical activity of an individual neuron. Either acoustic stimuli or electrical stimuli are then presented and the electrical response of the auditory-nerve fiber, in the form of action potentials, is recorded from the individual neuron. These responses are usually counted or used to generate histograms that represent the fiber's activity over time. These response patterns are thought to be primarily from the larger Type I afferent fibers synapsing on inner hair cells (since activity from larger diameter cells are easier to isolate).

The response of auditory-nerve fibers in impaired ears can be quite variable, depending on the type and degree of sensorineural damage.

No effort is made here to be comprehensive, but only to discuss some general properties of impaired ears. The reader is referred to a text by Harrison (1988) for a more detailed analysis of pathological responses.

The response of the auditory-nerve fibers to electrical stimulation are quite different than the response of the same fibers to acoustic versions of the same stimulus. Direct electrical stimulation of the auditory nerve bypasses the processing of the acoustic stimulus by the middle ear, the mechanical tuning of the basilar membrane, and the transduction process of hair cells. Consequently, the responses of neurons to electrical stimulation do not reflect the filtering properties of the middle ear, the tuning properties of the cochlea, or the synaptic properties of the hair cells.

Electrical stimulation in most of the experiments that are described below is accomplished through electrodes placed either on the round window, within the cochlea fluid, or within the modiolus of the cochlea. Electrical current is effective in stimulating an action potential within an afferent neuron of the auditory nerve, although the site of initiation of the action potential (along the length of the fiber) may vary with stimulus waveform or current level (Finley, Wilson, & White, 1989; van den Honert & Stypulkowski, 1984). Responses have been characterized in response to analog stimulation (sinusoidal or slowly time-varying stimuli) and to pulsatile stimulation. Pulsatile stimulation can be either biphasic (a short positive pulse followed by an equal negative pulse) or monophasic.

SPONTANEOUS ACTIVITY

With no stimulation of the ear, the neurons of the auditory nerve generally discharge with a series of action potentials referred to as spontaneous activity. The rate of spontaneous activity can be high in some neurons (on the order of 100 spikes/s) or close to zero spikes/s in other neurons (Kiang, Watanabe, Thomas, & Clark, 1965). Spontaneous activity is related to the sensitivity of individual fibers in the normal ear. Neurons with high spontaneous activity typically have low-response thresholds (Liberman, 1978). In certain situations, the rate of spontaneous activity of auditory-nerve fiber can be affected by hair-cell damage. Liberman and Dodds (1984) observed that spontaneous activity rate in fibers from noise-traumatized ears tended to be lower than that in normal ears, particularly those fibers where the stereocilia of inner hair cells were damaged. A normal distribution of spontaneous activity levels is observed in ears where only outer hair cells are damaged (Robertson & Wilson, 1991). Spontaneous activity is absent in ears devoid of both inner and outer hair cells (Hartmann & Klinke, 1989).

TUNING PROPERTIES

Single fibers generally respond with an increase in the rate of action potentials in response to pure-tone stimuli. This discharge rate carries information about the frequency and intensity of the tone. At low levels, the discharge rate of action potentials is low and a relatively narrow range of frequencies is effective in eliciting a response from a particular fiber or place. At higher levels, the discharge rate increases and the range of effective frequencies also increases. The threshold of response as a function of frequency is called a **tuning curve** or **frequency-threshold curve** (Kiang et al., 1965; Liberman & Kiang, 1978). Schematic examples are shown in Figure 7–1a. The characteristic frequency of a specific nerve fiber (i.e., the frequency to which it is most sensitive) depends on the location on the basilar membrane of the hair cell with which the neuron synapses. Low characteristic frequency fibers innervate hair cells close to the apex of the cochlea; high characteristic frequency fibers innervate hair cells near the base. The tuning curve of an individual neuron reflects the tuning properties of the mechanical traveling wave at the place of its source in the cochlea (Liberman, 1982; Sellick, Patuzzi, & Johnstone, 1983).

Responses of auditory-nerve fibers with experimentally induced sensorineural hearing impairment show several changes in tuning properties. The most consistent observation has been that the threshold in the sharply tuned tip of the tuning curve is higher than normal, making the fiber less sensitive to sound. In many cases, the thresholds at low frequencies are not affected. The result in these cases is a tuning curve distorted in shape with decreased frequency selectivity (Kiang, Moxon, & Levine, 1970; Liberman & Kiang, 1978). Examples of such a change are illustrated in Figure 7–1b. These changes may be permanent or reversible depending on the specific cochlear insult (Cody & Johnstone, 1980; Evans, 1974; Liberman & Dodds, 1984).

The frequency tuning properties in response to electrical stimulation are relatively broad. The threshold of response to sinusoidal electrical stimulation varies little as stimulus frequency is changed (Figure 7–1c). For all fibers, threshold is lowest at approximately 100 Hz and increases gradually with frequency (Hartmann, Topp, & Klinke, 1984; Kiang & Moxon, 1972). Also, threshold across fibers is relatively uniform, with a range on the order of 12 dB (van den Honert & Stypulkowski, 1984, 1987a). These observations contrast greatly with the normal sharp tuning to acoustic stimuli, where fibers have different characteristic frequencies that are a function of place along the basilar membrane. The similarity in threshold across fibers that is observed when electrical stimulation is used, is in contrast to the large differences in sensitivity to acoustic stimuli observed between low and high spontaneous rate fibers (Liberman, 1978).

Although the frequency tuning of fibers to electrical stimulation does not approach that obtained with acoustic stimulation, some semblance of place-specific stimulation can be accomplished by placing electrodes in different parts of the cochlea. The threshold of electrical stimulation of neurons of the auditory nerve is highly dependent on the position and

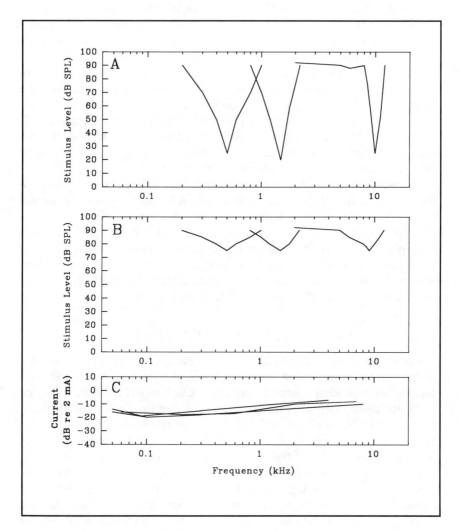

Figure 7–1. Schematic drawing of tuning curves of auditory nerve fibers in response to acoustic stimulation of a normal ear (a), of an impaired ear (b), and in response to electrical stimulation (c). Threshold sound pressure or current level is plotted as a function of stimulus frequency. (Adapted from Kiang & Moxon, 1972, and Evans, 1974.)

orientation of the stimulating electrodes. With monopolar intracochlear stimulation (one electrode within the cochlea and the second electrode outside), the threshold of all fibers are similar, that is, there is little change in threshold with fiber characteristic frequency (Hartmann & Klinke, 1989; van den Honert & Stypulkowski, 1987a). Bipolar electrodes placed longitudinally (along the length of the basilar membrane) demonstrate lower response thresholds for fibers in the region of electrodes than for fibers remote to the electrodes. The most highly place-specific responses are seen with bipolar electrodes arranged in a radial direction (at the same location but one placed farther away from the modiolus). With that configuration, the response threshold for fibers near the electrode place were substantially lower than fibers at adjacent locations (Finley et al., 1989; van den Honert & Stypulkowski, 1987a). Other studies in which recordings have been made from the inferior colliculus have also shown a high degree of place-specific responses with bipolar stimulation (Black & Clark, 1980; Merzenich & White, 1979; Schindler, Merzenich, White, & Bjorkroth, 1977).

The fact that place-specific neural responses can be obtained with electric stimulation of the cochlea means that, at least in ears with a normal complement of nerve fibers, different electrodes can be expected to stimulate different populations of nerve fibers and consequently transmit multiple channels of information to the nervous system. These observations are important because they suggest that multichannel implant arrays can be designed such that different nerve populations can be stimulated independently (see also Shannon, Chapter 8).

GROWTH OF RESPONSE WITH STIMULUS LEVEL

Other experiments have measured the changes in discharge rate that accompany changes in stimulus level. When a fiber is stimulated with pure tones at its characteristic frequency, discharge rate increases as the intensity of the stimulus increases over a dynamic range of approximately 30 dB. Above that level, the discharge rate shows saturation, that is, there is no further increase in discharge rate with increasing stimulus level. Both the growth of the response and the dynamic range are dependent on frequency of stimulation. Stimulus frequencies lower than fiber characteristic frequency produce steep growth functions and small dynamic ranges; stimulus frequencies higher than fiber characteristic frequencies produce more shallow growth functions with wider dynamic ranges obtained (Sachs & Abbas, 1974). Schematized examples of such functions are illustrated in Figure 7–2a.

The growth functions obtained from nerve fibers innervating impaired regions of the cochlea tend to have a steeper slopes than those in normal regions (Harrison, 1981). The changes in slope of the growth functions that are obtained when different stimulus frequencies are used to stimulate normal fibers are not evident in impaired fibers. Impaired fibers show uniformly steep slopes for each stimulus frequency as illustrated in Figure 7–2b. The responses of both normal and impaired auditory-nerve fibers are nonlinear in nature; they demonstrate a threshold effect and a saturation with increasing stimulus level. However, fibers innervating impaired regions of the cochlea lose many of their nonlinear properties, particularly the properties that have been attributed to basilar-membrane mechanics.

When electrical stimulation is used, auditory-nerve fibers show a fast growth of response with increases in stimulus level compared to fibers of either normal or hearing-impaired ears that are stimulated acoustically (Figure 7–2c). When electrical stimulation is used, dynamic range is reduced (2–6 dB) and the maximum discharge rate of action potentials is typically much greater than when acoustic stimulation is used (Hartmann et al., 1984; Javel, Tong, Shepherd, & Clark, 1987; Kiang & Moxon, 1972). These differences are at least in part attributable to the absence of the nonlinear compression introduced by the basilar membrane vibrations and the hair-cell transduction process.

TEMPORAL RESPONSE PROPERTIES

The auditory hair cells are polarized; stereocilia movement in one direction is **excitatory,** and movement in the other is **inhibitory.** Therefore, the timing of action potentials follows the vibration of the basilar membrane. This pattern can be observed in the period histogram, which is generated by recording the timing of action potentials relative to the beginning of a cycle of a periodic stimulus. Figure 7–3a shows a schematized example of a period histogram plotting the number of action potentials that occur as a function of time across one period of the pure-tone stimulus. There is a peak in the histogram, indicating that action potentials tend to occur at a preferred phase of the stimulus (phase locking). This **phase locking** does not necessarily indicate entrainment of action potentials to the cyclic stimulus, that is, an action potential may not occur during each stimulus cycle. Rather, when action potentials occur they do so with a greater probability at a specific phase of the stimulus.

The timing of the responses to electrical stimulation tends to be more precise and repeatable than with acoustic stimulation. The period histogram in Figure 7–3b characterize these response patterns to a sinusoidal current stimulus. This histogram shows a narrower peak indicating greater synchrony than that observed for acoustic stimulation (Hartmann et al.,

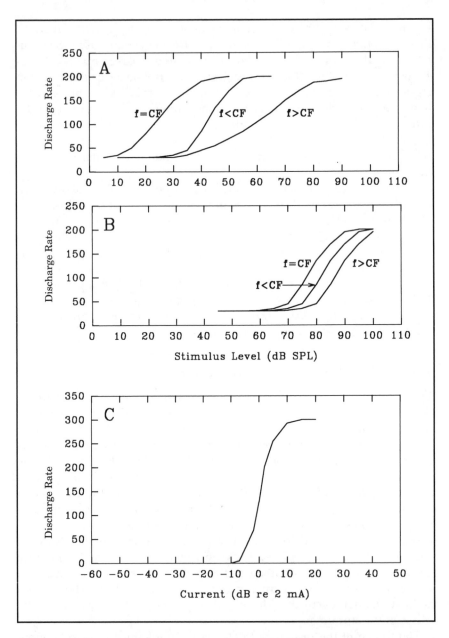

Figure 7–2. Schematic drawing of discharge rate versus stimulus level functions of auditory nerve fibers in response to acoustic stimulation from a normal ear (a), impaired ear (b), and in response to electrical stimulation (c). Frequency of pure-tone stimulation relative to fiber characteristic frequency is indicated in (a) and (b). (Adapted from Sachs & Abbas, 1974, Harrison, 1981, and Kiang & Moxon, 1972.)

1984; Kiang & Moxon, 1972). The responses to square waves or pulsatile stimuli also demonstrate a high degree of synchrony relative to acoustic stimuli (Parkins, 1989; van den Honert & Stypulkowski, 1987b). When electrical stimulation of the cochlea is used, the growth of synchrony with current level is also relatively steep. In animals that have been deafened with

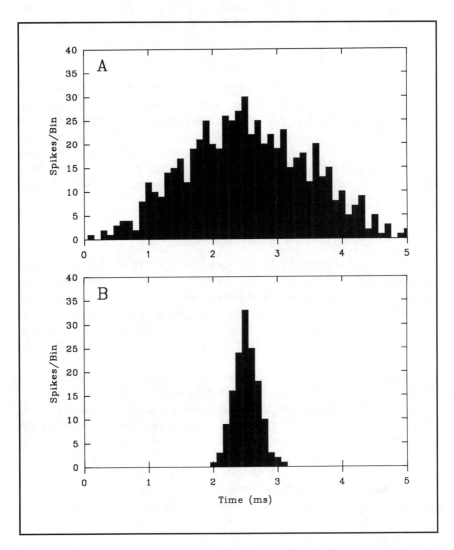

Figure 7–3. Schematic drawing of period histograms of auditory nerve fibers in response to acoustic stimulation (a) and electrical stimulation (b). Number of spikes or action potentials is plotted as a function of time relative to the phase of a pure tone stimulus at 200 Hz. (Adapted from Kiang & Moxon, 1972.)

ototoxic drugs, there is no spontaneous activity in the auditory-nerve fibers. In those cases, the growth of synchrony is particularly steep, reaching nearly perfect synchrony at levels just above threshold (Hartmann et al., 1984; Javel, 1989).

These observations indicate that the neural responses to electrical stimulation are much more repeatable across stimulus presentations than responses to acoustic stimulation. This difference is most likely due to the fact that electrical stimulation bypasses the synaptic mechanism at the hair cell. The lack of time jitter in response to electrical stimulation is a major difference in that there is no statistical independence in the response among fibers in the population (Javel, 1989). The extent to which this may be helpful or detrimental to stimulus encoding is not clear. In some ways, the greater synchrony may be advantageous, since timing changes may be more precisely transmitted to the central nervous system. Certainly, results from some of the better cochlear-implant users suggest that "natural" (probabilistic) stimulation of nerve fibers may not be a necessary prerequisite for good performance (see Dorman, Chapter 4; Tyler, Moore, & Kuk, 1989).

POST-STIMULUS-TIME HISTOGRAMS

A post-stimulus-time (PST) histogram is used to measure the time course of the neural response relative to the onset of a stimulus. In this case, instead of measuring the timing relative to the phase of a periodic stimulus (as described above), the timing is measured relative to the onset of a gated stimulus, usually a click or tone burst and usually represents a longer time epoch. The PST histogram of a fiber's response to a click (Figure 7–4a) shows a series of peaks which reflect the underlying ringing of the basilar membrane in response to the impulse-like stimulus (Kiang et al., 1965). This histogram is typical of low characteristic frequency fibers. Because the traveling wave requires greater travel time to the apex of the cochlea, response latency is longer for fibers with low characteristic frequency. The time intervals between peaks in the histogram reflect the vibration of the cochlea at the place in the cochlea innervated by the fiber. Higher characteristic frequency fibers display shorter latency responses with smaller intervals between peaks in the histogram. Fibers with characteristic frequency above 4 kHz show only a single peak with a latency of about 1.5 ms (Figure 7–4b) (Kiang et al., 1965).

Many cochlear implants use pulsatile stimulation; accordingly, several studies have detailed the neural responses to both monophasic and biphasic electrical pulses. A schematized example of a PST histogram obtained in response to a monophasic current pulse is shown in Figure

7–4c. It shows a shorter latency of response and relatively little spread over time compared to the multi-peaked responses seen with acoustic-click stimulation. The electrically evoked responses reflect the lack of "ringing" due to basilar membrane tuning and lack of delay due to bypassing the synapse between the hair cell and neuron. The responses consist of up to three components characterized by different latencies. Moxon (1971) termed the shortest latency response the α component. It is highly synchronous with a latency on the order of 0.5 ms, and is thought to be the result of direct stimulation of the auditory-nerve fibers. A longer latency response (> 1 ms), termed the β component, appears as a series of peaks that are similar to those obtained with acoustic stimulation. These longer latency peaks, the "electrophonic" component, are thought to originate from the mechanical excitation of the basilar membrane, likely caused by the action of the outer hair cells. The basilar membrane vibration results in excitation of the hair cells and nerve fibers through normal transduction channels. The electrophonic response is seen only in ears with functioning hair cells and probably is not important in stimulation of ears with no functional hearing (van den Honert & Stypulkowski, 1984). A third component, termed the δ response, shows a latency intermediate to the α and β components (approximately 1 ms) and relatively poor synchrony. Van den Honert and Stypulkowski (1984) suggest that the δ response may also be the result of hair-cell excitation. Neither the β nor δ responses are observed in animal preparation in which the hair cells are destroyed (van den Honert & Stypulkowski, 1984).

With biphasic stimulation of the nerve, a separate α response peak can be observed in response to each phase of the stimulus. Each α peak has a slightly different response latency. These observations suggest that the same neuron can be stimulated by different polarity of stimulus current, but that the place of spike initiation is different as indicated by the difference in response latency (Stypulkowski & van den Honert, 1984). As a result, period histograms in response to sinusoidal electrical stimulation can also show two peaks within one period of the stimulus, that is, one in response to each phase of the stimulus (van den Honert & Stypulkowski, 1987b). These cases differ from observations with acoustic stimulation in that the rectifying feature of the hair cell is bypassed, resulting in effective response for both polarities of stimulation.

Threshold of single-fiber response with pulsatile electrical stimuli is highly dependent on the duration of the pulse. Neuron cell membranes have properties such that stimulus current is integrated over time, so that levels for long duration pulses are lower than for short-duration pulses (Colombo & Parkins, 1987; Loeb, White, & Jenkins, 1983; Parkins

& Colombo, 1987; van den Honert & Stypulkowski, 1984). Frequency of stimulation on pulse rate can also have a significant effect on threshold. Parkins and Colombo (1987) showed lower threshold for high rates (625 or 2500 Hz) of pulsatile stimulation than for low rates (156 Hz).

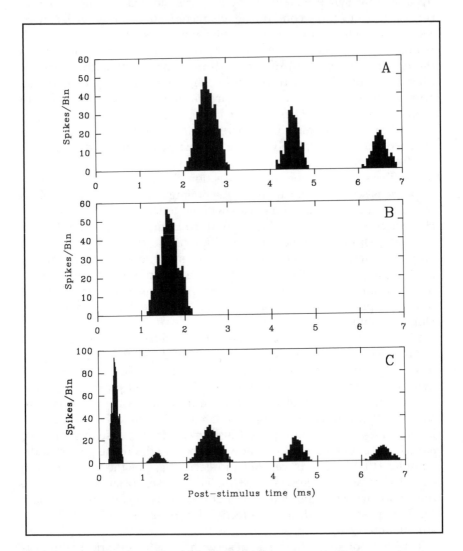

Figure 7–4. Schematic PST histograms of auditory-nerve fiber responses to a click or pulsatile stimulus. Responses of a low characteristic-frequency fiber (a) and a high characteristic-frequency fiber (b) are shown in response to an acoustic click. PST histogram in response to an electrical pulse is shown in (c). (Adapted from Kiang et al., 1965, and van den Honert & Stypulkowski, 1984.)

ADAPTATION

For acoustic tone-burst stimuli (Figure 7–5a), PST histograms show a high probability of generating an action potential at the stimulus onset, which decreases within several hundred ms to a steady-state discharge rate. This phenomenon is termed **adaptation** and is attributable in part to properties of the hair cell-neuron synapse (Smith & Brachman, 1982). In ears with no functioning hair cells, electrical stimulation is thought to bypass this synapse. Nevertheless, several investigators have observed decreases in the responses to electrical stimulation over time similar to those observed with acoustic stimulation. Javel (1989) used trains of biphasic clicks and observed a decrease in the response over approximately 150 ms (Figure 7–5b). These adaptation-like properties, however, were only observed over a narrow intensity range (2–3 dB). At higher stimulus levels, where the response reached saturation, no decrease in responsiveness over time was observed. Van den Honert and Stypulkowski (1987b) observed decreases over several seconds in response to sinusoidal stimulation, particularly for high-frequency stimuli (> 1 kHz). Parkins (1989) used short (20 ms) tone-burst stimuli and noted that electrical stimulation produced more action potentials near signal onset. In comparing the results to those with acoustic stimulation, however, he demonstrated quite different patterns of responses. He attributed the changes over time with electrical stimulation to be due to the neuron responding to the repetitive stimulus many times with a single pulse only the first phase of the tone burst.

Auditory-nerve fibers also demonstrate refractory effects in which the response to one stimulus can affect the generation of an action potential in response to subsequent stimuli. With two-pulse stimuli, such effects are typically limited to stimuli occurring with interpulse intervals of less than 8 ms (Brown & Abbas, 1990; Hartmann et al., 1984; van den Honert & Stypulkowski, 1984). In general, although adaptation-like effects are observed with electrical stimulation, changes in response over time are different than those observed with acoustic stimulation.

SPEECH-LIKE STIMULI

The responses of auditory-nerve fibers to speech-like stimuli have received a great deal of attention in recent years. Much of the research has focused on how certain features of the speech stimulus are encoded in the discharge patterns of auditory-nerve fibers. Studies with steady-state vowels have used stimuli with a fixed fundamental frequency but with varying formant-frequency patterns so that each has different areas of maximal energy in the frequency domain (Sachs & Young, 1979). Responses from fibers in response to speech stimuli presented acousti-

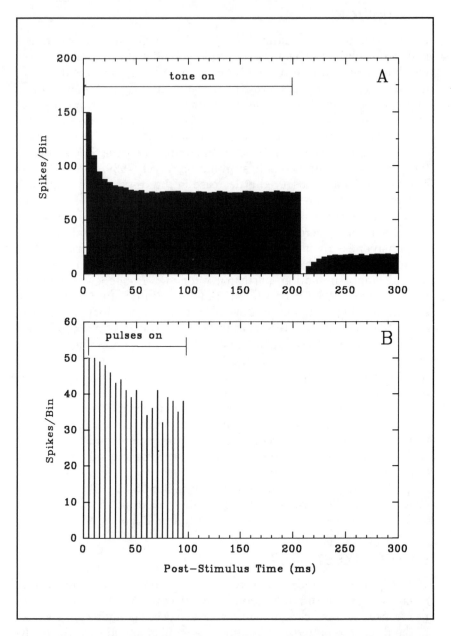

Figure 7–5. Schematic PST histograms of auditory nerve fiber responses. In (a), the stimulus is a acoustic tone burst 200 ms in duration. In (b), the stimulus is a train of electrical pulses at a rate of 200 pulses/s. (Adapted from Kiang et al., 1965, and Javel, 1989.)

cally at low levels have demonstrated that a "place" code may carry significant information. Fibers with characteristic frequencies near frequencies which have significant energy tend to have the highest discharge rates while those fibers with characteristic frequencies between the formant frequencies tend to have lower discharge rates. At moderate to high stimulus levels, the pattern is not as clear. At these levels, neural discharge rate tends to be more similar across fiber characteristic frequency, due in part to the fact that many fibers may be in saturation. Thus, at low stimulus levels, the profile of discharge rate across fiber characteristic frequency carries information concerning formant frequencies of synthesized vowels, but at higher levels, still within the range of conversational speech, this effect is not clear.

These observations led Young and Sachs (1979) to examine the response to the same stimuli in a different way, measuring the phase-locking properties of the response. The vowel stimulus contains energy at the fundamental frequency of vibration of the larynx and at each harmonic of the fundamental frequency. The amplitude of the harmonic frequencies are large near the formant frequencies, the resonant frequencies of the vocal tract. A frequency analysis of the period histogram shows the response of each fiber to the different frequency components present in the complex stimulus. Young and Sachs (1979) found that the responses of auditory-nerve fibers tend to phase-lock to one of the formant frequencies or to a harmonic component near the fiber's characteristic frequency. They then described an index called the averaged localized synchronized response, a measure of phase-locked activity at frequencies near fiber characteristic frequency. The averaged localized synchronized response provided an assessment of the degree of phase-locked response at the stimulus component closest to its characteristic frequency. When this phase-locked measure is used, the response versus fiber characteristic frequency functions show a peak for fibers near the formant frequencies. This response pattern is consistent across stimulus level and has been shown to be consistent under different levels of background masking noise (Voigt, Sachs, & Young, 1981). From data such as these we can conclude that information concerning formant frequencies of speech-like stimuli can be transmitted to the central nervous system via the neural discharge pattern on auditory-nerve fibers.

Responses to consonant-like stimuli have also been examined in a similar way, measuring both discharge rate and phase-locked response. Miller and Sachs (1983) observed responses to the frequency transitions characteristic of voiced stop consonants. The average localized synchronized response was calculated at different time windows throughout the formant-frequency transition period. The frequencies at which the peak response occurred followed the same time course as the changes of formant frequencies. For voiceless-fricative consonants, the profile of discharge rate across fiber characteristic frequency corresponds well with the spectrum of the stimulus (Delgutte & Kiang, 1984). For these stimuli, discharge rate provides spectral information for both low and high stimulus levels. An analysis of phase-locked activity similar to that successful in representing vowel stimuli could not distinguish fricative consonant responses. Thus, depending on the particular phoneme, an analysis of both the synchronized response and a discharge-rate profile are required to transmit phonemic information to higher centers.

There have not been extensive measures of responses to speech-like electrical stimuli. Nevertheless, related to the above data is the observation described earlier that the electrically evoked response does not reflect the tuning or nonlinear properties of the cochlea. Consequently, complex electrical stimuli, which have multiple frequency components, generally result in a much different response than those elicited by acoustic stimuli (Javel, 1989). Electrically evoked responses primarily reflect the waveform peaks (and troughs) in the stimulus rather than a spectrally based representation of the signal.

FAR-FIELD RECORDINGS

The compound whole-nerve action potential (CAP) is a measure of summed activity of the population of auditory-nerve fibers. It is typically measured from an electrode placed on or near the round window, although it can be measured from an electrode placed directly on the nerve trunk (Derbyshire & Davis, 1935). Although the CAP does not reflect the activity in individual neurons, it is of particular interest because it can be recorded in human subjects as well as in experimental animals. When the CAP is measured in humans it is usually called electrocochleography. Electrocochleography is usually conducted in humans by placing electrodes through the tympanic membrane onto the promontory or in the external auditory meatus (Eggermont, 1974; Montandon, Megill, Kahn, Peake, & Kiang, 1975).

The source of the CAP has been fairly well documented through a number of experiments. Kiang, Moxon, and Kahn (1976) measured the voltage waveform produced by an action potential in an auditory-nerve fiber with an electrode placed at the round window; each action potential produced a very small-amplitude bipolar pulse. Action potentials from different fibers in the nerve resulted in a similar recorded potential at the round-window recording electrode. Thus the action potentials discharging across the entire population are essentially summed to produce the far-field potential at the round window. Continuous stimulation of the cochlea produces a continuous sequence of action potentials from many different nerve fibers. In this case there is little synchrony across individual fiber action potentials. The effects of each action potential tend to cancel one another, resulting in essentially no measurable CAP. In contrast, transient stimuli produce synchronized action potentials in a number of fibers, which tend to sum with one another to produce a measurable CAP (Dolan, Teas, & Walton, 1983; Goldstein & Kiang, 1958).

In recording the CAP, responses to several stimuli are typically averaged in time to enhance the stimulus-evoked response potential relative to the random background noise. Figure 7–6a shows CAP responses measured in response to a click stimuli at different levels. The response has the form of a series of one to three negative peaks. The first peak, termed N_1, is caused by the synchronous discharge of auditory-nerve fibers. The amplitude of the N_1 peak increases monotonically with stimulus level and its latency decreases monotonically with level. Teas, Eldredge, and Davis (1962) measured the response to click stimuli in the presence of band-pass masking noise in order to eliminate the contribution of specific regions of the cochlea to the CAP. They demonstrated that the response to a click stimulus is composed primarily of the discharging of high-characteristic frequency, basal-turn fibers.

Electrodes placed into the brain, on its surface, or on the skin around the cranium can be used to measure neural activity from higher levels of the auditory pathway. These evoked potentials are typically measured in humans using electrodes placed on the skin. Specific electrode configuration can vary; many experimenters use an electrode at the vertex (top of the head) as the positive input and a mastoid electrode as the reference to their recording apparatus. Response potentials occurring within 10 ms of a click or tone burst stimulus are known as the auditory brainstem response (ABR). The ABR consists of a series of positive peaks (measured vertex positive) whose source is the auditory nerve and brainstem nuclei (Figure 7–6b). In the human, the first two peaks with latencies on the order of 1½–3ms have been shown to arise from auditory-nerve activity (Moller & Janetta, 1985). Later peaks in the ABR are attributed to activity in brainstem nuclei and the inferior colliculus. Longer latency responses can be also be recorded. Activity with latency 30-100 ms are usually called the middle latency response (MLR); responses with latency up to 300–400 ms are referred to as late components. These longer latency response are thought be primarily cortical in nature (Fifer & Sierra-Inzarry, 1988; Hall, 1992).

There has been a great deal of work with both humans and animals recording electrically evoked brain potentials, particularly the electrically evoked auditory brainstem response (EABR). An example of an EABR waveform is shown in Figure 7–6c. When the auditory system is stimulated by electrical current, the response waveform of the EABR is similar to that evoked by an acoustic stimulus, but the peaks are shorter in latency (Starr & Brackmann, 1979). The interpeak latencies, however, are similar to those observed using acoustic stimulation since the subsequent sequence of ascending brainstem activation is similar in either case (van den Honert & Stypulkowski, 1986).

The amplitude of the peaks in the response grow very quickly with increases in stimulus current level in comparison to the growth rate observed using acoustic stimulation, but the latency of each peak of the EABR changes little as stimulus current is increased. The large changes in EABR amplitude are consistent with single-neuron responses to electric stimulation which show less jitter and steeper growth functions as compared to acoustic stimulation (see above). The small latency changes with intensity that are observed in the EABR are also consistent with single-unit

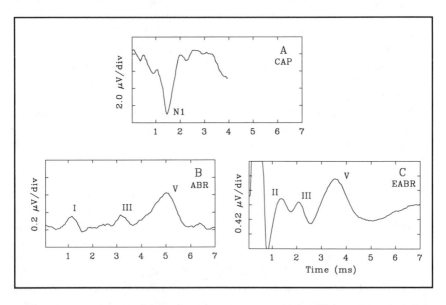

Figure 7–6. Evoked responses from humans in response to acoustic and electrical stimulation of the auditory system. In (a), the compound whole-nerve action potential is measured in response to an acoustic click from an electrode placed on the eardrum. N1 indicates the auditory nerve response shown as a negative peak. In (b), the auditory brainstem response is recorded in response to an acoustic click from electrodes placed on the skull. Response peaks of waves I, III, and V are indicated. In (c), the auditory brainstem response is recorded from a deaf subject in response to electrical stimulation via a cochlear implant. Waves II, III, and V are evident. Stimulus artifact at the beginning of the trace obscures any measurement of wave I in this case.

data and can be attributed to the lack of delays characteristic of the traveling wave in the cochlea.

Starr and Brackmann (1979) have observed the effects of changing rate
of stimulus presentation on the EABR. Latency of wave V changed little
for pulse rates up to 100/s. Amplitude of wave V decreased above rates
of 50/s; at rates of 200/s, the response was not detectable. In contrast, the
ABR in response to acoustic clicks in normal listeners shows greater
changes with changes in stimulation rate (Hall, 1992; Pratt & Sohmer,
1976). The difference between electrical and acoustic stimulation likely
reflects the results of bypassing the peripheral synaptic mechanisms with
electrical stimulation.

When the ABR is measured using electrical stimulation, there are
two issues of particular concern. The first is the elimination or reduction of the large stimulation artifact that is inevitably recorded, and the
second is the concern that the ABR may be contaminated by responses
from structures other than those of the auditory nervous system. These
two issues will be addressed in the following paragraphs.

The EABR is typically elicited by a biphasic current pulse. Since the
stimulus is electric current, the electrodes used to record the EABR will
also record the potentials that result from the stimulus presentation. The
stimulus artifact that is recorded is generally much larger than the
recorded neural potential. Several methods can be used to reduce the
contamination of the EABR by the stimulus artifact. The choice of the
positions of the stimulating and recording electrodes is critical in determining the amplitude of the stimulus artifact (Gardi, 1985). Since the
EABR is recorded differentially, if the orientation is such that each
recording electrode picks up a similar potential from the stimulating
electrodes, the artifact should be minimal. Also, if the duration of the
biphasic stimulus is kept relatively short (< 0.5 ms), later response
potentials can be recorded relatively unaffected by the stimulus artifact.
This can be accomplished by using filtering with the widest pass-band
possible. With wideband filtering, the stimulus artifact will "ring" for
only a short time and consequently the stimulus artifact will be confined
to the very beginning of the recording epoch. In subsequent analysis of
the averaged waveform, the artifact can be eliminated and the waveforms digitally filtered to eliminate noise. Some investigators (Black,
Clark, Shepherd, O'Leary, & Walters, 1983) have used a sample-and-
hold circuit to essentially turn off the amplifier during stimulation. Such
a device will avoid overloading the amplifier during stimulation, allowing better isolation of the response. Another procedure that can be used
to minimize stimulus artifact is to alternate the polarity of the stimulus
on sequential presentations (Abbas & Brown, 1988; Hall, 1990). Since the
artifact produced by each alternating pulse is opposite in phase, in the

average the artifact will tend to cancel. Using a combination of these techniques, one can usually reduce the stimulus artifact sufficiently to adequately record electrically evoked brainstem potentials.

The second important factor to consider when measuring electrically evoked potentials is the source of the potentials. When electrical stimulation is used, nonauditory neural and muscular systems may be stimulated. The form of the EABR that is recorded with intracochlear electrical stimulation is consistent across subjects and is similar to that evoked with acoustic stimulation. Experiments with such stimulation in monkeys have indicated that the response is primarily from the auditory system rather than from the facial or vestibular systems (Dobie & Kimm, 1980; Starr & Brackmann, 1979; Yamane, Marsh, & Potsic, 1981). Van den Honert and Stypulkowski (1986) measured potentials vestibular in origin which temporally overlapped the response peaks of the EABR. These vestibular potentials are distinguishable from those of auditory origin in that they are opposite in polarity and quite different in form. Muscle activity tends to be longer in latency, but can also be differentiated from the auditory potentials by its large amplitude and rapid rate of growth with stimulus current. Additionally, measures of activity in experimental animals have demonstrated an electrophonic response in ears with normal hair-cell populations. This response arises from electromechanical stimulation of the basilar membrane rather than via direct nerve stimulation. Electrophonic potentials have a lower threshold, longer latency and slower growth of response than electrically evoked potentials (Black et al., 1983; Lusted & Simmons, 1988). In general, a good criterion for use in determining whether the recorded potentials are auditory in origin, is that the form of the response and its amplitude are similar to that recorded to acoustic stimulation.

The source of the response is especially important to consider when measures of the EABR are made using a middle-ear stimulation site. A number of animal studies have demonstrated that different electrode placements in the cochlea and middle ear can result in different amplitude and waveform of the electrically evoked response (Clopton & Bosma, 1982; Lusted, Shelton, & Simmons, 1984; Marsh, Yamane, & Potsic, 1981; Yamane et al., 1981). Electrode placements outside the cochlea usually require higher levels of current to effectively stimulate the nerve than intracochlear placements. Consequently, there is greater likelihood of stimulating other structures such as vestibular or facial nerve. In our experience with human implant users (Abbas & Brown, 1991b), intracochlear stimulation produces consistent response waveforms across subjects. In a similar population of subjects in which preimplant, round-window stimulation was used, we recorded a response only from approximately one-half of the subjects. Of those subjects for whom we were able to record a response, the morphology of the potentials that were recorded were quite variable.

SUMMARY

The responses of auditory-nerve fibers to electrical stimulation differ from those to acoustic stimulation in a number of important ways. With electrical stimulation, the frequency analysis of the cochlea is bypassed, resulting in poorer frequency tuning and a smaller dynamic range of response. The temporal response properties with electrical stimulation are more precise and adaptation at the level of the auditory nerve is less than with acoustic stimulation. Many of these properties are demonstrable using far-field potentials in humans. Thus, these responses can be evaluated in individuals who have received cochlear implants. These physiological responses have potential uses in a number of situations which are described below.

PREDICTING NERVE SURVIVAL

The performance of individuals with cochlear implants can be quite variable. An important clinical issue concerns whether and to what extent a given candidate will benefit from a cochlear implant (see also Shannon, Chapter 8; Dorman, Chapter 4; Tyler, Chapter 5). One of many parameters that may affect performance is the status of the auditory nerve, in particular, the number of surviving neurons and their physiological responsiveness to electrical stimulation. A method of assessing the viability of the population of neurons in a reliable and quantitative fashion could be helpful in making decisions, not only about whether to implant a patient, but also in selection of the type of electrode array to implant and the optimal stimulation parameters for the subject. Several of the physiological measures described above may be useful in assessing nerve viability.

Experiments with both animals and implanted humans have attempted to evaluate the usefulness of specific physiological measures. Animal experiments have the advantage of being able to assess nerve population directly from histological preparations of the cochlea. Experiments with human cochlear-implant users have relied on preimplant, intraoperative, and postimplant stimulation. Obviously the most direct application of a predictive measure employs preimplant stimulation. Nevertheless, postimplant measures tend to be more consistent; that is, the latency and amplitude of evoked response waveforms are more stable over time and less contaminated by artifact. Postimplant measures also allow for more flexibility in choosing stimulation parameters. Information on the utility of specific postimplant tests may be useful in determining tests worth modifying so that they can be recorded preoperatively. Research on both test regimes are discussed below.

ELECTRICALLY EVOKED AUDITORY BRAINSTEM RESPONSE

Several experiments have been published in which experimental animals were used to investigate the effects of cochlear nerve survival on the EABR. The EABR has been used to monitor physiological changes in cats with chronically implanted electrodes (Miller, Duckert, Malone, & Pfingst, 1983; Walsh & Leake-Jones, 1982). Both bony growth and loss of nerve fibers resulted in decreased EABR amplitudes. Smith and Simmons (1983) measured threshold and growth of the EABR in cats with different degrees of experimentally induced neural degeneration. Threshold proved to be a poor predictor of the number of surviving ganglion cells; however, the slope of the amplitude-current function was shown to be a better predictor. Lusted et al. (1984) compared electrode sites and demonstrated that a scala tympani placement resulted in clearer changes in growth of amplitude for different degrees of neuron loss than electrodes placed outside the cochlea. Hall (1990) has reported on measures of the EABR of rats in which he demonstrated a correlation between growth of response magnitude and nerve-fiber survival. Wave I, the auditory nerve response, showed the strongest correlation, while later peaks of the EABR showed poorer correlations. In contrast to the above findings, there have been several studies in which a strong relationship between evoked potential measures and nerve survival have not been demonstrated (Cazals, Aran, & Charlet de Sauvage, 1983; Shepard, Clark, & Black, 1983; Steel & Bock, 1984; van den Honert & Stypulkowski, 1986).

In work with human subjects, several groups have included the recording of EABR to stimulation of the middle ear prior to cochlear implantation in an effort to evaluate the usefulness of such a measure in predicting success with the implant (Black, Lilly, Fowler, & Stypulkowski, 1987; Game, Gibson, & Pauka, 1987; Gantz et al., 1988; Meyer, Drira, Gegu, & Chouard, 1984; Simmons, Lusted, Meyers, & Shelton, 1984; van den Honert & Stypulkowski, 1986). In general, measures of the EABR made preoperatively have been quite variable and no clear correlation has been found between EABR preimplant data and postimplant performance. Kileny (1991) has described a preoperative procedure using EABR measures to aid in the selection of the ear to implant in children who are cochlear-implant candidates. With patients anesthetized before surgery, promontory stimulation is accomplished in both ears and EABR recorded. The relative sensitivity of the EABR, along with other criteria, then can serve as a basis of choosing an ear to implant.

A number of investigators have used postimplant intracochlear stimulation to measure EABR responses (Abbas & Brown, 1988, 1991; Gardi, 1985; Starr & Brackmann, 1979; van den Honert & Stypulkowski, 1986; Waring, Don, & Brimacombe, 1985). The responses in these cases are much more consistent, both across both studies and implant types. The differences between preimplant and postimplant studies are likely related to the proximity of the electrodes to the nerve and the consistency of electrode placement in cases of intracochlear stimulation. An example of EABR data collected postoperatively is shown in Figure 7–7. The amplitude (7–7a) and latency (7–7b) of the peak of the EABR analogous to wave V of the acoustic ABR is plotted as a function of current level. The amplitude of the response generally increases with increasing stimulus level, and the latency of the peak tends to decrease slightly. Stimulation of different electrodes within the Ineraid implant can result in different sensitivity, but all show similar changes of amplitude and latency with current level. We have recently investigated the correlation of these measures to speech-perception performance with the implant (Abbas & Brown, 1991a). Measures of threshold and growth of response showed at best only modest correlation to scores on tests of word recognition.

ELECTRICALLY EVOKED MIDDLE AND LATE POTENTIALS

The limited success of the EABR as a predictor of implant performance in humans has lead some researchers to investigate other physiological responses. Kileny and Kemink (1987) have used the electrically evoked middle latency response (EMLR) in their measures of preimplant stimulation. The advantage of this technique is that stimulus artifact problems are reduced because the neural response occurs at a much longer latency than the earlier EABR which is more prone to contamination by stimulus artifact. With response latencies on the order of 30 ms, there is little chance that the stimulus artifact will overlap the neural response. A disadvantage of the middle latency responses is that it is not consistently recorded in young children (Stein & Kraus, 1987). Similar to EABR, EMLRs have slightly shorter latencies than its acoustically derived version (Kileny, Kemink, & Miller, 1989). In addition, thresholds are similar to behavioral threshold for the same stimuli (Kileny, 1991; Kileny & Kemink, 1987). Jyung, Miller, and Cannon, (1989) have recently reported on EMLR measures made in experimental animals in which a good correlation to nerve survival was found.

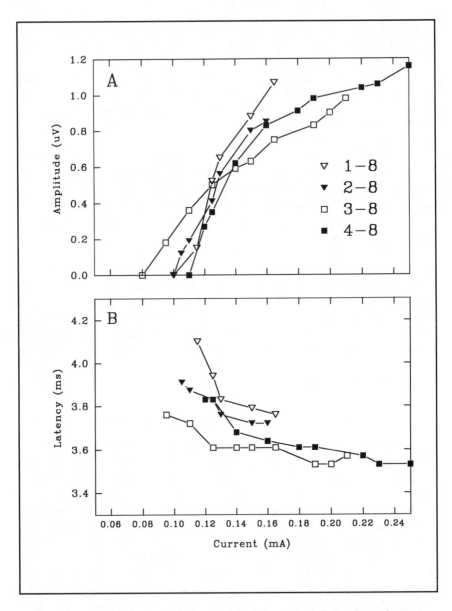

Figure 7–7. Amplitude (a) and latency (b) of wave V of the auditory brainstem response to electrical stimulation via a cochlear implant in a deaf subject. Responses are plotted as a function of current level of a biphasic pulse 100 μs in duration. Responses to different electrode pairs in the Ineraid cochlear implant are indicated in the legend. Electrode 1 to 4 are intracochlear, with electrode 1 the most basal. Electrode 8 is placed in the temporalis muscle.

The latency of the positive peak of the MLR is approximately 30 ms. Potentials with latencies on the order of 300 ms are termed event-related potentials. To evoke the latter potential, stimuli are usually presented in an "oddball" paradigm, that is, a novel stimulus is presented infrequently, interspersed within a repetitive series of a more common signal. The presence of the late response is thought to be indicative of subjects' discrimination of the rare signal from the common signal (Duncan-Johnson & Donchin, 1982; Squires & Hecox, 1983). The advantage of this later response is that it is indicative of a degree of recognition of the signal by the subject, implying a higher degree of processing than is evident in the measurement of shorter latency responses.

Oviatt and Kileny (1991) compared these late event-related potentials in cochlear-implant users and normal-hearing subjects. They used frequent-and-rare signal pairs of 500 and 1000 Hz, 500 and 2000 Hz, and 500 and 3000 Hz. The latency of the response for the 1000 Hz stimulus was greatest, indicating that discrimination was most difficult. Also, the latencies tended to be longer in the cochlear-implant users than in normal listeners. These results show some promise in using these responses to provide not only detection, but also information on users' discrimination of signals. Event-related potentials have also been recorded in children with cochlear implants (Kileny, 1991).

ELECTRICALLY EVOKED COMPOUND ACTION POTENTIAL

An alternate approach taken by Brown, Abbas, and Gantz (1990) is the recording of the electrically evoked compound action potential (EAP), a potential whose source is the summed action potentials in auditory nerve fibers. This method has the disadvantage that artifact problems are compounded by the short latency of the response (< 0.4 ms), but has the advantage that the response is a direct measure of the nerve activity and consequently may more directly correlate with the state of the nerve (Hall, 1990). Several measures of the EAP have been conducted in experimental animals (Nagel, 1974; Prijs, 1980; Stypulkowski & van den Honert, 1984). The latency of the peak of the response ranged between 0.35 and 0.55 ms across several animal species. Van den Honert and Stypulkowski (1984) observed two peaks attributed to the auditory nerve having different latencies. They suggested that the later, more sensitive peak was initiated at the peripheral, dendritic process and the earlier, less sensitive peak was initiated at the central axonal process. They further suggested that the presence or absence of the later peak may be indicative of the stimulability of peripheral dendrites in cochlear-implant users.

   Charlet de Sauvage, Cazals, Erre, and Aran (1983) used a noise masker
and a subtraction technique to eliminate stimulus artifact and record
EAP in guinea pigs. The technique, adapted by Brown et al. (1990) to
record EAP in human implant users, is illustrated in Figure 7–8. Two
biphasic current pulses are presented in a forward-masking paradigm.
Responses are recorded in three different stimulating conditions. The
first is the probe-alone condition (Figure 7–8a), in which the recorded
response includes both stimulus artifact and the neural response. The
second is a masker-plus-probe condition (Figure 7–8b), in which two
current pulses are presented separated by a short interstimulus interval.
The recorded response in this case consists of two stimulus artifacts with
an overlying neural response to the masker and a reduced or absent
neural response to the probe due to the refractory properties of the stimulated neurons. The third condition (Figure 7–8c) is that of the masker
alone. The recording in this condition contains both stimulus artifact and
neural response to the masker. Subtracting the second response condi-

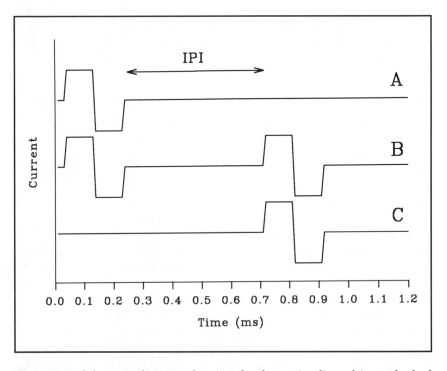

Figure 7–8. Schematic diagram showing the three stimuli used in method of
extracting the neural response form stimulus artifact. (Adapted from Brown et
al., 1990.) Interpulse interval (IPI) is the time between the offset of the first pulse
(masker) and the onset of the second pulse (probe).

tion (B) from the first (A) eliminates the stimulus artifact to the probe and leaves the neural response. Adding the third response (C) to the above subtraction eliminates the masker artifact and response, leaving a voltage trace with only the EAP elicited by the probe current pulse.

To date, there have been no measures of the EAP in humans before implantation, but the measures of the EAP made using intracochlear stimulation through the implant have shown promising results. Brown et al. (1990) measured EAP growth functions by changing the level of the probe pulse using the two-pulse stimulation paradigm described above. They also measured recovery from the refractory state by varying the interpulse interval. The graphs in Figure 7–9 illustrate growth functions (amplitude-versus-current level) and recovery from the refractory state (normalized amplitude-versus-interstimulus interval). In the right-hand graph, a normalized value of 1 indicates no response to the second pulse in the two-pulse sequence; a value of 0 indicates a normal (unadapted) response. Each curve is the result of stimulating a different pair of intra-cochlear electrodes in the Ineraid cochlear implant. Electrode 1 is the most apical and electrodes 5 the most basal. There are differences among electrodes in sensitivity, growth of response, and rate of recovery. Preliminary data from similar measures across users suggest that they may be indicative of performance with the implant. Both slope of the growth function and the time necessary to recover from the refractory state showed a modest correlation to word-recognition scores. We interpret these findings to mean that both numbers of neurons and the refractory

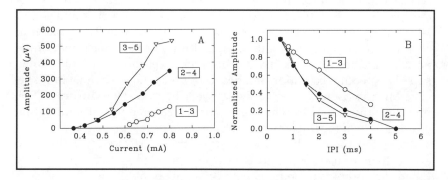

Figure 7–9. Amplitude of the EAP measured using an intracochlear electrode in a subject with the Ineraid cochlear implant. Amplitude of the response as function of current level is shown in (a). In (b), the normalized amplitude (normalized to the amplitude in response to the probe presented alone) is plotted as a function of interpulse interval (see Figure 7–8) with current level fixed. Responses from several stimulating electrode pairs were measured and are indicated in the legend. Electrode 1 is the most basal and electrode 5 is the most apical.

properties of those surviving neurons may be related to the user's ability to understand speech with the implant.

These measures of EAP using intracochlear stimulating and recording electrodes have not yet been measured preoperatively, but we are presently making similar measures using a temporary electrode array placed during implantation surgery (Abbas, Purdy, & Gantz, 1990). Waveforms and growth functions are similar to measures made through the implant. Correlations to performance are not yet available.

IMPLICATIONS FOR THE PROCESSING OF SPEECH

There are several important issues involving the response properties of single fibers relative to the processing of speech information (see also Wilson, Chapter 2). The lack of sharp frequency tuning, particularly, the lack of differences in tuning across the population of nerve fibers, is important. That feature of normal cochlear processing can be simulated by placing electrodes along the length of the cochlea and independently stimulating different populations of neurons. To a great extent, the processing of speech in multichannel implants attempts to replace some of the normally present spectral analysis properties. Filtering of the incoming signal for each stimulation channel can partially simulate the filtering properties of the normal cochlea. The Ineraid cochlear implant uses four independent bandpass filters, the output of each stimulating a different electrode pair depending on the pass band of the filter. The Nucleus cochlear implant performs a more complex feature analysis of the speech signal, still based primarily on spectral properties and stimulates a sequence of electrode pairs based on this analysis. The number of channels of stimulation in either implant does not approach that of the normal ear. Results from users of multichannel implants have shown superior speech recognition abilities to those of single-channel implants (Tye-Murray, Gantz, Kuk, & Tyler, 1988; Tyler & Tye-Murray, 1991); however, the extent to which more or fewer channels of stimulation affects utility of the implant is not clear (see Wilson, Chapter 2).

Bypassing the cochlear processing with electrical stimulation also affect the neural response to electrically encoded speech signals. The range of thresholds of neurons with different spontaneous rate, the nonlinear growth of response with stimulus level, and the tuning properties of the cochlea all contribute to the ability of the normal auditory system to encode changes in intensity over a wide intensity range. Electrical stimulation results in steep growth functions, limited dynamic range, similar thresholds across fibers, and broad tuning properties. The speech processor needs to compensate in some way for these properties. Compression and "noise-reduction" circuits may help in overcoming some of these limitations inherent with electrical stimulation, but these problems can be particularly difficult in noisy listening situations where the response to one stimulus may dominate the neural responses.

Finally, the temporal properties in response to electrical stimulation show greater synchrony than those obtained in response to acoustic stimulation. Experimental data indicate that the responses to electrical stimulation may preserve the time structure of the signal to a greater extent than is possible through acoustic stimulation. Given the limitations of a spectral representation through an implant, the temporal response properties may be particularly important. The extent to which the brain can take advantage of this unnatural mode of stimulation, in combination with other information, is yet to be determined. Data from implant users indicate that very high levels of performance are possible using pulsatile stimuli, which can provide almost complete entrainment (Wilson, Finley, & Lawson, 1989). Also, speech-perception data from some "star" users with single-channel cochlear implants certainly suggest that a great deal of information can be extracted from temporal aspects of the neural response alone (see also Dorman, Chapter 4; Banfai, Karczag, & Luers, 1984; Hochmair & Hochmair-Desoyer, 1983, 1985).

OBJECTIVE MEASUREMENTS TO DETERMINE STIMULATION PARAMETERS

In addition to using the evoked neural response as a predictive measure, there is also the possibility of its use in setting the parameters for signal processing. With multichannel cochlear implants, there are several adjustments that can be made in the stimulation parameters to set the device for an individual (Tyler & Tye-Murray, 1991). Minimally, the range of current levels over which stimulation will occur is determined by psychophysical measurements of threshold, most comfortable stimulation level, and maximum comfort level on each electrode pair. Some implant systems allow for other choices such as pulse duration, active electrode combinations, and bandwidth of filtering of the incoming signal. The choice of stimulation parameters can be customized to the particular user's needs. These choices are generally made on the basis of perceptual testing, but as increasingly more young, and prelingually deafened children are implanted, additional information gained from physiological measures may prove to be useful.

Auditory-evoked brain potentials have proved to be a useful correlate of perceptual threshold in response to the same stimuli (Gorga, Worthington, Reiland, Beauchaine, & Goldgar, 1985; Stapells, Picton, Percy-Abalo, Read, & Smith, 1985). In our studies with cochlear-implant patients, threshold of response varied across patient and across stimulating electrode within a patient. Across this population of patients, the detectable level of the EABR is correlated with behavioral threshold measures for the same stimuli and electrode pair (Abbas & Brown, 1991a). Shallop, Beiter, Goin, and Mischke (1990) and Shallop, Goin, Van Dyke, and Mischke (1991) have noted that EABR detection thresholds in Nucleus cochlear-implant users tend to be higher than behavioral measures which are typically used to set the implant stimulation parameters. They attribute these differences in part to an incomplete temporal integration of the low-rate pulse presentation used for EABR (10–14 pulses/s) compared to the higher rate (200/s) in behavioral testing. Shannon (1985) demonstrated psychophysical threshold decreases with pulse rate for rates above 100/s.

Allum, Shallop, Hotz, and Pfaltz (1990) have also noted correlations between the current level at which the maximum amplitude of the response is achieved and the maximum level at which the stimulation was comfortable for the subject. The correlations were poor when compared with behavioral maximum comfort levels measured at a faster pulse rate (250/s). In our experience (Abbas & Brown, 1988, 1991a), when the EABR is recorded using stimuli ranging up to the highest current levels tolerable to the subject, no clear saturation in the growth functions are obtained. However, there are significant differences in slope of the growth functions for different stimulating electrodes within an implant. These differences do not correlate with perceptual dynamic range or maximum comfort level. Miller, Duckert, Sutton, Pfingst, and Malone (1985) and Miller (1991) have reported that threshold of the evoked potential in experimental animals can be reversibly affected by moderately high levels of electrical stimulation. They suggest that the observation of such changes in an individual may provide a practical limit to safe stimulation levels, particularly for young children. No data are yet available from human implant users, however.

The correlations that are observed may be to some extent affected by the time at which the evoked response measures are made. Most of the measures of EABR and EAP in humans have been made after the electrode array has been implanted for a month or more. Several measures have also shown moderate correlations between the intraoperative measures of EABR and subsequent threshold and maximum comfort levels (Allum et al., 1990; Shallop et al., 1990). In studies of implanted monkeys, thresholds have been shown to vary significantly over time after implantation (Pfingst, 1990). In human implant patients, initial hook-up of the implant usually does not take place until several weeks after implantation at which time behavioral thresholds are generally slightly higher than after several months of implant use (Dorman, Smith, Dankowski, McCandless, & Parkin, in press). After implantation, thresholds can be stable over several years (Eddington, Dobelle, Brackmann, Mladejousky, & Parkin, 1978; Hochmair-Desoyer & Burian, 1985; Waltzman, Cohen, & Shapiro, 1986).

Multichannel implants are designed so that each channel delivers electrical current to a different portion of the cochlea. Regardless of the specific speech-processing strategy employed in an implant, the benefits of a multichannel system are dependent on the degree to which independent populations of neurons are stimulated by different channels of the implant. The degree to which specific electrode pairs within an implant stimulate independent neuron populations could be instrumental in choosing appropriate electrode pairs for stimulation through its speech processor. Single-cell responses in animals have demonstrated that stimulation of independent neuron populations is possible with longitudinal and particularly with radially oriented electrodes (van den Honert & Stypulkowski, 1987a). Individual human patients with different spatial patterns of neural loss may vary significantly in their ability to make use of multiple channels of stimulation (see Wilson, Chapter 2). Information concerning the independence of stimulated electrode channels could prove useful in programming the implant for an individual (see also Shannon, Chapter 8).

White, Merzenich, and Gardi (1989) and Gardi (1985) have used a stimulus paradigm in which two channels are stimulated simultaneously to demonstrate interaction effects. Abbas and Brown (1988) performed a similar experiment in subjects with an Ineraid multichannel implant. The responses from two electrode pairs being stimulated simultaneously with current pulses in phase and the same electrode pairs being stimulated with current pulses inverted relative to one another were compared. If the field of current from each electrode pair is stimulating the same group of neurons, then when the two are presented in phase, the current will tend to add and the response will be greater. Alternately, when the current pulses on the two electrodes are presented out of phase or inverted, the current at the stimulated neurons will tend to cancel and the response will be less. Therefore, the difference in amplitude or threshold of response between these two stimulating conditions (in phase and inverted) should be indicative of the degree of overlap in the stimulated neural populations. Monopolar stimulation (the normal mode used in the Ineraid implant) resulted in significant differences between the two conditions; when stimulation was accomplished between two nonoverlapping pairs of intracochlear electrodes (such as 1 to 2 and 3 to 4), little difference was observed. The results of this test also show some differences among users, which may be indicative of differences in the surviving ganglion-cell population in the field of the stimulating electrode pairs.

Simultaneous stimulation of two electrode pairs is impossible in certain implant systems, such as the Nucleus multichannel implant. In these cases, it is possible to use a forward masking or an adaptation paradigm to assess channel interaction. Lim, Tong, and Clark (1989) have measured psychophysical forward masking effects in Nucleus implant users and observed that the spread of masking tends to be greater toward more basal electrodes than to more apical electrodes (see also Shannon, Chapter 8). Abbas and Purdy (1990) used pairs of pulses (one on each electrode pair) to assess the effects of stimulation from one channel on the subsequent EABR in response to stimulation of another channel. Individual users showed differences in the spread of masking across electrode pairs. They interpreted these differences to be indicative of differences in the overlap of the stimulated neurons. Both of these tests are probably limited in their clinical usefulness because of the testing time necessary to acquire results for channel interaction on several pairs of electrodes. Based on our experience, the testing time would be prohibitive to evaluate all pairs of electrodes within a 22-electrode implant.

MEASUREMENTS OF DEVICE FUNCTION

As discussed above, in measuring the EABR or EAP, the stimulating current generally produces a large artifactual potential on the recording electrodes. In general, this potential can interfere with measurements of short-latency peaks in the evoked response, but its measurement can be useful under certain circumstances. For example, some implants (such as the Nucleus, Figure 7–10) transmit a code from the external processor to an internal (implanted) receiver which, in turn, produces current pulses for stimulation of the appropriate electrodes. This internal receiver is an electronic circuit that decodes the series of pulses transmitted across the skin and, based on a prescribed code, chooses specific electrode pairs, current level, and pulse duration for stimulation. If the internal electronics fail, then measurement of the stimulus artifact (the current pulse produced by the internal electrodes) can be an objective test of the integrity of the internal circuitry. Heller, Brehm, Sinipoli, and Shallop (1991) have outlined a procedure for taking such measurements. If one presents the activating sequence of pulses to the transmitting coil and no current pulses are measured, then one can deduce that there is a failure of the internal electronics.

Device failure may not necessarily be complete when a problem occurs. By making measurement of the EABR at regular time intervals,

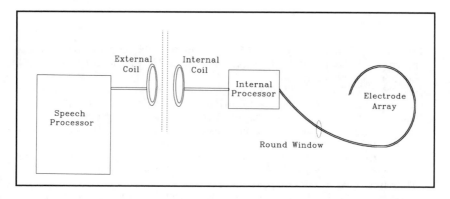

Figure 7–10. Schematic diagram of the parts of the Nucleus cochlear implant.

any changes in the physiological response may be indicative of changes in the auditory nervous system, the environment around the stimulating electrodes, or of the internal electronics. Having some history of both the physiological responses measured with surface electrodes can be useful in detecting changes in the stimulability of the nervous system. Having the measurement of stimulating artifact in the same ear over time can help to isolate the problem to either the device or to changes within the users' physiological responsiveness. Presently, these measures are used to confirm implant failure. Regular measures in young children receiving implants may be particularly important to ensure the integrity of the system.

SUMMARY

Data from physiological experiments with both electrical and acoustic stimuli suggest that electrical stimulation can mimic some of the response properties with acoustic stimulation, but there are usually some very important differences. Despite these differences, many cochlear-implant users can achieve high levels of performance with their devices. Improvements in implant design may take advantage of knowledge of both limitations and the flexibility of electrical stimulation of the auditory nerve using various electrode arrays and stimulation parameters. The particular areas in which physiological measures may be most useful in present and prospective implant users are the prediction of nerve survival, setting implant parameters and in monitoring device and nervous system functioning over time.

REFERENCES

Abbas, P. J., & Brown, C. J. (1991b). Assessment of the status of the auditory nerve. In H. Cooper (Ed.), *Practical aspects of cochlear implants* (pp. 109–124). London: Whurr Publishers Ltd.

Abbas, P. J., & Brown, C. J. (1991a). Electrically evoked auditory brainstem response: Growth of response with current level. *Hearing Research, 51*, 123–138.

Abbas, P. J., & Brown, C. J. (1988). Electrically evoked brainstem potentials in cochlear implant patients with multi-electrode stimulation. *Hearing Research, 36*, 153–162.

Abbas, P. J., & Purdy, S. J. (1990). *Use of forward masking of the EABR to evaluate channel interaction in cochlear implant users.* Paper presented at the ARO Midwinter Research Meeting, Miami, FL.

Abbas, P. J., Purdy, S. L., & Gantz, B. J. (1990, June). *Electrically evoked whole-nerve action potential in Nucleus implant users and intraoperative measures.* Paper presented at the Second International Cochlear Implant Symposium, Iowa City, IA.

Allum, J. H. J., Shallop, J. K., Hotz, M., & Pfaltz, C. P. (1990). Characteristics of electrically evoked 'auditory' brainstem responses elicited with the Nucleus 22-electrode intracochlear implant. *Scandinavian Audiology, 19*, 263–267.

Banfai, P., Karcza, A., & Luers, P. (1984). Clinical results: The rehabilitation. *Acta Otolaryngologica* (Stockholm), (Suppl. 411), 183–194.

Black, F. O., Lilly, D. J., Fowler, L. P., & Stypulkowski, P. H. (1987). Surgical evaluation of candidates for cochlear implants. *Annals of Otology, Rhinology, and Laryngology, 96*(Suppl. 128), 96–99.

Black, R. C., & Clark, G. M. (1980). Differential electrical excitation of the auditory nerve. *Journal of the Acoustical Society of America, 67*, 868–874.

Black, R., Clark, G., Shepherd, R., O'Leary, S., & Walters, C. (1983). Intracochlear electrical stimulation: Brainstem response audiometric and histopathological studies. *Acta Otolaryngologica*, (Suppl. 399), 1–18.

Brown, C. J., & Abbas, P. J. (1990). Electrically evoked whole-nerve action potentials II. Parametric data from the cat. *Journal of the Acoustical Society of America, 88*(5), 2205–2210.

Brown, C. J., Abbas, P. J., & Gantz, B. (1990). Electrically evoked whole-nerve action potentials I. Data from Symbion cochlear implant users. *Journal of the Acoustical Society of America, 88*, 1385–1391.

Cazals, Y., Aran J–M., & Charlet de Sauvage, R. C. (1983). Artificial activation and degeneration of the cochlear nerve in guinea pigs. *Archives of Otorhinolaryngologica, 238*, 1–9.

Charlet de Sauvage, R., Cazals, Y., Erre, J. P., & Aran, J. M. (1983). Acoustically derived auditory nerve action potential evoked by electrical stimulation: An estimation of the wave form of single unit contribution. *Journal of the Acoustical Society of America, 73*, 616–627.

Clopton, B. M., & Bosma, M. M. (1982). Effectiveness of middle ear electrical stimulation for activating central auditory pathways. *Annals of Otology, Rhinology, and Laryngology, 91*, 285–291.

Cody, A. R., & Johnstone, B. M. (1980). Single auditory neuron responses during acute acoustic trauma. *Hearing Research, 3*, 3–16.

Colombo, J., & Parkins, C. W. (1987). A model of electrical excitation of the mammalian auditory-nerve neuron. *Hearing Research, 31*, 287–312.

Delgutte, B., & Kiang, N.Y.–S. (1984). Speech coding in the auditory nerve III. Voiceless fricative consonants. *Journal of the Acoustical Society of America, 75*, 887–896.

Derbyshire, A. J., & Davis, H. (1935). Action potential of the auditory nerve. *American Journal of Physiology, 113,* 476–504.

Dobie, R. A., & Kimm, J. (1980). Brainstem responses to electrical stimulation of the cochlea. *Archives of Otolaryngology, 106,* 673–537.

Dolan, D. F., Teas, D. C., & Walton, J. P. (1983). Relation between discharges in auditory nerve fibers and the whole-nerve action potential: An empirical model for the AP. *Journal of the Acoustical Society of America, 73,* 580–591.

Dorman, M. F., Smith, L. M., Dankowski, K., McCandless, G., & Parkin, J. L. (in press). Long-term measures of electrode impedance and auditory thresholds for the Ineraid cochlear implant. *Journal of Speech and Hearing Research.*

Duncan-Johnson, C., & Donchin, E. (1982). The P300 component of the event-related brain potential as an index of information processing. *Biological Psychology, 14,* 1–52.

Eddington, D., Dobelle, W., Brackmann, D., Mladejousky, M., & Parkin, J. (1978). Auditory prosthesis research with multiple channel intracochlear stimulation in man. *Annals of Otology, Rhinology, and Laryngology, 87,* 1–39.

Eggermont, J. J. (1974). Basic principles for electrocochleography. *Acta Otolaryngologica* (Stockholm), (Suppl. 316), 7–16.

Evans, E. F. (1974). Auditory frequency selectivity and the cochlear nerve. In E. Zwicker & E. Terhardt (Eds.), *Facts and models in hearing* (pp. 118–129). New York: Springer-Verlag.

Fifer, R. C., & Sierra-Inzarry, B. (1988). Clinical application of the auditory middle latency response. *The American Journal of Otolaryngology, 9,* 47–56.

Finley, C. C., Wilson, B. S., & White, M. W. (1989). Models of neural responsiveness to electrical stimulation. In J. M. Miller & F. A. Spelman (Eds.), *Cochlear implants: Models of the electrically stimulated ear.* New York: Springer-Verlag.

Game, C. J. A., Gibson, W. P. R., & Pauka, C. K. (1987). Electrically evoked brain stem auditory potentials. *Annals of Otology, Rhinology, and Laryngology, 96* (Suppl. 128), 94–95.

Gantz, B. J., Tyler, R. S., Knutson, J. F., Woodworth, G., Abbas, P., McCabe, B. F., Hinrichs, J., Tye-Murray, N., Lansing, C., Kuk, F., & Brown, C. J. (1988). Evaluation of five different cochlear implant designs: *Audiologic assessment and predictors of performance. Laryngoscope, 98,* 1100–1106.

Gardi, J. N. (1985). Human brainstem and middle latency responses to electrical stimulation: Preliminary observations. In R. A. Schindler & M. M. Merzenich (Eds.), *Cochlear implants* (pp. 351–363). New York: Raven Press.

Goldstein, M. H., Jr., & Kiang, N.Y.-S (1958). Synchrony of neural activity in electric response evoked by transient acoustic stimuli. *Journal of the Acoustical Society of America, 30,* 107–114.

Gorga, M. P., Worthington, D. W., Reiland, J. K., Beauchaine, K.A., & Goldgar, D. E. (1985). Some comparisons between auditory brain stem response thresholds, latencies, and the pure-tone audiogram. *Ear and Hearing, 6,* 105–112.

Hall, J. W. (1992). *Handbook of auditory evoked responses.* Boston: Allyn and Bacon.

Hall, R. D. (1990). Estimation of surviving spiral ganglion cells in the deaf rat using the electrically evoked auditory brainstem response. *Hearing Research, 45,* 123–136.

Harrison, R. V. (1981). Rate-versus-intensity and related AP responses in normal and pathological guinea pig and human cochleas. *Journal of the Acoustical Society of America, 70,* 1036–1044.

Harrison, R. V. (1988). *The biology of hearing and deafness.* Springfield, IL: Charles Thomas.

Hartmann, R., & Klinke, R. (1989). Auditory nerve impulse pattern by electrical stimulation. In J. M. Miller & F. A. Spelman (Eds.), *Cochlear implants: Models of the electrically stimulated ear* (pp. 135–160). New York: Springer-Verlag.

Hartmann, R., Topp, G., & Klinke, R. (1984). Discharge patterns of cat primary auditory fibers with electrical stimulation of the cochlea. *Hearing Research, 13,* 47–62.

Heller, J. W., Brehm, N., Sinopoli, T., & Shallop. J.K. (1991, October). Characterization of surface-measured potentials from implanted cochlear prostheses. Proceedings of the Annual International conference IEEE, *Engineering in Biology and Medicine, 13,* 1907–1908.

Hochmair, E. S., & Hochmair-Desoyer, I. J. (1985). Aspects of sound signal processing using the Vienna intra-aid extracochlear implants. In R. A. Schindler & M. M. Merzenich (Eds.), *Cochlear implants* (pp. 101–110). New York: Raven Press.

Hochmair, E. S., & Hochmair-Desoyer, I. J. (1983). Percepts elicited by different speech-coding strategies. *Annals of New York Academy of Sciences, 405,* 268–279.

Hochmair-Desoyer, I. J., & Burian, K. (1985). Reimplantation of a molded scala tympani electrode: Impact on psychophysical and speech discrimination abilities. *Annals of Otology, Rhinology, and Laryngology, 94,* 65–70.

Javel, E. (1989). Acoustic and electrical encoding of temporal information. In J. M. Miller & F. A. Spelman (Eds.), *Cochlear implants: Models of the electrically stimulated ear* (pp. 247–296). New York: Springer-Verlag.

Javel, E., Tong, Y. C., Shepherd, R. K., & Clark, G. M. (1987). Responses of cat auditory nerve fibers to biphasic electrical current pulses. *Annals of Otology, Rhinology, and Laryngology, 96*(Suppl. 128), 26–80.

Jyung, R. W., Miller, J. M., & Cannon, S. C. (1989). Evaluation of eighth nerve integrity using the electrically evoked middle latency response. *Otolaryngology and Head and Neck Surgery, 101,* 670–682.

Kiang, N.Y.-S., & Moxon, E.C. (1972). Physiological considerations in artificial stimulation of the inner ear. *Annals of Otology, Rhinology, and Laryngology, 81,* 714–730.

Kiang, N.Y.-S., Moxon, E.C., & Kahn, A.R. (1976). The relationship of gross potentials recorded from the cochlea to single unit activity in the auditory nerve. In R. J. Ruben, C. Elberling, & G. Salomon (Eds.), *Electrocochleography* (pp. 95–115). Baltimore: University Park Press.

Kiang, N.Y.-S., Moxon, E. C., & Levine, R. A. (1970). Auditory-nerve activity in cats with normal and abnormal cochleas. In G.E.W. Wolstenholme & J. Knight (Eds.), *Sensorineural Hearing Loss* (pp. 241–268). London: Churchill.

Kiang, N.Y.-S., Watanabe, T., Thomas, E.C., & Clark, L.F. (1965). Discharge patterns of single fibers in the cat's auditory nerve. *Research Monographs, 35.* Cambridge, MA: M. I. T. Press.

Kileny, P. R. (1991). Use of electrophysiologic measures in the management of children with cochlear implants: Brainstem, middle latency, and cognitive (P300) responses. *The American Journal of Otology, 12,* 37–42.

Kileny, P. R., & Kemink, J. L. (1987). Electrically evoked middle latency auditory evoked potentials in cochlear implant candidates. *Archives of Otolaryngology–Head and Neck Surgery, 113,* 1072–1077.

Kileny, P. R., Kemink, J. L., & Miller, J. M. (1989). An intrasubject comparison of electric and acoustic middle latency responses. *American Journal of Otology, 10,* 23–27.

Liberman, M. C. (1978). Auditory-nerve responses from cats raised in a low–noise chamber. *Journal of the Acoustical Society of America, 63,* 442–459.

Liberman, M. C. (1982). The cochlear frequency map for the cat: Labeling auditory-nerve fibers of known characteristic frequency. *Journal of the Acoustical Society of America, 72,* 1441–1449.

Liberman, M. C., & Dodds, L. W. (1984). Single-neuron labeling and chronic cochlear pathology II. Stereocilia damage and alterations of spontaneous discharge rates. *Hearing Research, 16*, 43–59.

Liberman, M.C., & Kiang, N.Y.-S. (1978). Acoustic trauma in cats. *Acta Otolaryngologica* (Stockholm), (Suppl. 358), 1–63.

Lim, H. H., Tong, Y. C., & Clark, G. M. (1989). Forward masking patterns produced by intracochlear electrical stimulation of one and two electrode pairs in the human cochlea. *Journal of the Acoustical Society of America, 86*, 971–980.

Loeb, G. E., White, M. W., & Jenkins, W. M. (1983). Biophysical considerations in electrical stimulation of the auditory nervous system. *Annals of the New York Academy of Science, 405*, 123–136.

Lusted, H. S., Shelton, C., & Simmons, F. B. (1984). Comparison of electrode sites in electrical stimulation of the cochlea. *Laryngoscope, 94*, 878–882.

Lusted, H. S., & Simmons, F. B. (1988). Comparison of electrophonic and auditory-nerve electroneural responses. *Journal of the Acoustical Society of America, 83*, 657–661.

Marsh, R. R., Yamane, H., & Potsic, W. P. (1981). Effect of site of stimulation on the guinea pig's electrically evoked brainstem response. *Otolaryngology–Head and Neck Surgery, 89*, 125–130.

Merzenich, M. M., & White, M. W. (1979). Cochlear implant. The interface problem. *Biomedical Engineering Instrumentation, 3*, 321–340.

Meyer, B., Drira, M., Gegu, D., & Chouard, C. H. (1984). Results of the round window electrical stimulation in 400 cases of total deafness. *Acta Otolaryngologica*, (Suppl. 411), 168–176.

Miller, J. M. (1991). Physiologic measures of electrically evoked auditory system responsiveness: Effects of pathology and electrical stimulation. *The American Journal of Otology, 12*, 28–36.

Miller, J., Duckert, L., Malone, M., & Pfingst, B. (1983). Cochlear prostheses: Stimulation-induced damage. *Annals of Otology, Rhinology, and Laryngology, 92*, 599–609.

Miller, J. M., Duckert, L., Sutton, D., Pfingst, B. E., Malone, M. (1985). Animal models: Relevance to implant use in humans. In R. A. Schindler and M. M. Merzenich (Eds.), *Cochlear Implants* (pp. 35–54). New York: Raven Press.

Miller, M. I., & Sachs, M. B. (1983). Representation of stop consonants in the disharge patterns of auditory nerve fibers. *Journal of the Acoustical Society of America, 74*, 502–517.

Moller, A. R., & Jannetta, P. J. (1985). Neural generators of the auditory brainstem response. In J. T. Jacobson (Ed.), *The auditory brainstem response*. Boston: College-Hill Press.

Montandon, P. B., Megill, N.D., Kahn, A.R., Peake, W.T., and Kiang, N.Y.-S. (1975). Recording auditory-nerve potentials as an office procedure. *Rhinology and Laryngology, 84*, 2–9.

Moxon, E. C. (1971). *Neural and mechanical responses to electrical stimulation of the cat's inner ear*. Unpublished doctoral dissertation, Massachusetts Institute of Technology, Cambridge, MA.

Nagal, D. (1974). Compound action potential of the cochlear nerve evoked electrically. *Archives of Otology, Rhinology, and Laryngology, 206*, 293–298.

Oviatt, D. L., & Kileny, P.R. (1991). Auditory event-related potentials elicited from cochlear implant recipients and hearing subjects. *American Journal of Audiology, 1*, 48–55.

Parkins, C. W. (1989). Temporal response patterns of auditory nerve fibers to electrical stimulation in deafened squirrel monkeys. *Hearing Research, 41*, 137–168.

Parkins, C. W., & Colombo, J. (1987). Auditory-nerve single-neuron thresholds to electrical stimulation from scala tympani electrodes. *Hearing Research, 31,* 267–286.

Pfingst, P. E. (1990). Changes over time in thresholds for electrical stimulation of the cochlea. *Hearing Research, 50,* 225–236.

Pratt, H., & Somer, H. (1976). Intensity and rate functions of cochlear and brainstem responses (ABR). *American Journal of Otology, 4,* 226–234.

Prijs, V. F. (1980). On peripheral auditory adaptation II. Comparison of electrically and acoustically evoked action potentials in the guinea pig. *Acoustica, 45,* 1–13.

Robertson, D., & Wilson, S.A. (1991). Changes in cochlear sensitivity do not alter relative thresholds of different spontaneous rate categories of primary auditory-nerve fibers. *Hearing Research, 51,* 29.

Sachs, M. B., & Abbas, P. J. (1974). Rate versus level functions for auditory-nerve fibers in cats: Tone-burst stimuli. *Journal of the Acoustical Society of America, 56,* 1835–1847.

Sachs, M. B., & Young, E. D. (1979). Encoding of steady-state vowels in the auditory nerve: Representation in terms of discharge rate. *Journal of the Acoustical Society of America, 66,* 470–479.

Schindler, R. A., Merzenich, M. M., White, M. W., & Bjorkroth, B. B. (1977). Multi-electrode intracochlear implants. *Archives of Otolaryngology, 103,* 691–699.

Sellick, P. M., Patuzzi, R., & Johnstone, B. M. (1983). Comparison between tuning properties of inner hair cells and basilar membrane motion. *Hearing Research, 10,* 93–100.

Shallop, J. K., Beiter, A. L., Goin, D. W., & Mischke, R. E. (1990). Electrically evoked auditory brainstem responses (EABR) and middle latency responses (EMLR) obtained from patients with the nucleus multichannel cochlear implant. *Ear and Hearing, 11,* 5–15.

Shallop, J. K., Goin, D. N., Van Dyke, L., & Mischke, R. E. (1991). Prediction of behavioral threshold and comfort values for Nucleus 22-channel implant patients from electrical auditory brainstem response test results. *Annals of Otology, Rhinology, and Laryngology, 100,* 896–898.

Shannon, R. V. (1985). Threshold and loudness functions for pulsatile stimulation of cochlear implants. *Hearing Research, 18,* 135–143.

Shepard, R. K., Clark, G. M., & Black, R. C. (1983). Chronic electrical stimulation of the auditory nerve in cats. *Acta Otolaryngologica,* (Suppl. 399), 19–31.

Simmons, F. B., Lusted, H., Meyers, T., & Shelton, C. (1984). Electrically induced auditory brainstem response as a clinical tool in estimating nerve survival. *Annals of Otology, Rhinology, and Laryngology, 93*(Suppl. 112), 97–100.

Smith, L., & Simmons, F. B. (1983). Estimating eighth nerve survival by electrical stimulation. *Annals of Otology, Rhinology, and Laryngology, 92,* 19–25.

Smith, R. L., & Brachman, M. L. (1982). Adaptation in auditory-nerve fibers: A revised model. *Biological Cybernetics, 44,* 107–120.

Spoendlin, H. (1973). The innervation of the cochlear receptor. In A. R. Moller and P. Boston (Eds.), *Basic mechanisms in hearing.* New York: Academic Press.

Squires, K. C., & Hecox, K. E. (1983). Electrophysiological evaluation of higher level auditory processing. *Seminars in Hearing, 4,* 415–433.

Stapells, D. R., Picton, T. W., Percy-Abalo, M., Read, D., & Smith, A. (1985). Frequency specificity in evoked potential audiometry. In John T. Jacobson (Ed.), *The auditory brainstem response.* San Diego: CollegeHill Press.

Starr, A., & Brackmann, D. E. (1979). Brainstem potentials evoked by electrical stimulation of the cochlea in human subjects. *Annals Otology, 88,* 550–560.

Steel, K. P., & Bock, G. R. (1984). Electrically evoked responses in animals with progressive spiral ganglion degeneration. *Hearing Research, 15,* 59–67.

Stein, L., & Kraus, N. (1987). Maturation of the middle latency response. *Seminars in Hearing, 8,* 93–102.

Stypulkowski, P. H., & van den Honert, C. (1984). Physiological properties of the electrically stimulated auditory nerve I. Compound action potential recordings. *Hearing Research, 14,* 205–223.

Teas, D. C., Eldredge, D. H., & Davis, H. (1962). Cochlear responses to acoustic transients: An interpretation of whole-nerve action potentials. *Journal of the Acoustical Society of America, 34,* 1438–1459.

Tye-Murray, N., Gantz, B. J., Kuk, F., & Tyler, R. S. (1988). Word recognition performance of patients using three different cochlear implant designs. In P. Banfai (Ed.), *Proceedings of the Third International Conference on Cochlear Implants.*

Tyler, R. S., Moore, B. C. J., & Kuk, F. K. (1989). Performance of some of the better cochlear-implant patients. *Journal of Speech and Hearing Research, 32,* 887–911.

Tyler, R. S., & Tye-Murray, N. (1991). Cochlear implant signal processing strategies and patient perception of speech and environmental sounds. In H. Cooper (Ed.), *Cochlear implants: A practical guide.* London: Whurr Publishers.

van den Honert, C., & Stypulkowski, P. H. (1986). Characterization of the electrically auditory brainstem response (ABR) in cats and humans. *Hearing Research, 21,* 109–126.

van den Honert, C., & Stypulkowski, P. H. (1984). Physiological properties of the electrically stimulated auditory nerve. II. Single fiber recordings. *Hearing Research, 14,* 225–243.

van den Honert, C., & Stypulkowski, P. H. (1987a). Single fiber mapping of spatial excitation patterns in the electrically stimulated auditory nerve. *Hearing Research, 29,* 195–206.

van den Honert, C., & Stypulkowski, P. H. (1987b). Temporal response patterns of single auditory nerve fibers elicited by periodic electrical stimuli. *Hearing Research, 29,* 207–222.

Voigt, H. F., Sachs, M. B., & Young, E. D. (1981). Effects of masking noise on the representation of vowel spectra in the auditory nerve. In J. Syko and L. Aitkins (Eds.), *Neuronal Mechanisms of Hearing.* Prague: Plenum.

Walsh, S. M., & Leake–Jones, P. A. (1982). Chronic electrical stimulation of auditory nerve in cat: Physiological and histological results. *Hearing Research, 7,* 281–304.

Waltzman, S., Cohen, N., & Shapiro, W. (1986). Long-term effects of cochlear implant usage. *Laryngoscope, 96,* 1083–1087.

Waring, M., Don, M., & Brimacombe, J. (1985). ABR assessment of stimulation in induction coil implant patients. In R. Schindler & M. Merzenich (Eds.), *Cochlear implants* (pp. 375–378). New York: Raven Press.

White, M. W., Merzenich, M. M., & Gardi, J. N. (1989). Multichannel cochlear implants. Channel interactions and processor design. *Archives of Otolaryngology, 110,* 493–501.

Wilson, B. S., Finley, C. C., & Lawson, D. T. (1989). Representations of speech features with cochlear implants. In J. M. Miller and F. A. Spelman (Eds.), *Cochlear implants: Models of the electrically stimulated ear.* New York: Springer-Verlag.

Yamane, H., Marsh, R. R., & Potsic, W. P. (1981). Brainstem response evoked by electrical stimulation of the round window of the guinea pig. *Otolaryngology–Head and Neck Surgery, 89,* 117–124.

Young, E. D., & Sachs, M. B. (1979). Representation of steady-state vowels in the temporal aspects of the discharge patterns of populations of auditory-nerve fibers. *Journal of the Acoustical Society of America, 66,* 1381.

CHAPTER 8

Psychophysics

ROBERT V. SHANNON

Psychophysics is the discipline of relating quantitative perceptual capabilities to the properties of the physical stimulus. In the normal auditory system psychophysics usually refers to the measurement of loudness and pitch, for example, and relating these perceptual quantities to the acoustic stimulus properties. When a sensory system is artificially stimulated, as in cochlear implants, psychophysics relates familiar auditory percepts, such as loudness and pitch, to the physical properties of the electrical stimulus. We must be careful that we are not mislead by our familiarity with the normal auditory system and misunderstand the function of cochlear implants because of poor or inappropriate analogies with acoustic hearing.

To ensure objectivity, imagine that a person with a cochlear implant is like a person with an entirely new sensory system that is unfamiliar to us. How can we understand what the person with this new sensory system is perceiving? What are the basic perceptual capabilities of this new sensory system? What complex patterns can be percieved and reliably differentiated using this new sensory system? Can the new sensory system be used to convey complex linguistic information at a high rate? Although cochlear implants are stimulating the auditory system of people, it is often useful to remind ourselves that the mechanism of its stimulation is completely different from that of normal acoustic hearing and must be approached as if it were a completely new sensory system. Only after we understand the basic capabilities of electrical stimulation should we attempt to reconcile our knowledge with what we know of the normal auditory system.

Psychophysical measurements can serve three purposes in characterizing cochlear implants:

1. To quantify the biophysical limitations of electrical stimulation,
2. To compare basic perceptual performance of electrical and acoustic hearing, and
3. To understand the brain's capability for processing complex auditory patterns.

This information will help us customize the device for the individual patient and to predict performance. In the long run, understanding at all three levels will allow the design of better speech processors that take advantage of the strengths and compensate for the weaknesses of the electrically stimulated system.

In normal hearing the mechanics of the external ear, middle ear, and the cochlea determine the pattern of neural response produced by an acoustic stimulus. In electrical stimulation the neural response pattern is determined by the extent of the electrical field, by the electrical stimulus parameters, and by the neural survival. We will compare quantitative psychophysical measurements to physiological data and models to understand how the perception depends on the biophysics of the electrode/neuron interface.

One of the first questions in comparing acoustic hearing and implant hearing is: How do the listeners' basic perceptual capabilities compare? Some basic perceptual capabilities are surely determined by cochlear mechanisms and so will be impaired in implanted listeners, but which ones will be affected most? We can answer these questions only by comparing careful quantitative measurements of basic perceptual capabilities with electrical and acoustic stimulation using similar methods.

Although basic perceptual capabilities are important for understanding the function of the electrically stimulated system, most important speech sounds are complex patterns of changing time-intensity cues and spectral cues. Thus, to understand cochlear implant function we must also measure implant listeners' ability to detect and discriminate complex patterns of stimulation.

BIOPHYSICAL CHARACTERIZATION

The smallest amount of physical energy detectable by any sensory system is primarily determined by the biophysical properties of the sensory end organ and transducer cells. In vision, it is estimated that a single photon falling on a single photoreceptor can produce a visible sensation. In general, threshold functions for any sensory system reflect the physical limitations of the sensory end organ to convert the physical energy of the sensory modality into nerve impulses.

THRESHOLDS FOR ELECTRICAL CURRENT

In acoustic stimulation, threshold is probably determined by the mechanical sensitivity of the basilar membrane and hair cells. Recently, attention has been focused on the active mechanism in the cochlea, called the cochlear amplifier (Davis, 1983), which is thought to be associated with the outer hair cells.

With electrical stimulation the relevant biophysical properties are determined by the activation of a neuron by an induced electrical field. Psychophysical measures of threshold can be compared with known electrical properties of auditory neurons (e.g., Hartmann, Topp, & Klinke, 1984; van den Honert & Stypulkowski, 1984) to see if the perceptual threshold for electrical stimulation is a simple reflection of the biophysics of this "new" type of sensory end organ.

Care must be taken, however, that the stimulation level does not produce damage to the tissue surrounding the electrode, from electrolytic dissolution of the electrode, from evolution of gases, or from overstimulation of neurons (see Shannon, 1992b, for a discussion of safe stimulation levels). Current levels that produce electrode dissolution and gas evolution are well defined from electrochemistry (Roblee & Rose, 1990). Current levels that produce neural damage have received considerable study, but have not resulted in clear definitions of safe levels (Leake, Kessler, & Merzenich, 1990; McCreery, Agnew, Yuen, & Bullara (1988).

Figure 8–1 presents thresholds measured on an apical monopolar electrode stimulated with biphasic pulses or sinusoids as a function of the pulse rate or sinusoidal frequency. Note that the sinusoidal threshold functions show impressive sensitivity to electrical current at low frequencies. Detection thresholds for frequencies below 100 Hz are typically less than 1 μA.[1] As stimulus frequency is increased, the current required for threshold increases rapidly from 100 to 300 Hz and then flattens to about 3–4 dB/octave above 300 Hz (see Fourcin et al., 1979; Pfingst, 1984; Pfingst, De Hahn, & Holloway, 1991; Shannon, 1983a, 1985; Simmons, 1966). The general shape of these threshold functions are remarkably similar across subjects and electrodes (Shannon, 1983a), while the absolute current level can vary from one subject to another and even from one electrode to another in the same subject.

One caution about the interpretation of electrical threshold functions is: The relative sensitivity across frequency cannot be interpreted in the same manner as an acoustic frequency-threshold function. Acoustic threshold curves indicate the relative sensitivity across frequency. In a normal cochlea, the acoustic stimulus is processed into independent frequency regions. Thus, if acoustic sensitivity is poor in one frequency region, the amplitude of that frequency region can be increased to compensate without affecting the processing in other frequency regions. However, in electrical stimulation on a single electrode the stimulus is not analyzed separately into different frequency regions, but the instantaneous waveform is the effective stimulus to the nerve. In this case, altering the balance of amplitudes across frequency bands alters the instantaneous time waveform. This alteration can improve or deteriorate the quality of the sound depending on the phase relations of the spectral components. This is one case where our knowledge of the normal auditory system impairs our ability to interpret the meaning of the electrical threshold function. Our intuitions based on normal and impaired acoustic hearing can be completely misleading when applied to electrical hearing, due to the lack of electrical spectral processing. *Threshold functions for*

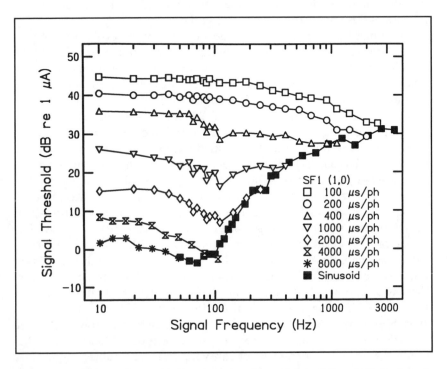

Figure 8–1. Typical threshold functions for sinusoidal (solid) and biphasic pulsatile stimulation. (Replotted from Shannon, 1989.)

electrical hearing should not be interpreted by analogy to similar acoustic threshold functions.

Physiological data and models (Columbo & Parkins, 1987; Hartmann et al., 1984; Kiang & Moxon, 1972; Parkins & Colombo, 1987; van den Honert & Stypulkowski, 1984) show sinusoidal thresholds that are shallow, bowl-shaped functions of frequency. These physiological functions match the absolute level and shape of the behavioral curves above 300 Hz. The physiological data and models do not show the low-frequency sensitivity of the human and monkey behavioral threshold functions. There seems to be an additional factor contributing to the low behavioral thresholds at low frequencies that is not yet understood in terms of the physiological response.

It is possible that we do not adequately understand the biophysics of electrical stimulation of the auditory nerve and so are overestimating the low-frequency behavioral thresholds. For example, it is possible that the low-frequency sensitivity represents stimulation of a different neural population than the rest of the threshold function. It is known that the normal auditory nerve contains at least two subpopulations of high and low spontaneous units (Liberman, 1991). If one of these neuronal populations has different physical characteristics than the other, it is possible that the composite behavioral threshold function is composed of the lowest thresholds from each subpopulation. If this were the case, low-frequency thresholds could indicate the relative survival of one subpopulation of neurons, while the high-frequency thresholds might indicate the relative survival of another subpopulation. Although two populations are known in acoustic stimulation, all physiological data with electrical stimulation have indicated only a single population response (see Abbas, Chapter 7).

A second possibility is that we do adequately understand the peripheral physiology and biophysical models. In this case, the low-frequency behavioral sensitivity is due to unknown central mechanisms that are able to integrate peripheral information at low frequencies. Central mechanisms could combine information from the periphery to achieve lower behavioral thresholds than we might expect from the peripheral physiology. There is presently not enough physiological data to resolve this issue.

Many speech processing strategies for cochlear implants use short, biphasic pulses to convey speech information to the electrodes (see Wilson, Chapter 2). Figure 8–1 also presents threshold data from biphasic pulses of different pulse durations. The same low-frequency sensitivity is observed in the pulse thresholds, although it is now present in terms of lower thresholds for long pulse durations. In all cases, thresholds for pulses are essentially equal to the sinusoidal threshold when the pulse rate is equal to the reciprocal of the pulse duration, resulting in a square wave stimulus. For example, in Figure 8–1, observe the threshold function for 1000 μs/phase biphasic pulses. The highest repetition rate at which this pulse can be presented is 500 Hz because the duration of both phases of the biphasic pulse is 2 ms which is the period of 500 Hz. The threshold for a 500 Hz, 1000 μs/phase biphasic pulse is similar to the threshold of a 500 Hz sinusoid. The pulse threshold is slightly lower because a 500 Hz square wave has slightly more charge per phase than the same sinusoidal frequency. When this difference in charge per phase is taken into account, the thresholds are essentially the same for sinusoidal and square wave stimulation at the same frequency.

Figure 8–2 presents threshold data for biphasic pulses in terms of charge per pulse. The amount of charge in each biphasic pulse is calculated as the pulse amplitude times the pulse duration. For example, a 100 μA pulse of 100 μs/phase would contain 10 nanoCoulombs/phase. Note that thresholds for different pulse durations do not correspond to constant charge (also see Shannon, 1985a). Constant charge would imply that threshold would drop 6 dB as the pulse duration is doubled. In Figure 8–2 constant charge would be indicated by a horizontal line. However, as pulse duration increases the threshold charge first increases then for long pulse durations threshold charge decreases. Thus, threshold is not determined by constant amount of charge per pulse and, in fact, threshold charge is a nonmonotonic function of pulse duration. Physiological data and models (Colombo & Parkins, 1987; Parkins & Colombo , 1987) show only the increasing portion of this same function. Again, the behavioral thresholds show a sensitivity to low sinusoidal frequencies and long pulse durations that is not present in physiological data.

The pattern of thresholds for sinusoidal and pulsatile stimuli is a complex one, both as a function of frequency and as a function of pulse duration. Mathematical models can be useful to provide a simple equation or set of equations that can account for a large array of complicated data. A model has been proposed to account for the sinusoidal and pulsatile threshold functions (Shannon, 1989b). This model proposes two mechanisms, which essentially reflect the low-frequency and high-frequency portion of the threshold functions, respectively. These two mechanisms could correspond to the two neural subpopulations discussed above or to two central mechanisms. It is not clear at this time if the two mechanisms in the model have any physiological counterparts.

In summary, threshold functions for electrical stimulation are complicated functions of stimulus frequency and waveform. At present the behavioral threshold functions cannot be predicted from the physiological threshold functions. These functional relations must be understood to properly adjust the pulse duration or frequency response in a cochlear implant speech processor.

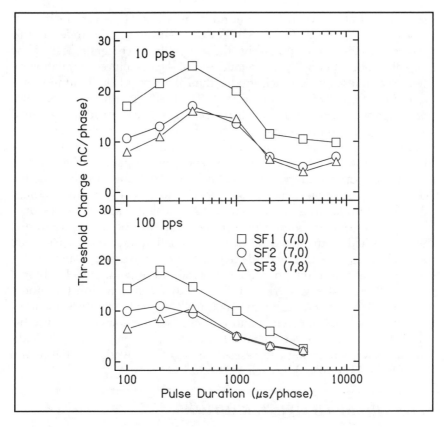

Figure 8–2. Absolute threshold for biphasic pulse stimuli as a function of pulse duration. Threshold level is expressed in terms of charge per phase of each pulse. (Replotted from Shannon, 1985a.)

CHANNEL INTERACTION

Another psychophysical measure that is important for understanding the biophysics of electrical stimulation is the interaction between stimulation on different electrodes. When two electrodes are simultaneously stimulated their electrical fields can add together and potentially cause an undesirable stimulation pattern and highly undesirable perceptual effects. Consider one case in which the electrodes are close to the target neurons. In this case, the individual electrical fields might each stimulate a localized region of neurons and cause a loud sensation at a relatively low stimulus level. This stimulus level could be below the level at which the electrical fields sum in an undesirable manner, that is, each electrode stimulates only its own local neural population. However, a different case exists if the neurons are a larger distance from the electrodes. In this case, some neurons would receive the sum of the electrical fields from the two electrodes. In this case, the loudness of the combined stimulation on two electrodes can be much louder than the sum of the loudness produced on each electrode individually. The excess loudness can produce undesirable effects in a speech processor and can produce reduced speech-recognition performance. The difference between these two cases can result from differences in the position of the electrode relative to the target neurons, or as a result of differences in the pattern of nerve survival. Psychophysical measurements should be made to determine the degree of interaction, which should then determine the relative settings of the amplitude levels on channels of a multichannel speech processor.

Two types of interactions can occur between two stimulated electrodes: electrical-field interactions and neural-population interactions. There are several psychophysical methods that can be used to assess channel interaction: threshold interaction (Cotter, 1986; Eddington, Dobelle, Brachman, Mladevasky, & Parkin, 1987), loudness summation (Shannon, 1983b, 1985b), and forward masking (Lim, Tong, & Clark, 1989; Shannon, 1983b). Threshold interaction and loudness summation can measure the degree of summation of the simultaneously presented electrical fields, while forward masking can assess the degree of overlap in the neural populations stimulated by each electrode.

ELECTRICAL-FIELD INTERACTIONS

Electrical field interactions can occur when the electrical fields generated by the two electrodes add together prior to activating neurons. In this case, the threshold on the two electrodes stimulated together could be considerably lower than the threshold level on either electrode stimulated alone. Consider a case in which a neuron is activated by 100 μA of current and where the electrical fields of the two electrodes add. The neuron will be activated by 100 μA presented on either electrode alone, or 50 μA presented on both electrodes. If the waveforms on the two electrodes are out of phase the current fields will largely cancel, and the threshold for the combined stimulation will be much higher than the threshold for each electrode individually. On the other hand, if two electrodes are stimulated simultaneously in phase, the current fields would add. Loudness functions in electrical stimulation are a steep function of stimulus level, so if the electrical fields add, the result could produce a loudness far louder than the sum of the two constituent loudnesses from the individual electrodes. Thus, electrical-field interaction can produce undesirable loudness interactions in a multichannel cochlear implant.

In contrast, if no electrical field interactions occur so that the two electrodes are exciting two distinct neural populations, then the threshold and loudness on one electrode should be independent of the current presented on the other electrode. In this case, there would be no significant electrical field interactions and two electrodes could be stimulated simultaneously with no undesirable perceptual consequences.

The degree of electrical-field interaction can be measured at threshold (Cotter, 1986; Shannon, 1983b) or at supra-threshold loudness levels (Shannon, 1985b) with simultaneous stimuli delivered to the two electrodes. The difference observed in the threshold or loudness when the stimuli are presented in-phase or out-of-phase indicates the degree of electrical field overlap. A large phase effect indicates large interactions, while the lack of a phase effect indicates independence between the two electrodes.

NEURAL-POPULATION INTERACTIONS

One method used in speech processors to avoid simultaneous channel interactions is to present the stimulation in brief biphasic pulses and present those pulses nonsimultaneously on different electrodes. These processor designs have been called interleaved-pulsatile processors and continuous interleaved sampler processors (see Wilson, Chapter 2). However, even nonsimultaneous stimulation on two electrodes can produce interactions if the two electrodes stimulate the same neural population.

For example, consider the case where two electrodes each carry a 100-Hz pulse train and are interleaved so that no two pulses occur at the same time on the two electrodes. If the two electrodes stimulate the same neural population, the neurons would "see" a combined stimulus of 200 Hz because the neurons would not be able to separate the stimuli from the two electrodes. On the other hand, if the two electrodes stimulated different neural populations each electrode would produce a 100-Hz response in its respective population. Intermediate cases can also arise in which the electrodes stimulate overlapping but not identical populations. Shannon (1983b) proposed the use of forward masking to measure the overlap of neural populations, and a modified form of this procedure was elegantly demonstrated by Lim et al. (1989). Figure 8–3 presents forward masking interaction patterns measured by Lim et al. (1989) across 22 electrodes as a function of masker level. As the masker level increased, more interaction was observed, indicating that the masker was stimulating a broader neural population, as expected. An interesting observation in this one patient is that of apparent "upward spread of masking," that is, as masker level increased, the masking increased more in the basal direction than in the apical direction. Although this appears similar to the acoustic masking phenomenon it probably results from a quite different mechanisms. Lim and collegues speculate that this spread toward the base is the result of the geometry of the spiral ganglion, in that a major current-flow path for cochlear stimulation is down the modiolus. Thus, stimulation of one position in the cochlea results in a current field that spreads basally more than apically. Again, psychophysical measures can be used to quantify a biophysical phenomenon, such as the asymmetric spread of the current field.

In summary, psychophysics can be used in some cases to measure effects that can be related to the underlying electrical fields and biophysics of electrical stimulation. Once the underlying biophysical properties are understood, electrical thresholds and channel interaction measures could provide behavioral measures of neural survival and accuracy of electrode placement. These psychophysical measures could potentially be streamlined and applied as clinical tests that could have implications for speech processor design and fitting.

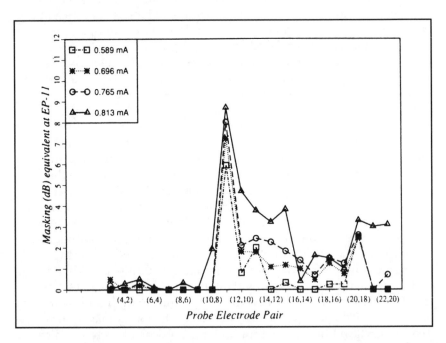

Figure 8–3. Channel interaction across the electrode array measured by forward masking. Interaction curves are shown for a masker on electrodes (11,13) at three masker levels. (Reprinted from Lim, H.H., Tong, Y.C., & Clark, G.M., 1989. Forward masking patterns produced by intracochlear stimulation of one and two electrode pairs in the human cochlear. *Journal of the Acoustical Society of America*, *86*, 971–980, with permission.)

BASIC PERCEPTUAL CAPABILITIES

Psychophysical measures can also be used to characterize the basic perceptual abilities of patients with cochlear implants. To design effective speech processors we need to know which dimensions of electrical stimuli are relevant for perception. It makes no sense to design a speech processor to preserve a fine detail of the acoustic waveform if the patient cannot distinguish that feature when presented electrically. Speech processor design should take into consideration the basic perceptual capabilities of implant listeners: exploiting stimulus features that can be perceived and discriminated and de-emphasizing distinctions that are not discriminable by patients. Important speech features that implant patients cannot receive directly must be recoded into an electrical dimension in which the patient can make the proper distinction. In addition, it is probably important to understand the individual differences in basic perceptual capabilities to optimally adjust a speech processor specifically for a given patient.

Basic perceptual capabilities can be divided into those that involve temporal processing, intensity processing, and spectral resolution. We will first review psychophysical data on temporal processing, using forward masking, gap detection, temporal integration, modulation detection, and rate discrimination as measures.

TEMPORAL PROCESSING

Temporal processing refers to the perceptual ability to detect and discriminate changes in a stimulus in time. For example, television and movies depend on the fact that our visual system has relatively slow temporal processing. Two static pictures presented rapidly give the sensation of movement because the temporal response of our eye is slow and smears the individual frames together in time. We do not notice the interval between the two frames because of the long temporal integration time of the eye. In general, hearing can process information much faster than vision and the following section describes several methods for quantifying the electrically stimulated ears' temporal response capabilities.

Forward Masking

One psychophysical measure of temporal resolution is forward masking, which measures the recovery from prior stimulation. Forward masking describes the recovery of perceptual sensitivity following the offset of a preceding masker. An intense masking stimulus is presented and then turned off. The threshold of a brief signal (10–20 ms) is then measured as a function of the time delay from the masker offset to signal onset. Immediately following the masker, the signal threshold is elevated from its quiet threshold. The longer the signal delay the smaller the shift in threshold. At some long signal delay the signal threshold will return to its quiet threshold level, indicating no residual effect of the masker.

Figure 8–4 presents a comparison of forward masking for normal-hearing listeners and implant listeners (Shannon, 1990). Threshold of a brief signal is plotted as a function of the time delay following masker offset. The amplitude scale has been normalized to allow comparison across different thresholds and different dynamic ranges. Masking is plotted from the masker level (100 arbitrary units) to quiet threshold (0 units). The cochlear implant data have been normalized in terms of μA, and the acoustic data have been normalized in terms of dB (see Shannon, 1990, for details of the normalization). Note that both sets of data show that signal thresholds recover linearly on these axes so that little masking is evident by 300–500 ms following the masker. When compared in these terms the recovery from adaptation is similar between implant and acoustic listeners. This result indicates that implant listeners have the same recovery time from adaptation as normal-hearing listeners.

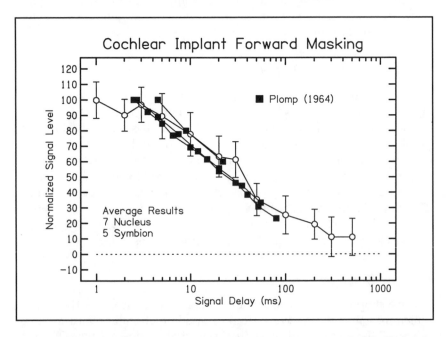

Figure 8–4. Forward masking recovery functions on a normalized amplitude scale. Solid symbols present data from acoustic listeners (Plomp, 1964) at three masker levels with the data normalization in dB.

The cochlea normally compresses the amplitude of the acoustic stimulus into a smaller range of neural firing rates. The acoustic dynamic range of amplitudes span a range of more than 1,000,000 to 1, while neurons increase their firing rate from a spontaneous rate of 20–50 spikes/s to a saturated firing rate of only 300 spikes/s, a ratio of only 10 to 1. This compression is approximately logarithmic, in that, within the dynamic range of the neuron, equal changes in dB produce equal changes in firing rate. Electrical stimulation stimulates the nerve directly, without a logarithmic compression, so that an increase in electrical stimulus amplitude produces a proportional increase in neural firing rate. Therefore, it is not unreasonable to compare acoustic dB and electrical μA. Once this difference in intensity scale is normalized, the recovery from adaptation in implants is normal.

Gap Detection

Another psychophysical measure of temporal resolution is gap detection, which measures the ability to detect a brief interruption in an ongoing stimulus. Figure 8–5 (after Shannon, 1989a) presents average gap thresholds from implant listeners as a function of the level of the stimulus. In general, the louder the stimulus, the shorter the gap-detection threshold. When the stimulus is soft, near threshold, listeners required gaps of 20–50 ms for detection, while for loud stimuli listeners required gaps of only 2–5 ms for detection (see also Dobie & Dillier, 1985; Moore & Glasberg, 1988; Preece & Tyler, 1989). No significant differences are observed between subjects in gap detection. These values are similar to gap-detection thresholds of normal acoustic listeners, indicating that implant listeners can detect brief interruptions as well as normal acoustic listeners. Gaps of 10–20 ms duration are often important in discriminating speech sounds and implant listeners should be able to detect gaps of that duration (see Dorman, Chapter 4).

Temporal Integration

Temporal integration measures the time over which the auditory system integrates stimulus energy. If there is an auditory mechanism integrating the stimulus representation over time, then long-duration stimuli should have lower thresholds than short-duration stimuli. The stimulus duration at which threshold no longer changes is called the limit of temporal integration or temporal-integration time. Normal acoustic listeners have temporal-integration times of 100–200 ms and appear to integrate the stimulus power. This means that when a stimulus duration is shortened by half, the stimulus power must be doubled (3 dB increase) to keep the signal at threshold.

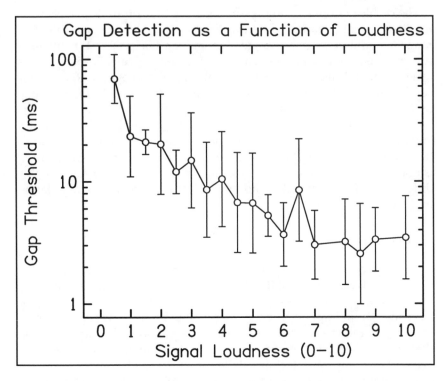

Figure 8–5. Gap detection as a function of stimulus level. The listeners were asked to estimate the loudness level of the stimulus on a scale of 0–10.

Figure 8–6 presents thresholds as a function of stimulus duration for implant listeners. The solid line indicates constant power integration typical of normal listeners. Note that for implant listeners thresholds increase only slightly as stimulus duration is decreased from 100 to 1 ms. Although this appears to indicate that implant listeners have less temporal integration than acoustic listeners, we must keep in mind the greatly reduced dynamic range of electrical hearing. An increase in threshold of a few dB might constitute as much integration in perceptual terms as 15–20 dB of threshold change in acoustic listeners over the same range. Although no model presently exists to allow direct comparison of the magnitude of the integration effect, it is possible that the implant data indicates similar temporal integration to acoustic listeners. If thresholds could be normalized in a manner similar to the normalization used in Figure 8–3 for forward masking, temporal integration functions might be more comparable between normal-hearing and implant listeners. Unfortunately, insufficient dynamic range data exist to perform this normalization for the present temporal integration functions.

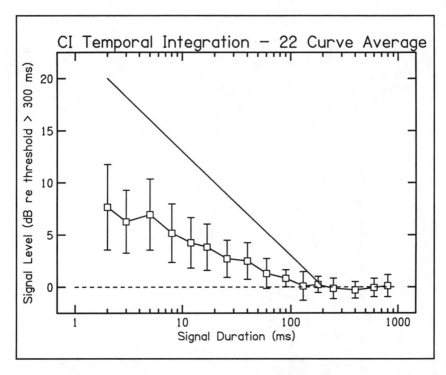

Figure 8–6. Temporal integration functions for implant listeners. Solid line presents prediction of an equal energy detector for comparison. The equal energy prediction is similar to temporal integration in acoustic listeners.

Modulation Detection

A widely used psychophysical method for quantifying temporal resolution is the temporal modulation transfer function (Bacon & Viemeister, 1985). This technique measures the listener's threshold for detecting amplitude modulation as a function of the modulating frequency. Figure 8–7 compares modulation detection for acoustic listeners (dashed line) and listeners with two types of cochlear implants. The curves from implant and acoustic listeners are low-pass functions, showing best sensitivity to low modulation frequencies. Sensitivity to modulation decreases as modulation frequency increases, that is, larger modulation amplitudes are necessary for detection. Although implant modulation detection appears to be better than acoustic performance, this apparent difference is probably due to differences in the carrier stimulus used in the two experiments. There are no obvious differences between acoustic and implant modulation detection, indicating that implant listeners can detect amplitude modulation as well as acoustic listeners (Shannon, 1992a).

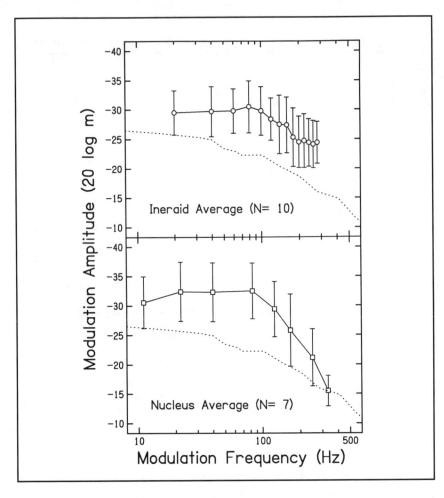

Figure 8–7. Detection thresholds for amplitude modulation as a function of modulation frequency. Dashed curve presents data from normal acoustic listeners.

Several implant processors use amplitude-modulated carriers to present speech information to patients (Fretz & Fravel, 1985; Wilson, Finley, Lawson, & Wolford, 1989; Wilson et al., 1991; see Wilson, Chapter 2). The data in Figure 8–7 indicate that implant patients can detect modulation as well as normal-hearing listeners, but it is not clear if comparable performance on a basic psychophysical task translates into comparable performance on envelope features in speech that are conveyed by envelope fluctuations. Preliminary results indicate that implant listeners can make full use of temporal envelope cues if the amplitude is mapped properly from acoustic to electrical domains (Shannon, Zeng, & Wygonski, 1992).

Rate Discrimination

Acoustic listeners can detect the difference between stimulus frequencies by resolving the stimuli into different frequency regions along the cochlea. In this case, different frequencies activate different neural populations. However, when spectral information is removed by modulating a wide-band noise, acoustic listeners can only discriminate pitches based on modulation rate up to 300–500 Hz (Burns & Viemeister, 1976, 1981). Figure 8–8 presents measures of pitch as a function of pulse rate for cochlear implant listeners (Shannon, 1983a). Listeners were instructed to rate the pitch of the stimulus on a scale of 0–100 arbitrary units, where 1 was a very low pitch like a fog horn or deep bass note and 100 was a very high-pitch screech, like a fingernail scratched on a blackboard. Note that as the stimulus frequency was increased from 100–300 Hz the pitch increased substantially. However, the pitch estimate did not change appreciably for stimulus frequencies above 300 Hz. The asymptotic pitch reached at stimulus frequencies above 300 Hz was dependent on the cochlear location of the electrode. Apical electrodes sounded lower in pitch than basal electrodes, in agreement with the general tonotopic organization of the cochlea. These data are representative of similar measures by others of pitch as a function of pulse rate and rate discrimination

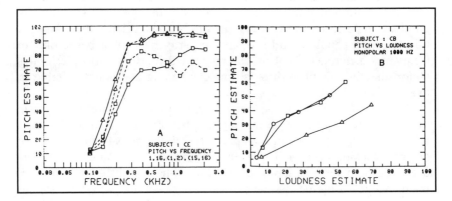

Figure 8–8. Pitch rating as a function of pulse rate for several electrode positions. (Reprinted from Shannon, R.V., 1983a. Multichannel electrical stimulation of the auditory nerve in man: I. Basic psychophysics. *Hearing Research, 11,* 157–189, with permission.)

(Dobie & Dillier, 1985; Muller, 1983; Pfingst & Rush, 1987; Tong, Blamey, Dowell, & Clark, 1983; Townshend, Cotter, van Compernolle, & White, 1987). It appears that implant listeners can discriminate rate information and use rate-based pitch in approximately the same manner as acoustic listeners for whom all spectral cues have been eliminated. This result is also consistent with the modulation detection data (Figure 8–7). Thus, stimulus rate information above 300 Hz must be conveyed in implants by the tonotopic location of the electrode.

Pitch perception can also be inferred from the patient's ability to discriminate frequency. In this method, two stimuli are presented that differ in frequency and the patient is required to indicate which of the two is higher in pitch. The frequency difference is reduced to find the point at which patient can just detect the frequency difference. However, loudness can be a strong confounding cue in these experiments because threshold and loudness functions for electrical stimulation change significantly as a function of frequency. Pitch can change dramatically with loudness in some implant listeners (Shannon, 1983a; Townshend et al., 1987), so that unless loudness cues are adequately counterbalanced, loudness can be a confounding variable in rate or frequency discrimination measures. One approach to this problem is to balance stimuli for loudness before measuring rate or frequency discrimination. However, the error in adjustment for balancing loudness is larger than the discrimination threshold. Thus, any two stimuli may be easily discriminable in loudness, even though the stimulus set as a whole is balanced for equal loudness.

Pfingst and Rush (1987) proposed a method for removing loudness as a confounding cue when measuring rate discrimination. They measured the discrimination of two frequencies over a range of loudness levels. The combination of amplitudes that produced the poorest frequency discrimination performance was assumed to be the level at which the stimuli were most equal in loudness, and so performance was based only on frequency differences, not on the combined loudness and pitch cues. Unfortunately, this procedure is time-consuming and is not suitable for use in a clinical setting.

The limit of pitch change associated with purely temporal rate appears to be 300–500 Hz for both normal and implant listeners. Although temporal information is present in auditory nerve discharge patterns in the form of phase locking up to 4–5 kHz, this information does not appear to be useful in the determination of pitch. Normal-hearing listeners can detect pitch changes at higher frequencies because the auditory system changes frequency information into a place-specific spatial representation. Electrical stimulation can simulate this spatial distribution by stimulating electrodes positioned tonotopically along the cochlea, but on any one electrode pitch and rate discrimination are only possible up to about 300 Hz.

Overall, the pattern of results on temporal resolution indicates that implant listeners can detect and discriminate temporal changes about the same as acoustic listeners. Cochlear implant listeners' temporal resolution appears to be relatively normal even though they have no remaining cochlear mechanisms.

LOUDNESS

In designing a speech processor for a cochlear implant one of the most important factors lies in the transformation of acoustic amplitude to electrical amplitude. The range of stimulus amplitudes between threshold and the loudness discomfort level (or uncomfortable level) is called the dynamic range. Normal acoustic hearing can process sounds that vary over a range of 1,000,000 to 1 in terms of amplitude. Even speech sounds in normal conversation can vary over a range of 1000 to 1 in acoustic amplitude. However, implant listeners can have a dynamic range as small as 3 to 1, or as large as 30 to 1. The large range of acoustic amplitude variation must be compressed to the considerably smaller range of electrical stimulation. To maximize the transmission of speech information, this transformation should be done in a way that preserves the important intensity relationships between phonetic elements.

Loudness functions have generally been measured using rating methods and classical magnitude estimation scaling techniques. All of these techniques require subjective responses in which the patient is instructed to give a numerical response to indicate the loudness of the stimulus. While this appears to be a straightforward task, considerable evidence has shown that people do not assign numbers in the same way. Thus, it may not be possible to compare loudness growth functions across patients. Some patients show linear loudness growth as the electrical current (in μA) increases linearly, while others show linear loudness growth as electrical current increases logarithmically. It is not yet clear whether these observed differences reflect actual variation in the form of the loudness function across listeners, or simply reflect the variation in the way individual patients use numbers to describe sensory magnitude. Additional studies are necessary to determine the actual loudness growth for electrical stimulation.

Figure 8–9 presents measures of the threshold and upper range of comfortable loudness for different pulse durations as a function of pulse rate. This figure demonstrates that the dynamic range is not simply related to the stimulus frequency and pulse duration. Note that as pulse duration increases the thresholds decrease and the dynamic range increases. The lower right panel summarizes the dynamic range measures for a 50-Hz pulse rate. Constant charge would be represented as a

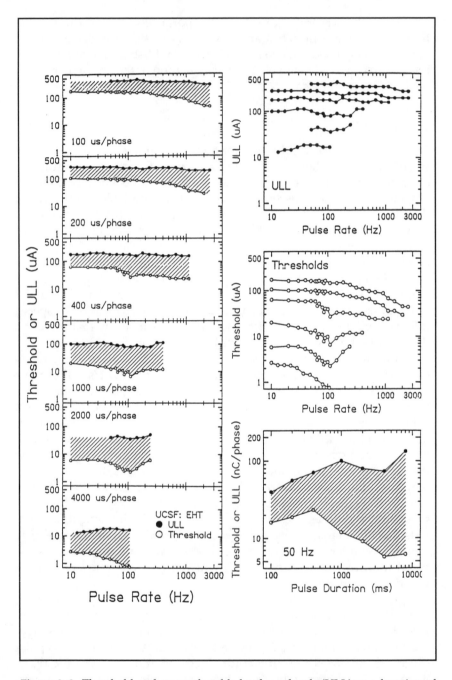

Figure 8–9. Threshold and uncomfortable loudness levels (ULL) as a function of pulse rate and pulse duration for one subject.

horizontal line in this figure. Note that neither threshold or uncomfortable loudness level are well described by constant charge. Thus, threshold, uncomfortable loudness level, and dynamic range are all complex functions of pulse duration.

One study (Shannon, 1985a) indicates that the loudness of an electrical stimulus is a complex function of the electrical waveform. Shannon measured loudness estimates on a 0–100 scale as a function of pulse duration. All stimuli were 100-Hz pulse trains with equal charge/phase in each pulse. Loudness was a nonmonotonic function of pulse duration first decreasing, then increasing to a local maximum before decreasing again, as pulse duration was increased. This result indicates that equal charge in a biphasic pulse does not produce equal loudness and, in fact, demonstrates that the relation between pulse duration and loudness is a complex one.

Eddington et al. (1978) matched loudness binaurally in a listener with normal acoustic hearing in one ear and a cochlear implant in the other ear. They found a linear relation between electrical microamps and acoustic dB. Recently, Zeng and Shannon (1992) replicated this finding in three patients with implants on the cochlear nucleus on one side and (temporary) residual hearing on the contralateral side (Figure 8–10). Based on the linear relation between the logarithm of acoustic amplitude and linear electrical amplitude, Zeng and Shannon derived an exponential loudness model for electrical stimulation. This exponential model provided an excellent fit to the Zeng and Shannon data as well as the data from Eddington et al. (1978). This model indicates that a logarithmic amplitude compression is necessary to match loudness between acoustic and electrical amplitudes. The surprisingly simple result is that, once the electrical threshold and uncomfortable loudness level are measured, the loudness of an electrical stimulus between these two levels in microamps is analogous to the loudness of an acoustic stimulus in dB SL.

INTENSITY DISCRIMINATION

Although implant patients have a smaller dynamic range than acoustic listeners, it is possible that they could also detect smaller intensity changes so that they would have the same number of discriminable steps in loudness within their smaller dynamic range. If this were the case then we might map acoustic intensity DLs to electrical intensity DLs to preserve loudness relations. Unfortunately, intensity discrimination in implant listeners is not significantly better than that of acoustic listeners. Implant listeners can detect 1–2 dB changes in intensity near threshold and improve to 0.25–0.5 dB at high intensities (Hochmair-Desoyer, Hochmair, Burain, & Stiglbrunner, 1983; Pfingst, 1984; Pfingst, Burnett, & Sutton, 1983; Pfingst et al., 1991; Shannon, 1983a). Although

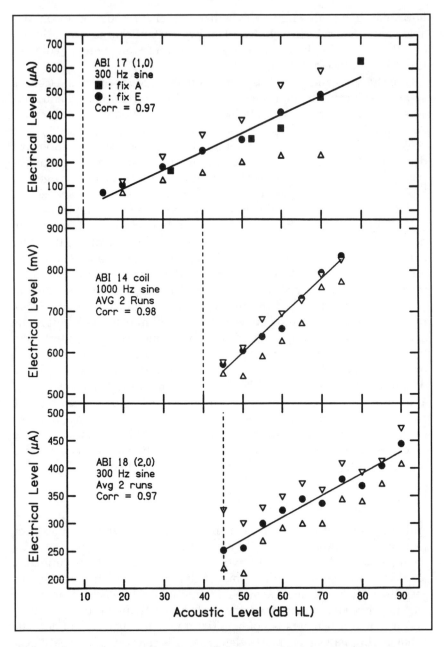

Figure 8–10. Loudness balances between an ear with residual acoustic hearing and electrical stimulation of the cochlear nucleus. (Reprinted from Zeng F.G. & Shannon, R.V. 1992. Loudness balance between acoustic and electric stimulation. *Hearing Research, 60*, 231–235, with permission.)

some implant listeners, might be able to detect slightly smaller intensity increments than acoustic listeners, the difference is not enough to offset the huge difference in dynamic range. Normal-hearing listeners have approximately 200 discriminable intensity steps in their 120-dB dynamic range, while implant listeners have only 10–30 discriminable intensity steps in their 10–20 dB dynamic range. Because of this mismatch in the number of discriminable steps in intensity, it is not clear how to compress the large acoustic range into the smaller electrical range. Even with amplitude compression, two acoustic stimuli that are discriminable could be compressed into two electrical stimuli that are not discriminable. If the lost distinction is an important phonetic cue, the speech distinction will also be lost in the compression process.

SPECTRAL RESOLUTION

In normal acoustic stimulation there is an inherent covariation between spectral cues and the location of neural stimulation. As we change the frequency of a stimulus, its representation in the cochlea shifts along the basilar membrane. We cannot deliver high-frequency information to the apical end of the cochlea. However, in electrical stimulation we can deliver a low-frequency electrical stimulus to an electrode in a basal part of the cochlea, or we can deliver a high-frequency electrical stimulus to an electrode in the apical part of the cochlea. Because there is no mechanism for spectrally resolving the electrical frequency, we can electrically stimulate high-frequency neurons with low-frequency stimuli and vice versa.

In acoustic hearing the cochlea performs an exquisite frequency analysis on the acoustic stimulus, resolving frequency components into a spatially distributed array of activity. However, electrical stimulation bypasses all mechanisms for spectrally separating acoustic stimuli. In electrical stimulation the electrical field spreads out from the electrode and activates nearby neurons. The electrical stimulus is not resolved into its spectral components because there is no physiological or biophysical mechanism to perform this spectral analysis. The effective stimulus to the neuron is the instantaneous electrical waveform, irrespective of its spectral content.

Psychophyscial experiments confirm that there is no spectral resolution in electrical stimulation. Shannon (1983a) measured the forward masking of a signal as a function of its frequency for a masker of fixed frequency and level. He observed equal threshold shift at all signal frequencies, that is, no additional masking near the masker frequency, indicating no spectral selectivity of electrical forward masking. In general, there are no biophysical or physiological mechanisms for spectrally resolving electrical stimuli and no perceptual effects of any such resolution have been observed.

Multichannel implants can crudely recreate some spatial distribution of activity along the cochlea that mimics some aspects of the normal acoustic spectral pattern, but the spectral resolution must be done externally in the speech processor and delivered to separate electrodes in different tonotopic locations. Most implant speech processors filter the speech signal into different frequency bands, each of which is further processed and presented to different electrodes (see Wilson, Chapter 2).

However, the number of electrodes that can be used as distinct "channels" is limited by the degree of channel interaction in an individual patient. For some patients, presumably those with good nerve survival and good electrode placement, each electrode may be usable as a distinct channel with which to represent speech information. Other patients who may have poor nerve survival and/or poor electrode placement may have many fewer effective information channels than the number of electrodes in their implant.

COMPLEX AUDITORY PATTERNS

Most biologically significant sounds are composed of complex patterns that change in time, intensity, and frequency. Speech, the most important sound pattern for human communication, consists of a complex pattern of changing spectral components and temporal fluctuations. Even if we understand the implant listener's perceptual ability to make simple acoustic discriminations, we may not be able to predict their performance at detecting and discriminating complex patterns like those found in speech.

Recent experiments in normal-hearing patients have demonstrated that psychophysical performance with complex stimuli cannot always be predicted from psychophysical performance with simple stimuli. For example, Hall and colleagues (e.g., Hall & Grose, 1990) have demonstrated that coherent amplitude modulation in remote frequency regions can improve detection of signals in another frequency region. The traditional concept of the "critical band" would predict that such modulation would have no effect on detection, as long as the additional masker was more than a critical band away.

Another example of psychophysics with complex acoustic sound patterns is an experiment of Zeng, Turner, and Relkin (1991), which demonstrated that intensity discrimination following a loud sound could be much poorer than intensity discrimination in quiet. Since speech consists of a complex temporal sequence of louder and softer segments, it is possible that intensity discrimination performance relevant for speech discrimination is not easily predictable from performance on basic psychophysical tasks, which are usually done with isolated sounds.

From these examples it is clear that psychophysical experiments, which quantify basic auditory capabilities, may not be applicable to complex patterns. More research is necessary to define basic detection and discrimination performance in complex patterns that represent speech. This direction is not only important in the study of cochlear implants, but in understanding normal and impaired acoustic hearing as well.

FREQUENCY/RATE TRANSITIONS

Tong, Clark, Blamey, Busby, & Dowell (1982) measured implant listeners' ability to detect changes in pulse rate that were intended to mimic transitions in fundamental frequency. Pulse rate was changed linearly with time from a variable starting rate to a fixed pulse rate of 150 Hz. The frequency extent of the rate transition and the duration of time over which the transition occurred were varied parametrically. The listener was presented with a constant pulse rate at 150 Hz and another stimulus, which was also constant or contained a change in the pulse rate. They were instructed to indicate if the two stimuli were the same or different. Figure 8–11 presents discrimination data of implant patients for different transition durations and different ranges of frequency change. When the transition duration was 50 ms or longer, listeners could distinguish the stimulus with the transition from the constant rate, and discrimination improved as the range of the transition increased. For 25 ms transition durations, discrimination was poor even for large transition ranges. However, transitions in fundamental voice frequency that provide phonetic information in speech should be discriminable.

ELECTRODE SWEEPS

One distinctive acoustic cue for discriminating phonemes is the trajectory of formant transitions, which reflect movement of the resonance cavities in the mouth during articulation. Cochlear-implant listeners are unable to discriminate frequency changes in the normal acoustic range of formant frequencies on a single electrode. Thus, such formant transition information must be conveyed by sweeping the electrical stimulus across electrodes. A stimulus to mimic a formant trajectory would thus be a constant electrical frequency moved across electrodes that stimulate neurons at different tonotopic locations. If each electrode produces a distinctive pitch sensation, a fixed-rate stimulus sweeping across electrodes should give the sensation of a sweeping pitch.

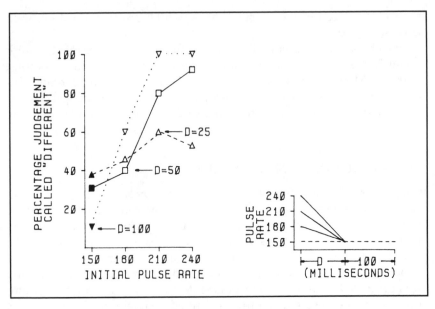

Figure 8–11. Percent correct performance at detecting a sweep in pulse rate as a function of the extent of the sweep, with duration of the sweep as a parameter. (Reprinted from Tong, Y.C., Clark, G.M., Blamey, P.J., Busby, P.A., & Dowell, R.C., 1982. Psychophysical studies evaluating the feasibility of a speech processing strategy for a multiple-channel cochlear implant. *Journal of the Acoustical Society of America, 71*, 153–160, with permission.)

Figure 8–12 presents data from an experiment of Tong et al. (1982) to measure implant patients' ability to detect and discriminate changes across electrode locations that were similar in time and tonotopic breadth to formant transitions in normal speech. Tong and colleagues presented the implant listeners with two stimuli. Each stimulus was either a fixed pulse rate on a single electrode, or the same fixed pulse rate swept across electrodes. Implant listeners were instructed to indicate if the two stimuli they heard were (a) the same constant rate presented twice on a single electrode or (b) one single-electrode stimulus and another stimulus swept across different electrodes. In general, listeners could easily distinguish if the pulses were presented to more than one electrode. In some cases, when the stimulus was only swept across two adjacent electrodes, patients could not distinguish this stimulus from a single-electrode stimulus. However, if the sweep trajectory spanned more than two electrodes, patients could always tell the difference from a single-electrode stimulus. This result indicates that implant patients should be able to discriminate phonemes that are distinguished by frequency transitions if they are properly converted to sweeps across electrodes.

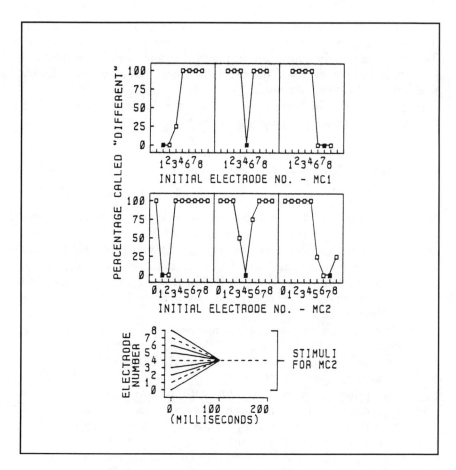

Figure 8–12. Detection of a stimulus swept across electrodes as a function of the number of electrodes in the sweep. (Reprinted from Tong, Y.C., Clark, G.M., Blamey, P.J., Busby, P.A., & Dowell, R.C., 1982. Psychophysical studies evaluating the feasibility of a speech processing strategy for a multiple-channel cochlear implant. *Journal of the Acoustical Society of America, 71*, 153-160, with permission.)

SUMMARY

We are only beginning to understand the basic perceptual capabilities of cochlear-implant patients through careful psychophysical experiments. Some measures can indicate the status of neural survival and the proximity of the electrode to the surviving neurons. Other measures indicate that implant patients' basic perceptual capabilities on temporal tasks are relatively unimpaired. We are only beginning to understand the perceptual capabilities of implanted patients on complex stimulus patterns that approximate speech patterns. Further psychophysical work is necessary in all three categories: biophysics, basic perception, and complex pattern perception, to fully understand the capabilities and limitations of auditory perception with electrical stimulation.

At present, we can draw the following conclusions about cochlear implants based on the psychophysical results:

1. Behavioral threshold functions are not simply related to the biophysics of electrical stimulation. The high sensitivity to low-frequency electrical current is not explained by presently understood biophysical mechanisms.
2. Perceptual interactions between electrodes may indicate the pattern of neural survival and placement of the electrode.
3. Once we compensate for the obvious differences in the dynamic range between electric and acoustic stimulation, all measures of basic temporal processing, including forward masking, temporal integration, gap detection, and modulation detection, are relatively normal.
4. On a single electrode, implant listeners can only detect temporal rate fluctuations up to about 300 Hz. Temporal fluctuations faster than 300 Hz cannot be detected and do not contribute to pitch sensation.
5. Perception of complex auditory patterns is not predictable from performance on simple psychophysical tasks. Additional experiments are necessary to quantify performance on complex temporal patterns that represent important speech patterns.
6. Psychophysical evidence predicts that implant patients should be able to normally receive envelope information and low-frequency rate information on a single electrode. Speech performance measures with specially designed speech processors on a single electrode validate this prediction.

IMPLICATIONS OF PSYCHOPHYSICS FOR CLINICIANS

Clinicians setting speech processors for cochlear implant patients should have a basic understanding of the basic psychophysical results. When the clinician encounters difficulties in fitting a processor, knowledge of basic perceptual capabilities and limitations of the patient will enable the clinician to efficiently modify the processor. One goal of cochlear implant psychophysics is to be able to predict the level of speech recognition by an individual patient. Eventually, psychophysical measures might be able to completely specify the optimal fitting of an implant speech processor, much like the fitting process used by an optometrist for new eye-glasses. While these goals are not presently close at hand, hearing professionals should always keep up with the latest research results so they can understand the potential clinical applications of laboratory research.

ACKNOWLEDGMENTS

Special thanks to the patients who participated in these experiments for their time and dedication. Thanks to Fan-Gang Zeng, Steve Otto, Chris Ahlstrom, and Vivek Kamath for help on earlier drafts of this chapter. Work described in this chapter was funded in part by NIH grants R29-DC00409 and R01-DC01526.

FOOTNOTE

[1]Electrical stimulation levels are presented in terms of microAmps peak amplitude, or in decibels computed relative to 1.0 μA. Thus, OdB on this scale would be a stimulus of 1 μA peak smplitude.

REFERENCES

Bacon, S. P., & Viemeister, N. F. (1985). Temporal modulation transfer functions in normal-hearing and hearing-impaired listeners. *Audiology, 24,* 117–134.

Burns, E. M., & Viemeister, N. F. (1976). Nonspectral pitch. *Journal of the Acoustical Society of America, 60,* 863–869.

Burns, E. M., & Viemeister, N. F. (1981). Played-again SAM: Further observations on the pitch of amplitude-modulated noise. *Journal of the Acoustical Society of America, 70,* 1655–1660.

Columbo, J., & Parkins, C. W. (1987). A model of electrical excitation of the mammalian auditory nerve. *Hearing Research, 31,* 287–312.

Cotter, N. E. (1986). *Modeling of auditory prostheses.* Doctoral dissertation, Stanford University, Stanford, CA. (Stanford Electronics Laboratories Technical Report No. G906-8.)

Davis, H. (1983). An active process in cochlear mechanics. *Hearing Research, 9,* 79–90.

Dobie, R. A., & Dillier, N. (1985). Some aspects of temporal coding for single-channel electrical stimulation of the cochlea. *Hearing Research, 18,* 41–55.

Eddington, D. K., Dobelle, W. H., Brachman, D. E., Mladevosky, M. G., & Parkin, J.L. (1978) Auditory prosthesis research with multiple channel intracochlear stimulation in man. *Annals of Otology, Rhinololgy, and Laryngololgy, 87*(Suppl. 53), 1–39.

Fourcin, A.J., Rosen, S.M., Moore, B.C.J., Doueck, E.E., Clarke, G.P., Dodson, H., & Bannister, L.H. (1979). External electrical stimulation of the cochlea: Clinical, psychophysical, speech-perceptual, and histological findings. *British Journal of Audiology, 13*, 85–107.

Fretz, R.J., & Fravel, R.P. (1985). Design and function: A physical and electrical description of the 3M House cochlear implant system, *Ear and Hearing, 6* (Suppl. 3), 14s–19s.

Hall, J.W., & Grose, J.H (1990). Comodulation masking release and auditory grouping. *Journal of the Acoustical Society of America, 88*, 119–125.

Hartmann, R., Topp, G., and Klinke, R. (1984). Discharge patterns of cat primary auditory fibers with electrical stimulation of the cochlea. *Hearing Research, 13*, 47–62.

Hochmair-Desoyer, I.J., Hochmair, E.S., Burian, K., & Stiglbrunner, H.K. (1983). Percepts from the Vienna cochlear prosthesis. In C.W. Parkins & S.W. Anderson (Eds.) Cochlear prostheses: An international symposium. *Annals of the New York Academy of Sciences, 405*, 295–306.

Hochmair-Desoyer, I.J., Hochmair, E.S., & Stiglbrunner, H.K. (1984). Psychocoustic temporal processing and speech understanding in cochlear implant patients. In R.A. Schindler and M.M. Merzenich(Eds.), *Cochlear implants: Current status and future* (pp. 291–304). New York: Raven Press.

Kiang, N.Y.S., & Moxon, E.C. (1972). Physiological considerations in artificial stimulation of the inner ear. *Annals of Otology Rhinology and Laryngology, 81*, 714–730.

Leake, P.A., Kessler, D.K., & Merzenich, M.M. (1990). Application and safety of cochlear prostheses, In W.F. Agnew & D.B. McCreery (Eds.), Neural prostheses: Fundamental studies (pp. 253–296). Englewood Cliffs: Prentice-Hall.

Liberman, M.C. (1991). Spatial segregation of auditory-nerve projections in the cochlear nucleus according to spontaneous discharge rates. *Abstracts of the ARO Midwinter Research Meeting*, 42.

Lim, H.H., Tong, Y.C., & Clark, G.M. (1989). Forward masking patterns produced by intracochlear stimulation of one and two electrode pairs in the human cochlea. *Journal of the Acoustical Society of America, 86*, 971–980.

McCreery, D.B., Agnew, W.F., Yuen, T.G.H., & Bullara, L. (1988). Comparison of neural damage induced by electrical stimulation with faradic and capacitor electrodes. *Annals of Biomedical Engineering, 16*, 463–481.

Moore, B.C.J., & Glasberg, B.R. (1988). Gap detection with sinusoids and noise in normal, impaired, and electrically stimulated ears. *Journal of the Acoustical Society of America, 83*, 1093–1101.

Muller, C.G. (1983). Comparison of percepts found with cochlear implant devices. In C.W. Parkins & S.W. Anderson (Eds.), Cochlear prostheses: An international symposium. *Annals of the New York Academy of Sciences, 405*, 412–420.

Parkins, C.W., & Colombo, J. (1987) Auditory-nerve single-neuron thresholds to electrical stimulation from scala tympani electrodes. *Hearing Research, 31*, 267–286.

Pfingst, B.E. (1984). Operating ranges and intensity psychophysics for cochlear implants. Implications for speech processing strategies. *Archives of Otolaryngology, 110*, 140–144.

Pfingst, B.E., Burnett, P.A., & Sutton, D. (1983). Intensity discrimination with cochlear implants. *Journal of the Acoustical Society of America, 73*, 1283–1292.

Pfingst, B.E., De Haan, D.R., & Holloway, L.A. (1991). Stimulus features affecting psychophysical detection thresholds for electrical stimulation of the cochlea. I:

Phase duration and stimulus duration. *Journal of the Acoustical Society of America, 90*, 1857–1866.

Pfingst, B.E., & Rush, N.L. (1987). Discrimination of simultaneous frequency and level changes in electrical stimuli. *Annals of Otology Rhinology and Laryngology, 96* (Suppl. 128), 34–37.

Plomp, R. (1964). Rate of decay of auditory sensation. *Journal of the Acoustical Society of America, 36*, 277–282.

Preece, J.P., & Tyler, R.S. (1989). Temporal-gap detection by cochlear prosthesis users. *Journal of Speech and Hearing Research, 32*, 849–856.

Roblee, L.S., & Rose, T.L. (1990). Electrochemical guidelines for selection of protocols and electrode materials for neural stimulation, In W.F. Agnew and D.B. McCreery (Eds.), Neural prostheses: Fundamental studies (pp. 25–66). Englewood Cliffs, Prentice-Hall.

Shannon, R.V. (1983a) Multichannel electrical stimulation of the auditory nerve in man: I. Basic psychophysics. *Hearing Research, 11*, 157–189.

Shannon, R.V. (1983b). Multichannel electrical stimulation of the auditory nerve in man: II. Channel interaction. *Hearing Research, 12*, 1–16.

Shannon, R.V. (1985a). Threshold and loudness functions for pulsatile stimulation of cochlear implants, *Hearing Research, 18*, 135–143.

Shannon, R.V. (1985b). Loudness summation as a measure of channel interaction in a multichannel cochlear implant. In R.A. Schindler & M.M. Merzenich (Eds.), Cochlear implants (pp. 323–334). New York: Raven Press.

Shannon, R.V. (1989a). Detection of gaps in sinusoids and biphasic pulse trains by patients with cochlear implants. *Journal of the Acoustical Society of America, 85*, 2587–2592.

Shannon, R.V. (1989b). A model of threshold for pulsatile electrical stimulation of cochlear implants. *Hearing Research, 40*, 197–204.

Shannon, R.V. (1990). Forward masking in patients with cochlear implants. *Journal of the Acoustical Society of America, 88*, 741-744.

Shannon, R.V. (1992a). Temporal Modulation Transfer Functions in Patients with Cochlear Implants. *Journal of the Acoustical Society of America, 91*, 1974–1982.

Shannon, R.V. (1992). A model of safe levels for electrical stimulation. *IEEE Transactions on Biomededical Engineering, 39*, 424–426.

Shannon, R.V, Zeng, F-G., & Wygonski, J. (1992). Speech recognition with only temporal cues. In M.E.H. Schouten (Ed.), *Speech processing: From the cochlea to language.* Berlin: Mouton-Gruyer.

Simmons, F.B. (1966). Electrical stimulation of the auditory nerve in man. *Archives of Otolaryngology, 84*, 2–54.

Tong, Y.C., Clark, G.M., Blamey, P.J., Busby, P.A., & Dowell, R.C. (1982). Psychophysical studies for two multiple-channel cochlear implant patients. *Journal of the Acoustical Society of America, 71*, 153–160.

Tong, Y.C., Blamey, P.J., Dowell, R.C., & Clark, G.M. (1983) Psychophysical studies evaluating the feasibility of a speech processing strategy for a multiple-channel cochlear implant. *Journal of the Acoustical Society of America, 74*, 73–80.

Townshend, B., Cotter, N., van Compernolle, D., & White, R.L. (1987). Pitch perception by cochlear implant subjects. *Journal of the Acoustical Society of America, 82*, 106–115.

Van den Honert, C., & Stypulkowski, P.H. (1984). Physiological properties of the electrically stimulated auditory nerve. II. Single fiber recordings. *Hearing Research, 14*, 225–243.

Wilson. B.S., Finley, C.C, Lawson, D.T., & Wolford, R.D. (1988). Speech processors for cochlear prostheses. *Proceedings of the I.E.E.E., 76,* 1143–1154.

Wilson. B.S., Finley, C.C, Lawson, D.T., Wolford, R.D., Eddington, D.K., & Rabinowitz, W.M. (1991). New levels of speech recognition with cochlear implants. *Nature, 352,* 236–238.

Zeng, F.G., & Shannon, R.V. (1992). Loudness balance between acoustic and electric stimulation. *Hearing Research, 60,* 231–235.

Zeng, F.G., Turner, C.W., & Relkin, E.M. (1991). Recovery from prior stimulation. II. Effects on intensity discrimination. *Hearing Research, 55,* 223–230.

Index

ABR. *See* Auditory brainstem response (ABR)

AB word list, 232

Acoupedic. *See* Speech skills, auditory-verbal

Acoustic cues
and connected discourse, 151–152
consonant and vowel, multiple, 146–147
consonant manner/voicing, envelope cues, 148–150
consonant place of articulation, frequency and envelope cues, 150–151
cues/features, 146
vowel, 147–148
word recognition, 151–152

American Sign Language (ASL), 19, 98, 246

ANT (Auditory Numbers Test), 206, 211–212

APAL (Auditory Perception of Alphabet Letters), 213, 223

ASL. *See* American Sign Language (ASL)

Assessment. *See also* Evaluation; Examination; Testing
auditory resolution, 10
auditory training, 120
DASL (Developmental Approach to Successful Listening Placement Test), 120
DAT (Discrimination After Training), 120
GASP (Glendonald Auditory Screening Procedure), 120
linguistic rules, child, 302–303

Audibility.
cochlear implant vs. hearing aid, 11

Audiologist
counseling expectation, 95–97
evaluation, formal, 100
evaluation/candidacy, 90–91

Audiovisual Feature Test, 208, 220, 224, 237, 239, 240

Auditory, general
capacity
and magnitude, hearing loss, 3
measure need, 10
performance vs. capacity, 6–7
resolution
assessment, 10
cochlear implant, 11–12
and speech perception, 4
training, 114–120
assessment, 120
materials/procedures, 117–120
objective/task design, 114–117

Auditory brainstem response (ABR), 333, 335, 339

Auditory function, physiological. *See* Electrophysiology

Bandwith. *See* Dynamic range

BKB (Bamford-Kowal-Bench) Sentences, 208, 218, 224, 232, 234

Blindness, 91, 250

Candidacy
audiological-medical criteria,

Candidacy (*continued*)
 audiological-medical criteria
  (*cont'd*)
  90–92
CAP. *See* Compound whole-nerve
 action potential (CAP)
CA prosthesis processing, 41–78
 channel interaction, 45
 CIS comparison, 46–47
 major steps employed, 43
 noise, interfering effects, 61–63
 speech features, extraction/rep-
  resentation, 47–50
 waveform representation vs. feature extraction, 73–78
CAT scan (computerized axial
 tomography), 100–101
Champus, 95
Change/No Change Test, 208,
 220–221, 235
Child. *See also* Education
 advocacy implant discourage
  ment, 98
 audiovisual enhancement,
  237–239, 240
 auditory training, 114–120
 aural rehabilitation, 110–113
 blindness, 250
 candidacy criteria, 91–92, 251
 as candidate, 16
 commitment need, 98
 communication mode, 99–100
 consonant feature perception,
  235–237
 environmental sound, 227–228
 evaluation, speechreading,
  127–128
 fitting, hearing aid, 4
 intellectual deficiency, 250
 linguistic rule assessment,
  302–303
 mainstreaming, 19–20, 99, 245
 multiple handicaps, 250

onset age, 15–16, 17
performance, function of time,
 239–242
performance prediction, 97,
 246–250
phonetic development, 268–270
postlingual, 114
 acquisition, 23–24
 speech production, 266–270
preimplant psychological evaluation, 101
prelingual, 24, 114
pure tone threshold, 9–10
rehabilitative needs, 16
sentence perception, 232–235
speech intelligibility, 292–293
speech-language evaluation,
 preimplant, 101
speech perception, 191–252,
 224–252
 testing considerations, 192–202
speech production characteristics, implant users, 279–303
 acoustics, 297–302
 elicited measures, 286–293
 imitative speech tasks,
  280–286
 phonetic analyses, 293–297
 spoken performance, 302–303
testing
 speech perception, 203–224
training, effects of, 242–244
vocal output and auditory feedback, 253
vowel feature perception,
 235–237
word recognition, 228–231,
 231–232
Childrens Vowel Perception Test,
 208, 221
CID (Central Institute for the Deaf)
 Everyday Sentences, 127–128,
 161–162, 181, 232, 234, 237

247, 249, 279–280
CIS processing, 41–78, 180
  CA comparison, 46–47
  channel interaction, 45–46
  channel number manipulations,
    59–61
  F0/F1/F2 comparison, 63–66
  major steps employed, 43
  Multipeak comparison, 63–66
  noise, interfering effects, 61–63
  single-channel comparison, 67
  speech features, extraction/rep
    resentation, 47–50
  speech perception, 169–171
  waveform representation vs.
    feature extraction, 73–78
Cochlear implant, general. *See also*
    Prostheses
  age, candidate, 16
  audibility, 11
  auditory resolution, 11–12
  bipolar/monopolar electrodes,
    38–39
  candidacy, 10, 12, 13–14, 16,
    90–92, 251
  child speech production charac-
    teristics, 279–303
  criteria, 2
  device function measure,
    electrophysiological, 348–349
  dynamic range, 11
  fitting, initial postsurgery,
    103–106
  and hearing aid, 27, 180
  high frequencies
    audibility, 11
    electrode placement, 37
  infection, 40
  low frequencies electrode place-
    ment, 37
  processors, 41–78
  severely deaf, 26
  speech perception

  vs. hearing aid, 11–12, 13–14
  speech production, effect on,
    271–303
    vs. hearing aid, 12
Cochlear nucleus implant, 181
Cochlear prosthesis. *See* Prostheses
Common Phrases Test, 218
Compound whole-nerve action
    potential (CAP), 332–333
Compressed analog (CA) proces-
    sors. *See* CA
Computerized axial tomography.
    See CAT scan (computerized
    axial tomography)
Connected Discourse Tracking
    Procedure, 128
Continuous interleaved sampling
    (CIS). *See* CIS
Continuous sampling processing.
    See CS processing
Cost, 89, 93–95
Craig Lipreading Inventory, 209,
    223–224
CS processing, 70–72, 73
Cultural identity, deafness, 20–21

DASL (Developmental Approach
    to Successful Listening
    Placement Test), 120
DAT (Discrimination After Train-
    ing), 120, 204
Deafness, general, 1. *See also*
    Hearing loss
  acquisition manner, 21, 23, 24
  advocacy implant discourage-
    ment, 98
  amplification advances, 1
  auditory capacity vs. perfor-
    mance, 6–7
  auditory resolution, 4
  characteristics, 2–4
  children, 4, 15–16
  conductive loss, 9

Deafness, general (*continued*)
  with considerable capacity, 7, 8
  as culture, 20–21
  and duration, 17–18
  dynamic range, 3–4, 5
  educational approach, 18–20
  fitting, hearing aid, 4–5
  implant applicability, 2
  nonauditory characteristics,
    14–25
  and onset age, 14–15, 17
  postlingual, 15–16, 17, 21–22,
    23–24, 91, 116
    speech production, 264–270
  prelingual, 15–16, 17, 22–23, 24
  profound and "total" loss, 1
  severe and cochlear implant, 26
  speech perception, 4–5
Devices
  assistive, 107–108
  research. *See* CIS; Research
    Triangle Institute
Dynamic range, 3–4, 5, 11

EABR. *See* Electrically evoked
    brainstem response (EABR)
EAP. *See* Electrically evoked com-
    pound action potential (EAP)
Education. *See also* Child
  American Sign Language (ASL),
    19, 246
  auditory-verbal approach, 18
  cued speech approach, 18, 245,
    246
  mainstreaming, 19–20, 99, 245
  oral approach, 18
  placement, 99–100, 244–246
  total communication (TC),
    18–19, 99, 239, 245, 246
Electrically evoked auditory brain
    stem response (EABR),
    338–339, 346–349
Electrically evoked brainstem

  response (EABR), 333–337
Electrically evoked compound
    action potential (EAP),
    341–344, 346–347, 348
Electrically evoked middle latency
    response (EMLR), 339–341
Electrocochleography, 332
Electrophysiology, 317–349. *See
    also* Psychophysics/electrical
    stimulation
  auditory brain stem response
    (ABR), 333, 335, 339
  auditory nerve fiber response
    properties, 318–349
  adaptation, 329
  compound whole-nerve
    action potential (CAP),
    332–333
  recordings, far-field, 332–337
  speech-like stimuli, 329–332
  spontaneous activity, 319
  stimulus level and response,
    322–323
  temporal, 323–326
  tuning, 320–322
  electrically evoked auditory
    brainstem response (EABR),
    338–339, 346–347, 348–349
  electrically evoked brainstem
    response (EABR), 333–337
  electrically evoked compound
    action potential (EAP),
    341–344, 346–347, 348
  electrically evoked middle
    latency response (EMLR),
    339–341
  electrocochleography, 332
    histograms, post-stimulus-
    time (PST), 326–329
  middle latency response
    (MLR), 333, 341
  nerve survival prediction,
    337–344

and speech processing, 344–348
EMLR. *See* Electrically evoked middle latency response (EMLR)
Environmental sound recognition, 173–175, 179–180, 227–228
ESP (Early Speech Perception) tests, 206, 213–214, 228
Evaluation. *See also* Assessment; Examination; Testing of candidacy, 90–91
  CID (Central Institute for the Deaf) Everyday Sentences, 127–128, 161–162, 181
  Connected Discourse Tracking Procedure, 128
  Iowa Media Consonant Test, 181
  preimplant, 100–102
  PSI (Pediatric Speech Intelligibility), 127
  psychological, preimplant, 101
  Repeated Sentence Frame Test, 129–130
  speechreading, 127–130
  WIPI (Word Intelligibility by Picture Identification), 127
Examination. *See also* Assessment; Evaluation; Testing
  medical, preimplant, 100–101

Family
  commitment, 97–98
  and fitting, 105–106
  questions by, 89
  questions for, preimplant, 102
  rehabilitation
    log, daily communication, 139–140
  and rehabilitation, 107, 108–113
F0/F1/F2 processing, 50, 63–66, 172, 307
  environmental sound recognition, 175

speech production, 283–284, 288–289
  vs. multipeak processing speech perception, 162–163
  waveform representation vs. feature extraction, 73–78
  word recognition scores, 161–162
F0/F2 processing, 49
  waveform representation vs. feature extraction, 73–78
Fitting
  activation, 105
  dynamic range, 103–104
  and electrodes, 104–105
  instruction, patient, 105–106
  loudness balancing, 104
  pitch, 104
Fundamental Speech Skills test, 279–280

GASP (Glendonald Auditory Screening Procedure), 120, 205, 210, 220, 231, 234
GOALS (Guide for Optimizing Auditory Learning Skills), 111–112

HAVE (Hoosier Auditory Visual Enhancement) Test, 224
Hearing aid. *See also* Prostheses; Tactile aids
  audibility, 11
  and cochlear implant, 180
  with cochlear implant, 27
  design, 4
  dynamic range, 11
  fitting, 4–5, 7
    children, 4
  gain need, 3
  high frequency audibility, 11
  speech production acoustics, 298–299

Hearing aid (*continued*)
  vs. implant, 10–12, 11–12, 13–14
Hearing loss. *See also* Deafness,
    general
  conductive and profound deaf-
    ness, 9
House device, 234–235, 245
  speech perception, 234–235, 236
  speech production, 282-283,
    293–297
House/3M device, 69–70

Implant. *See* Cochlear implant,
    general; Prostheses
IMSPAC (Imitative Speech Pattern
    Contrast) Test, 223, 235
Indiana Minimal Pairs, 221–222,
    237
Ineraid (Utah/Symbion/Richards)
    device, 38, 39–40, 42,
    53–55, 71, 74
  aural rehabilitation, 131
  and CA/CIS comparison, 46–47
  environmental sound recogni-
    tion, 173–175
  feature recognition, 178–179
  intelligibility and auditory nerve
    refractory state, 182–183
  music recognition, 175–176
  speech perception, 164–169
  speech production, 272
  speech recognition, 172–173
  word recognition, 177–178
Insurance, 93–95
Intellectual deficiency, 250
Interleaved pulses (IP) processing.
    See IP prosthesis processing
IP prosthesis processing, 51–55
  waveform representation
    vs. feature extraction, 73–78
Lipreading, 224–225, 237–239
Log, family daily communication,

139–140

MAC (Minimum Auditory Capa-
    bilities) battery, 152–153,
    179–180
Magnitude, 3
Mainstreaming, 19–20, 99, 245
Management, patient, 107–163
  child candidacy criteria, 91–92
  coordinator, clinical, 89–90
  counseling
    commitment, patient/family,
      97–98
    communication mode, 99–100
    cost/insurance, 93–95
    expectation, 95–98
    hardware, 92–93
    interactions, implant
      users/deaf adults, 100
    performance prediction, 96–97
    preliminary, 90–100
    evaluation, formal, 100–102
  implant fitting, 103–106
  initial contact, 88–90
  questions, by patient, common, 89
  questions for, 102
  rehabilitation, 106–113
  speech perception training,
    113–132
  surgery overview, 102–103
Matrix Test, 208, 218–219, 234–235,
    236
Medicaid, 94
Medicare, 94–95
Melbourne/Nucleus device. *See*
    Nucleus device
Meningitis, 91
Middle latency response (MLR),
    333, 341
MiniMed device, 39, 40, 171
Mini Speech Processor. *See* MSP
MLR. *See* Middle latency response

(MLR)
MSP, 56–57
MTS (Monosyllable-Trochee-
Spondee) Test, 204–205,
225–226, 228–230, 231–232,
233, 239, 241, 242–244, 247,
248, 249
Multichannel processing, 47–67
Multipeak processing, 55–57, 63–66
speech perception, 162–163
vs. F0/F1/F2 speech perception,
162–163
waveform representation vs.
feature extraction, 73–78
Multiple handicaps, child, 250
Music recognition, 175–176

Nerve survival prediction, 337–344
Nonspeech recognition. *See also*
Speech recognition
environmental sound, 173–175
music, 175–176
NU-CHIPS (Northwestern University Children's Perception
of Speech), 207
Nucleus device, 27, 38–39, 40, 74,
180–181, 232–233, 234,
235, 236, 237, 239, 242, 245,
247, 248–249, 348
auditory training, 115
aural rehabilitation, 131
CIS interface, 63–66
feature recognition, 178–179
Multipeak strategy, 55–57
music recognition, 175–176
speech intelligibility, 292–293
speech perception, 27, 40–41,
159–164, 232–233, 234, 235
speech perception training, 131,
132
speech production, 283–284,
288–289, 294–298,

299–300
speech recognition, 172

Parent. *See* Family
PBK (Phonetically Balanced
Kindergarten) Test, 207,
217, 231
Pediatric Speech Intelligibility Sentence Test, 220
Phonetic Level Speech Evaluation,
279–286
Phonetic Task Evaluation, 222,
235, 279–280, 286
Phonologic Level Speech Evaluation, 286–289
Postlingual
speech production, 264–270,
Post-Stimulus-Time (PST) histograms, 326–329
Processing, signal, 35–79
Processors
single-channel vs. multichannel,
72–73
Processors, cochlear implant, 41–78
Prostheses. *See also* CA prosthesis
processing; CIS processing;
F0/F1/F2 processing; F0/F2
processing; MSP; Multi-
peak processing; SMSP
prosthesis processing; WSP
analog vs. pulsatile, 73. *See also*
CS; Vienna/3M
electrodes, 37–39
IP prosthesis processing, 53–55
multichannel
speech perception, 158–171
strategies, 47–67
Multipeak strategy, 55–57
overview, 35–36
and patient, 40–41
processing, 41–78
single-channel

Prostheses *(continued)*
  single-channel *(cont'd)*
    speech perception, 153–158
    strategies, 67–71
  Spectral Maxima Sound Proces-
      sor (SMSP) strategy, 57–58
  speech features, 47–50, 75–77
    F0/F1/F2 strategy, 50
    F0/F2 strategy, 49
  and speech perception, 40–41
  transmission link, 39–40
PSI (Pediatric Speech Intelligibil-
    ity), 127
PST. *See* Post-Stimulus-Time his-
    tograms
Psychoacoustic measures, 183–185
Psychological preimplant evalua-
    tion, 101
Psychophysics/electrical stimula-
    tion, 357–385. *See also*
    Electrophysiology
  auditory pattern complexity,
      380–384
  biophysics, 358–366
  channel interaction, 363–364
  clinician implications, 384–385
  electrical current thresholds,
      359–363
  electrical field interactions,
      364–365
  intensity discrimination, 377–379
  loudness, 375–377
  neural population interactions,
      365–366
  perceptual capabilities, 367–380
  spectral resolution, 379–380
  temporal processing, 367–375

Rehabilitation, 98. *See also* Training
  adult, 107–110
  assistive devices, 107–108
  and auditory variables, 21–24
  child, 110–113

children's needs, 16
and family, 108–113
Repeated Sentence Frame Test,
    141–143
strategies, repair, 108, 109
structuring, listening environ
    ment, 108
Repeated Sentence Frame Test,
    129–130
Research Triangle Institute, 35–79,
    169
Retardation, mental, 91

Sensorineural loss
  extent and pure tone threshold, 9
SERT (Sound Effects Recognition
    Test), 205, 211
Signal processing, 35–79
Single-channel processing, 67–72
SMSP processing, 57–58
  speech perception, 163–164
  waveform representation vs.
      feature extraction, 73–78
Social worker, 102
SPAC (Speech Pattern Contrast)
    Test, 209, 222–223
Spectral Maxima Sound Processor.
    See SMSP prosthesis
    processing
Speech features, 47–50, 75–77
Speech-language pathologist
  preimplant evaluation, child, 101
  rehabilitation, aural, 112–113
Speech perception. *See also* Speech
    recognition
  adult, 145–185
  audiovisual, 237–239, 240
  and auditory resolution, 4
  child, 191–252
    age at onset, 202–203
    duration, 202–203
    tests, 203–224
  cochlear implant vs. hearing aid,

11–12, 13–14
consonant recognition, 156–157, 161, 166–167, 170
envelope/stress perception, 224–226
and gain, 5
House device, 234–235, 236, 245
multichannel prostheses, 158–171
Nucleus device, 27, 40–41, 232–233, 234, 235, 236, 237, 239, 242, 245, 247, 248–249
performance, function of time, 239–242
performance prediction, 246–250
profoundly deaf, 4–5
and prostheses, 40–41
sentence perception, 232–235
single-channel (Vienna) prostheses, 153–158
and speech production, 257–260
speech recognition acoustic cues, 146–153
training, 113–132
    auditory, 114–120
    benefits, 130–132
    effects of, 242–244
    speechreading, 120–130
vowel feature perception, 235–237
vowel recognition, 154–156, 160, 164–166, 169
word recognition, 228–232
word/sentence recognition, 157–158, 161–162, 167–169, 170
Speech processing and electro-physiology, 344–348
Speech production, 249–303. *See also* Vocal output and auditory feedback
adult users, 271–274

and age of onset, 259–260
child phonetic development, 268–270
cochlear implant, general, impact, 271–303
House device, 293–297
house implant, 282–283
implications, clinical, 303–307
Ineraid (Utah/Symbion/Richards) device, 272
Nucleus device, 283–284, 288–289, 292–300
postlingual adults, 264–266
postlingual child, 266–270
predictability, 259–260
and residual hearing, 259–260
and speech perception, 257–260
Speechreading, 5–6, 18
evaluation, 127–130
materials/procedures, 121–127
and tactile aids, 26
training, 120–130
Speech recognition. *See also* Non-speech recognition; Speech perception audiovisual, 171–173
patient-to-patient variation, 181–182
psychoacoustic measures, 183–185
reacquisition
    environmental sound recognition, 179–180
    feature recognition, 177–178
    word recognition, 177–178
tests, 152–153
word recognition, 183–184
Speech skills
American Sign Language (ASL), 19
auditory-verbal approach, 18
cued approach, 18
oral approach, 18
total communication (TC),

Speech skills *(continued)*
    18–19, 99, 239, 245, 246
Surgery overview, 102–103

Tactaid II, 294–297
TAC (Test of Auditory Compre-
    hension), 205, 211
Tactile aids, 25–26, 247, 298–299.
    See also Vibrotactile aids
Telephone use, 89, 107, 171
Television, 107–108
Testing. *See also* Assessment;
    Evaluation; Examination
    AB word list, 232
    ANT (Auditory Numbers Test),
        206, 211–212
    APAL (Auditory Perception of
        Alphabet Letters), 213, 223
    audiovisual enhancement,
        223–224
    Audiovisual Feature Test, 208,
        220, 237, 239, 240
    BKB (Bamford-Kowal-Bench)
        Sentences, 208, 218, 224, 232,
        234
    Change/No Change Test, 208,
        220–221, 235
    Childrens Vowel Perception Test,
        208, 221
    CID (Central Institute for the
        Deaf) Everyday Sentences,
        232, 234, 237, 247, 249,
        279–280
    consonant features, 208–209,
        220–223
    Craig Lipreading Inventory, 209,
        223–224
    DAT (Discrimination After Train-
        ing), 204
    device function measure, elec-
        trophysiological, 348–349
    envelope/stress perception,
        204–205, 210–211

environmental sound percep-
    tion, 205, 211
ESP (Early Speech Perception)
    tests, 206, 213–214, 228
Fundamental Speech Skills test,
    279–280
GASP (Glendonald Auditory
    Screening Procedure), 205,
    210, 220, 231, 234
HAVE (Hoosier Auditory Visual
    Enhancement) Test, 224
IMSPAC (Imitative Speech Pat-
    tern Contrast) Test, 223
Indiana Minimal Pairs, 221–222,
    237
MAC (Minimum Auditory
    Capabilities) battery,
    152–153,
    179–180
Matrix Test, 208, 218–219,
    234–235, 236
MTS (Monosyllable-Trochee-
    Spondee) Test, 204–205,
    225–226, 228–230, 231–232,
    233, 239, 241, 242–244, 247,
    248, 249
NU-CHIPS (Northwestern Uni-
    versity Children's Percep-
    tion of Speech), 207
NU-6 (Northwestern University-
    6), 232
PBK (Phonetically Balanced
    Kindergarten) Test, 207,
    217,231
Pediatric Speech Intelligibility
    Sentence Test, 220
Phonetic Level Speech Evalua-
    tion, 279–286
Phonetic Task Evaluation, 222,
    235, 279–280, 286
Phonologic Level Speech Evalu-
    ation, 286–289
Repeated Sentence Frame Test,

141–143
sentence perception, 208,
218–220
SERT (Sound Effects Recognition Test), 205, 211
SPAC (Speech Pattern Contrast) Test, 209, 222–223
speech perception, 11–12
considerations, child, 192–203
capability matching, 198
conversation, 194–195
equivalent lists, 196–197
features, 196
material selection, 198–199
recorded material, 199–200
repetition, 201
reporting, 201
sensory reception, 193–194
stimuli, 192–203
summarizing, 200–201
test-retest reliability, 196
variety, 202
vocabulary, 194
speech perception, child,
203–224
speech recognition, 152–153
TAC (Test of Auditory Comprehension), 205, 211
THRIFT (Three-Interval Forced-Choice Test of Speech Pattern Contrast Perception),
209, 223
Toy Discrimination Test,
215–216
vowel features, 208–209,
220–223
Wechsler Adult Intelligence Scale-Revised (WAIS-R), 97
WIPI (Word Intelligibility by Picture Identification),

207, 216–217, 224, 231,
237–238, 247, 248
word recognition, closed-set,
206–207, 211–217
word recognition, open-set, 207,
217
THRIFT (Three-Interval Forced-Choice Test of Speech Pattern Contrast Perception),
209, 223
Tinnitus, 89
Training. *See also* Rehabilitation
speech perception, 113–132

UCSF/Storz device, 39, 40, 42, 51,
52–55, 74
Utah/Symbion/Richards device.
See Ineraid

Verbo-tonal. *See* Speech skills,
auditory-verbal
Vibrotactile aid, 294–297. *See also*
Tactile aids
Vienna/3M device, 68–69, 70, 71, 73
auditory training, 115
Vocal output. *See* Speech production
Vocal output and auditory feedback
child, 253
deafness effect, animals, 261–264
influence of, 260–270, 274–279, 307

Wearable Speech Processor. *See*
WSP
Wechsler Adult Intelligence Scale-Revised (WAIS-R), 97
WIPI (Word Intelligibility by Picture Identification), 127,
207, 216–217, 224, 231,
237–238, 247, 248
WSP, 56, 57, 283–284, 288–289